SBAs and EMIs for the General Surgery FRCS

SBAs and EMIs for the General Surgery FRCS

Edited by

Richard G. Molloy
Consultant Colorectal Surgeon
Queen Elizabeth University Hospital, Glasgow UK

Graham J. MacKay
Consultant Colorectal Surgeon and Honorary Associate Professor,
Glasgow Royal Infirmary, UK

Campbell S. Roxburgh
Clinical Senior Lecturer and Honorary Consultant Colorectal Surgeon,
Institute of Cancer Sciences, College of Medical, Veterinary and Life Sciences,
University of Glasgow, UK

Martha M. Quinn
Consultant in Surgical Oncology
Glasgow Royal Infirmary, UK

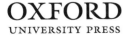

OXFORD
UNIVERSITY PRESS

OXFORD
UNIVERSITY PRESS

Great Clarendon Street, Oxford, OX2 6DP,
United Kingdom

Oxford University Press is a department of the University of Oxford.
It furthers the University's objective of excellence in research, scholarship,
and education by publishing worldwide. Oxford is a registered trade mark of
Oxford University Press in the UK and in certain other countries

Published in the United States of America by Oxford University Press
198 Madison Avenue, New York, NY 10016, United States of America

British Library Cataloguing in Publication Data
Data available

Library of Congress Control Number: 2018937423

ISBN 978–0–19–879415–8

Printed and bound by
CPI Group (UK) Ltd, Croydon, CR0 4YY

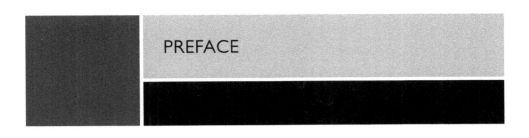

PREFACE

Our aim with *SBAs and EMIs for the General Surgery FRCS* is to provide high-quality sample questions for trainees in General Surgery preparing to sit the FRCS Section 1 examination. The Intercollegiate FRCS examination in General Surgery is the exit exam, which must be passed to qualify for the award of a Certificate of Completion of Training (CCT) by the General Medical Council Postgraduate Board. Candidates for the exam must hold a medical qualification recognized for registration by the General Medical Council of the United Kingdom or the Medical Council of Ireland and must be qualified for at least six years. They must also have evidence that they have reached the clinical competencies required for the award of a CCT.

The FRCS examination is divided in two sections. The Section 1 examination is a written test composed of Single Best Answer (multiple choice questions, choose one from five options) and Extended Matching Item questions (EMI). The examination is divided into two papers designed to cover the content of the curriculum as defined in the Intercollegiate Surgical Curriculum (<http://www.iscp.ac.uk>). Paper 1 consists of 110 SBA questions over 2 hours and Paper 2 consists of 135 EMI questions over 2 hours and 30 minutes. Successful completion of the Section 1 examination is required before being allowed to proceed to Section 2. The Section 2 examination consists of a series of structured clinical and oral interviews covering general surgery, emergency surgery, trauma and critical care, and specialty topics. Further information regarding the examination can be found on the website of the Joint Committee on Intercollegiate Examinations (<http://www.jcie.org.uk>).

This book contains sample questions laid out by sub-specialty and in the same format that candidates will be presented with in the Section 1 examination. The questions are mapped to specific areas of the surgical curriculum and mirror the level required for the successful award of an FRCS. Each question is accompanied by a detailed explanation of the answer and, where appropriate, signposts the reader to further resources. These features mean that the book not only helps you to assess your level of knowledge and practice completing MCQs but also adds depth to the learning experience and directs ongoing revision.

Many of the contributors to the book have successfully passed the FRCS in General Surgery within the last two to three years and so have an intimate knowledge of the examination in its current form. As an editorial group our aim has been to provide an accurate, high-quality, comprehensive resource of sample questions in an easily accessible format. We hope that you find the text useful in your preparations and wish you every success with both the examination and your further surgical career.

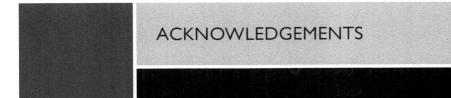

ACKNOWLEDGEMENTS

To Brigid, Niamh, and Jessica. As always, I couldn't do what I do without all your love and support.

Richard

To Catherine, Emily, Finlay, and Murdo. For your love and patience and for still being there when the computer is switched off.

Graham

To Tricia, Hamish, Annie, and Fraser. Thank you for all your help and support.

Campbell

To Stuart, Fraser, and Arran. Thank you for all your support, especially during my time away.

Martha

CONTENTS

ABBREVIATIONS

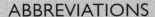

5-HIAA	5-hydroxyindoleacetic acid
A&E	Accident and Emergency
A–aO$_2$	alveolar–arterial gradient
AAA	abdominal aortic aneurysm
AAST	American Association for the Surgery of Trauma
ABCDE	Age, Blood pressure fall, Comorbidity, Diagnosis, and Evidence of bleeding
ABG	arterial blood gas
ABMR	antibody-mediated rejection
ABPI	ankle-brachial pressure index
ACE	angiotensin-converting enzyme
ACOT	acute coagulopathy of trauma
ACPGBI	Association of Coloproctology of Great Britain and Ireland
ACPO	acute colonic pseudo-obstruction
ACS	abdominal compartment syndrome
ACT	Anal Cancer Trial
ACTH	adrenocorticotropic hormone
ADH	antidiuretic hormone
AEN	acute oesophageal necrosis
AF	atrial fibrillation
AFP	alpha-fetoprotein
AI	aromatase inhibitor
AIDS	acquired immunodeficiency syndrome
AIN	anal intraepithelial neoplasia
AIP	autoimmune pancreatitis
AKI	acute kidney injury
ALS	afferent loop syndrome
AMR	antibody-mediated rejection
ANA	antinuclear antibody
ANC	acute necrotic collection
AP	acute pancreatitis
AP	anteroposterior/abdomino-perineal

APC	adenomatous polyposis coli
APFC	acute peri-pancreatic fluid collections
APP	abdominal perfusion pressure
APTT	activated partial thromboplastin time
APUD	amine precursor uptake and decarboxylation
ARDS	adult respiratory distress syndrome
ARR	absolute risk reduction
ASA	American Society of Anesthesiologists
ATG	anti-thymocyte globulin
ATLS	Advanced Trauma Life Support
ATP	adenosine triphosphate
AXR	abdominal X-ray
AVF	arteriovenous fistula
AVG	arteriovenous grafts
BAETS	British Association of Endocrine and Thyroid Surgeons
BMA	bone-modifying agents
BMI	body mass index
BP	blood pressure
bpm	beats per minute
BI-RADS	Breast Imaging and Reporting Data System
BSG	British Society of Gastroenterology
C&S	Culture and sensitivity/cerebrospinal
CABG	coronary artery bypass graft
cAMP	cyclic Adenosine Monophosphate
CBD	common bile duct
CCK	cholecystokinin
CD	Crohn's disease
CDC	complement-dependent cytotoxicity
CDI	*Clostridium difficile* infection
CFTR	cystic fibrosis transmembrane conductance regulator
CHRPE	congenital hypertrophy of the retinal pigment epithelium
CIPO	chronic intestinal pseudo-obstruction
CKD	chronic kidney disease
cm	centimetre
CMV	cytomegalovirus
CN	cranial nerve
CONSORT	CONsolidated Standards Of Reporting Trials
COPD	chronic obstructive pulmonary disease
CPAP	continuous positive airway pressure

CRC	colorectal cancer
CRF	calculated reaction frequency
CRLM	colorectal liver metastases
CRM	circumferential resection margin
CRP	C-reactive protein
CR-POSSUM	colorectal POSSUM
CT	computed tomography
CTT	Certificate of Completion of Training
CVS	critical view of safety
CXR	chest X-ray
DASH	disability of the arm, shoulder, and hand
DASS	dialysis-associated steal syndrome
DBD	donation after brain death
DCD	donation after cardiac death
DCI	distal contractile integral
DCIS	ductal carcinoma *in situ*
DFSP	dermatofibrosarcoma protuberens
DI	diabetes insipidus
DIC	disseminated intravascular coagulation
DIEP	deep inferior epigastric artery perforator
DNA	deoxyribonucleic acid
DNC	death using neurological criteria
DOAC	direct oral anticoagulant
DSA	donor-specific antibodies
DVT	deep venous thrombosis
EBL	endoscopic band ligation
EBV	Epstein–Barr virus
ECF	epirubicin, cisplatin, and 5-fluorouracil
ECG	electrocardiogram
ECMO	extracorporeal membrane oxygenation
EGFR	epidermal growth factor receptor
EHEC	enterohaemorrhagic *E. coli*
EIM	extra-intestinal manifestations
ELC	early laparoscopic cholecystectomy
EIM	extra-intestinal manifestation
ELC	early laparoscopic cholecystectomy
EMI	extended matching item
EMR	endoscopic mucosal resection
EPP	extraperitoneal pelvic packing

ER	oestrogen receptor
ERAS	enhanced recovery after surgery
ERCP	endoscopic retrograde cholangiopancreatography
ESD	endoscopic submucosal dissection
ESR	erythrocyte sedimentation rate
ESRD	end-stage renal disease
ETEC	enterotoxigenic *E. coli*
ETT	endotracheal tube
EUA	examination under anaesthetic
EUS	endoscopic ultrasound
FAP	familial adenomatous polyposis
FAST	Focused Assessment with Sonography for Trauma
FBC	full blood count
FC	flow cytometry
FDP	fibrin/fibrinogen degradation products
FDG	fluorodeoxyglucose
FEC	fluorouracil, epirubicin, cyclophosphamide
FES	fat embolism syndrome
FEV1	forced expiratory volume in one second
FFP	fresh frozen plasma
FGPD	fundic gland polyp with low-grade dysplasia
FMD	fibromuscular dysplasia
FNA	fine needle aspiration
FNAC	fine needle aspiration cytology
FNH	focal nodular hyperplasia
FOB	faecal occult blood
FRC	functional residual capacity
FRCS	Fellow of the Royal College of Surgeons
FSH	follicle-stimulating hormone
FU	fluorouracil
FVC	forced vital capacity
GBS	Glasgow–Blatchford score
GCA	giant cell arteritis
GCS	Glasgow Coma Scale
GCSF	granulocyte colony-stimulating factor
GES	gastric electrical stimulation
GFR	glomerular filtration rate
GH	growth hormone
GI	gastrointestinal

GIST	gastrointestinal stromal tumour
GMC	General Medical Council
GORD	gastro-oesophageal reflux disease
GOV	gastro-oesophageal varices
GP	General Practitioner
GPS	Glasgow Prognostic Score
GTN	glyceryl trinitrate
GSF	glomerular filtration rate
H2RA	H2 receptor antagonist
H&E	haemotoxylin and eosin
HA	hepatic adenoma
HAART	highly active antiretroviral therapy
Hb	haemoglobin
HBS	hungry bone syndrome
HBsAG	hepatitis B surface antigens
HBV	hepatitis B virus
HCC	hepatocellular carcinoma
HDGC	hereditary diffuse gastric carcinoma syndrome
HDU	high-dependence unit
HER	human epidermal growth factor receptor
HIPEC	hyperthermic intra-peritoneal chemotherapy
HIAA	hydroxyindoleacetic acid
HIPEC	hyperthermic intra-peritoneal chemotherapy
HIT	heparin-induced thrombocytopenia
HIV	human immunodeficiency virus
HLA	human leucocyte antigen
HNPCC	hereditary non-polyposis colorectal cancer
HPB	hepato-pancreaticobiliary
HPN	home parenteral nutrition
HPV	human papilloma virus
hr	hour
HSIL	high-grade squamous epithelial lesion
HTA	Human Tissue Authority
HTK	histidine–tryptophan–ketoglutarate
HUS	haemolytic uraemic syndrome
HVPG	hepatic venous pressure gradient
IA	independent assessor
IAH	intra-abdominal hypertension
IAP	intra-abdominal pressure

IBD	inflammatory bowel disease
ICA	intracranial carotid artery
ICU	Intensive Care Unit
IDCP	idiopathic duct-centric pancreatitis
IDDM	insulin-dependent diabetes mellitus
IGCLC	International Gastric Cancer Linkage Consortium Criteria
IGV	isolated gastric varices
IL	Interleukin
IMA	inferior mesenteric artery
IMPACT	Improved Protection Against CMV in Transplant
IMPDH	inhibitor of inosine monophosphate dehydrogenase
INR	international normalized ratio
IOC	intraoperative cholangiography
IPMN	intraductal papillary mucinous neoplasm
ITP	idiopathic thrombocytopenic purpura
IV	intravenous
IVC	inferior vena cava
LAMN	low-grade appendiceal mucinous neoplasms
LARS	low anterior resection syndrome
LCIS	lobular carcinoma *in situ*
LD	latissimus dorsi
LFT	liver function tests
LGV	lymphogranuloma venereum
LH	luteinizing hormone
LHM	laparoscopic Heller's myotomy
LICAP	lateral intercostal artery perforator
LIS	lateral internal sphincterotomy
LMWH	low molecular weight Heparin
LOS	lower oesophageal sphincter
LSIL	low-grade squamous intraepithelial lesion
LVEF	left ventricular ejection fraction
LVI	lymphovascular invasion
MALT	mucosa-associated lymphoid tissue
MAP	mean arterial pressure
MAPK	mitogen-activated protein kinase
MAST	military anti-shock trousers
MCN	mucinous cystic neoplasm
MCV	mean cell volume
MDT	multidisciplinary team

MELD	model for end-stage liver disease
MEN	multiple endocrine neoplasia
MI	myocardial infarction
mm	millimetre
MMC	mitomycin C
MMF	mycophenolate mofetil
MPA	mycophenolic acid
MPACT	Metastatic Pancreatic Adenocarcinoma Clinical Trial
MPSRUS	mucosal prolapse solitary rectal ulcer syndrome
MRCP	magnetic resonance cholangiopancreatography
MRI	magnetic resonance imaging
MRSA	methicillin-resistant staphylococcus aureus
MSI	microsatellite instability
mTOR	mammalian target of rapamycin
NAC	neo-adjuvant chemotherapy
NASH	non-alchoholic steatohepatitis
NET	neuroendocrine tumours
NG	nasogastric
NICE	National Institute for Health and Care Excellence
NK	natural killer
NNT	number needed to treat
NPI	Nottingham prognostic index
NPWT	negative pressure wound therapy
NRP	normothermic regional perfusion
NSAID	non-steroidal anti-inflammatory drugs
NST	no special type
OCP	oral contraceptive pill
OG	oesophagogastric
OGD	oesophagogastroduodenoscopy
OGJ	oesophago-gastric junction
OGTT	oral glucose tolerance test
O-POSSUM	oesophagogastric POSSUM
OPSI	overwhelming post-splenectomy infection
PARP	poly-ADP ribose polymerase
PCA	patient-controlled analgesia
PCB	primary biliary cirrhosis
PCC	prothrombin complex concentrate
PCL	primary colonic lymphoma
PCP	pneumocystis carinii pneumonia

pCR	pathological complete response
PCR	polymerase chain reaction
PD	pancreatico-duodenectomy/peritoneal dialysis
PE	pulmonary embolism
PEEP	positive end-expiratory pressure
PEG	polyethylene glycol
PET	positron emission tomography
PF	pancreatic fistula/platelet factor
PI	pulsatility index
PID	pelvic inflammatory disease
PMP	pseudomyxoma peritonei
PNEF	primitive neuroectodermal tumour
PNF	primary non-function
PPI	proton pump inhibitor
P-POSSUM	Portsmouth—Physiology and Operative Severity Score for the enUmeration of Mortality and Morbidity
PR	progesterone receptor
PRISMA	Preferred Reporting Items for Systematic Reviews and Meta-Analyses
PSA	persistent sciatic artery
PSC	primary sclerosing cholangitis
PT	partial thromboplastin/prothrombin time
PTC	percutaneous transhepatic cholangiography
PTDM	post-transplant diabetes mellitus
PTFE	polytetrafluoroethylene
PTH	parathyroid hormone
PTLD	post-transplant lymphoproliferative disease
PVE	portal vein embolization
QDS	*quarter die sumendus*/four times a day
rAAA	ruptured abdominal aortic aneurysm
RBC	red blood cell
RCT	randomized controlled trials
RFA	radio-frequency ablation
rhTSH	recombinant TSH
RIF	right iliac fossa
RLN	recurrent laryngeal nerve
RNA	ribonucleic acid
RR	respiratory rate
RRA	radioiodine remnant ablation
RRT	renal replacement therapy

RT	radiotherapy
RTA	road traffic accident
RUQ	right upper quadrant
SBA	single best answer/small bowel adenocarcinoma
SBLA	sarcoma breast leukaemia adrenal
SBO	small bowel obstruction
sc	subcutaneous
SC	sternoclavicular
SCA	serous cystadenomas
SCC	squamous cell carcinoma
SCD	sub-acute combined degeneration
SCFR	stem cell growth factor receptor
SD	standard deviation
SDD	selective decontamination of the digestive tract
SEMS	self-expanding metal stent
SFA	superficial femoral artery
SGAP	superior gluteal artery perforator
SIEA	superficial inferior epigastric artery
SIGN	Scottish Intercollegiate Guidelines Network
SIL	squamous intraepithelial lesion
SIRS	systemic inflammatory response syndrome
SIRT	selective internal radiotherapy
SLE	systemic lupus erythematosus
SMA	superior mesenteric artery
SMV	superior mesenteric vein
SNAP	Sepsis, Nutrition, Anatomy, and then a Plan
SPECT	single-photon emission CT
SPINK1	serine protease inhibitor Kazal-type 1
SPK	simultaneous pancreas and kidney
SPN	solid pseudopapillary neoplasm
SQUIRE	Standards for QUality Improvement Reporting Excellence
SRUS	solitary rectal ulcer syndrome
STI	sexually transmitted infection
STROBE	STrengthening the Reporting of OBservational studies in Epidemiology
TA	Takayasu's arteritis
TACE	trans-arterial chemoembolization
TB	tuberculosis
TBMR	T-cell-mediated rejection
TCMR	T-cell mediated rejection

TDAP	thoracodorsal artery perforator
TDS	*Ter die sumendum*/three times a day
TFT	thyroid function test
TG	thyroglobulin
TIA	transient ischaemic attack
TIPS	trans-jugular portosystemic shunt
TME	total mesorectal excision
TNF	tumour necrosis factor
TPN	total parenteral nutrition
TPO	thyroid peroxidase
TRAb	thyroid receptor antibodies
TRAM	transverse rectus abdominus myocutaneous
TRAS	transplant renal arterial stenosis
TRIPOD	Transparent Reporting of a multivariable prediction model for individual Prognosis or Diagnosis
TUG	transverse upper gracilis
U&E	urea and electrolytes
UC	ulcerative colitis
UFH	unfractionated heparin
UK	United Kingdom
US	ultrasound/United States
USS	ultrasound scan
UW	University of Wisconsin
VAP	ventilator-associated pneumonia
VEGF	vascular endothelial growth factor
VHL	Von Hippel–Lindau
V-POSSUM	vascular POSSUM
VQ	ventilation/perfusion
VTE	venous thromboembolism
WCC	white cell count
WLE	wide local excision
WHO	World Health Organization
Wnt	wingless type
WON	walled-off necrosis
YAG	yttrium aluminium garnet

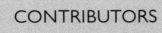

CONTRIBUTORS

Emma Aitken Specialty Registrar in General Surgery, Queen Elizabeth University Hospital, Glasgow, UK

Natasha Amiraraghi Specialty Registrar in ENT, Queen Elizabeth University Hospital, Glasgow, UK

Alexander Binning Clinical Director for Critical Care, NHS Greater Glasgow and Clyde, UK

David Chang Senior Lecturer in Surgery, Glasgow Royal Infirmary, UK

Robert Docking Consultant in Anaesthetics and Critical Care, Queen Elizabeth University Hospital, Glasgow, UK

Graeme Guthrie Specialty Registrar in Vascular Surgery, Ninewells Hospital, Dundee, UK

Omar Hilmi Consultant ENT surgeon, Queen Elizabeth University Hospital, Glasgow, UK

Andrew Jackson Specialist Registrar, Transplant and General Surgery, Queen Elizabeth University Hospital, Glasgow, UK

Nigel Jamieson Lecturer in Surgery, Glasgow Royal Infirmary, UK

Fiona Leitch Consultant General and Colorectal Surgeon, Forth Valley Royal Hospital, Larbert, UK

Graham J. MacKay Consultant Colorectal Surgeon & Honorary Associate Professor, Glasgow Royal Infirmary, UK

Fraser Maxwell Honorary Colorectal Fellow, Bankstown Hospital, Sydney, Australia

Donald McArthur Consultant General and Upper GI Surgeon, Queen Elizabeth University Hospital, Glasgow, UK

Andrew McCulloch Consultant Cardiologist and Physician, Inverclyde Royal Hospital, Greenock, UK

Jennifer McIlhenny Consultant Oncoplastic Breast Surgeon, Forth Valley Royal Hospital, Larbert, UK

Richard G. Molloy Consultant Colorectal Surgeon, Queen Elizabeth University Hospital, UK

Lisa Moyes Consultant General and Colorectal Surgeon, Queen Elizabeth University Hospital, Glasgow, UK

Gary Nicholson Consultant General and Colorectal Surgeon, Queen Elizabeth University Hospital, Glasgow, UK

Raymond Oliphant Consultant Colorectal Surgeon, Raigmore Hospital, Inverness, UK

Martha M. Quinn Consultant in Surgical Oncology, Glasgow Royal Infirmary, Glasgow UK

Lia Paton Consultant in Anaesthetics and Critical Care, Glasgow Royal Infirmary, UK

Thaven Ramachandren Vascular Registrar, The Royal Adelaide Hospital, Adelaide, South Australia

Judith Reid Consultant Breast Surgeon, Crosshouse Hospital, Kilmarnock, UK

Campbell S. Roxburgh Clinical Senior Lecturer and Honorary Consultant Colorectal Surgeon, Institute of Cancer Sciences, College of Medical, Veterinary and Life Sciences, University of Glasgow, UK

Sheila Stallard Consultant Breast Surgeon, Gartnavel General Hospital, Glasgow, UK

Karen Stevenson Consultant Transplant Surgeon, Queen Elizabeth University Hospital, Glasgow, UK

Brian Stewart Lecturer in Surgery, University of Glasgow, UK

Stuart Suttie Consultant Vascular Surgeon, Ninewells Hospital, Dundee, UK

Carol Watson Consultant General and Endocrine Surgeon, Queen Elizabeth University Hospital, Glasgow, UK

BASIC SCIENCE

Single Best Answers

1. **Dabigatran, a direct oral anticoagulant, may be best reversed by:**
   a) Vitamin K
   b) Beriplex
   c) Protamine
   d) Idarucizumab
   e) Fresh frozen plasma

2. **A patient planned for elective inguinal hernia repair is taking Apixaban for recurrent venous thromboembolism. How long before surgery should the patient stop the medication?**
   a) 12 hours
   b) 24 hours
   c) 48 hours
   d) Five days
   e) Seven days

3. **During preoperative workup, a patient's coagulation screen comes back with the following results: PT 12sec, APTT 47sec, Thrombin time 14sec. The most likely explanation is**
   a) Alcoholic liver disease
   b) Current low molecular weight heparin therapy
   c) Factor VII deficiency
   d) Lupus anticoagulant
   e) Warfarin therapy

4. **A patient reports a history of heparin-induced thrombocytopenia (HIT) whilst being treated with unfractionated heparin. Which of the following would be a suitable agent for prophylaxis of venous thromboembolism (VTE)?**
   a) Clopidogrel
   b) Dalteparin
   c) Enoxaparin
   d) Fondaparinux
   e) Tinzaparin

5. **Which of the following infections is a patient at increased risk of following an emergency splenectomy?**
   a) *Staphylococcus aureus*
   b) *Staphylococcus epidermidis*
   c) *Clostridium difficile*
   d) *Streptococcus pneumoniae*
   e) *Legionella pneumophila*

6. **An otherwise healthy 13 year old girl presents with bilateral leg swelling. What is the most likely diagnosis?**
   a) Congenital lymphoedema
   b) Lymphoedema praecox
   c) Congestive cardiac failure
   d) Lymphoedema tarda
   e) Bilateral deep venous thrombosis

7. **A patient with myasthenia gravis is referred for thymectomy. What is the embryological origin of the thymus gland?**
   a) First pharyngeal pouch
   b) Third pharyngeal pouch
   c) First pharyngeal arch
   d) Thyroglossal duct
   e) Rathke's pouch

8. **A 57 year old woman presents with squamous cell carcinoma of her anus. Which is the most likely aetiological agent?**
   a) Human papilloma virus
   b) Epstein–Barr virus
   c) Human Herpes virus 8
   d) Coxsackie virus
   e) Varicella Zoster virus

9. **A patient with multiple liver metastases from colonic carcinoma is discussed at the multidisciplinary team (MDT) meeting. Which of the following oncogenes might it be useful to test for?**
   a) p53
   b) HER-2
   c) KRAS
   d) BCR–ABL
   e) EGFR

10. **A 64 year old man with a permanent cardiac pacemaker is scheduled for elective laparoscopic cholecystectomy. He is known to be pacing-dependent. Which of the following strategies would deal best with the effect of diathermy on his pacemaker?**
    a) Monopolar diathermy
    b) Monopolar diathermy limited to short bursts
    c) Bipolar diathermy
    d) Clinical magnet secured on top of pacemaker
    e) Pacemaker reprogramming by cardiology department

11. **A 32 year old female patient is about to undergo an elective repair of a paraumbilical hernia. Which of the following skin preparation agents would be most appropriate to use?**
    a) 2% aqueous chlorhexidine
    b) 2% alcoholic chlorhexidine
    c) 0.5% alcoholic chlorhexidine
    d) Aqueous povidone-iodine solution
    e) Isopropyl alcohol

12. **When a patient is immobilized their body undergoes major changes to the cardiovascular and musculoskeletal systems and to the blood volume. Approximately how long after continued bed rest are these changes seen?**
    a) Three days
    b) Seven days
    c) 14 days
    d) 21 days
    e) 42 days

13. **Which of the following biochemical markers is least likely to show evidence of depletion in a patient who has nutrition reintroduced after 14 days of starvation?**
    a) Magnesium
    b) Phosphate
    c) Potassium
    d) Sodium
    e) Thiamine

14. **What is the mode of inheritance of Peutz–Jeghers syndrome?**
    a) Autosomal dominant
    b) Autosomal recessive
    c) Epigenetic
    d) Mitochondrial
    e) X-linked recessive

15. **During a sleeve gastrectomy the right gastroepiploic artery is divided. Which vessel does this artery arise from?**
    a) Gastroduodenal artery
    b) Hepatic artery
    c) Right gastric artery
    d) Splenic artery
    e) Superior pancreatico-duodenal artery

16. **A new chemotherapy regime for colorectal cancer was tested in 2000 patients with Dukes stage C. 1000 patients received the new regime while the other 1000 received standard therapy. Five-year survival in the standard therapy group is 65% versus 75% in the new regime group. What is the number needed to treat (NNT)?**
    a) 5
    b) 10
    c) 20
    d) 50
    e) 100

17. **A patient sustains a head injury in a road traffic accident. In the assessment of his cranial nerves, which is the most likely to have been injured?**
    a) I—Olfactory
    b) III—Oculomotor
    c) V—Trigeminal
    d) VI—Abducens
    e) VII—Facial

18. **An alternating magnetic field induced by a high-frequency alternating current may result in electrical currents in nearby conducting objects such as metal laparoscopic trochars. Such a phenomenon is known as:**
    a) Capacitance coupling
    b) Impedance
    c) Electromagnetic stimulation
    d) Bipolar diathermy
    e) Electrical arcing

19. **Which of the following treatment options is *not* advisable in the management of adult respiratory distress syndrome (ARDS)?**
    a) High-frequency oscillatory ventilation
    b) Prone-position ventilation
    c) Applying positive end expiratory pressure
    d) Use of diuretics
    e) Increasing ventilatory tidal volumes

20. **Which skin condition is associated with gastrointestinal (GI) malignancy and characterized by a thickened, pigmented, predominantly flexural rash?**
    a) Erythema ab igne
    b) Dermatitis herpetiformis
    c) Dermatomyositis
    d) Acanthosis nigricans
    e) Thrombophlebitis migrans

21. **Which of the following options is *not* a potential adverse effect of massive blood transfusion?**
    a) Coagulopathy
    b) Hypercalcaemia
    c) Hyperkalaemia
    d) Hypothermia
    e) Hypoxia

22. **The lower limit of the spinal cord in adults lies at the level of:**
    a) T11/12
    b) L1/2
    c) L3/4
    d) L5/S1
    e) S4/5

23. **A 34 year old welder arrives in the resuscitation room after an apparent industrial accident. He has a large laceration in his proximal right thigh. The paramedics report considerable blood loss at the scene. He appears pale and is obviously agitated, shouting inappropriately. His pulse is 133bpm and his blood pressure is 80/58mmHg. Which class of haemorrhagic shock is he likely to fall into, allowing an estimation of blood loss?**
    a) Class I, <750ml, 15% of total volume
    b) Class II, 750–1500ml, 15–30% of total volume
    c) Class III, 1500–2000ml, 30–40% of total volume
    d) Class IV, >2000ml, >40% of total volume
    e) Class V, >3000ml, >60% of total volume

24. **Regarding intra-abdominal hypertension and abdominal compartment syndrome, which of the following statements is true?**
    a) Diagnosis of abdominal compartment syndrome requires an intra-abdominal pressure of >25mmHg.
    b) Normal intra-abdominal pressure is 15–19mmHg.
    c) The reference standard for intra-abdominal pressure measurement is via the bladder with a maximum volume of 100ml sterile saline.
    d) Abdominal compartment syndrome is defined as an intra-abdominal pressure >20mmHg with associated organ dysfunction.
    e) Abdominal perfusion pressure = mean arterial pressure + intra-abdominal pressure

25. **Exogenous injury to cells resulting in denaturing of proteins and degradation by proteolytic enzymes is known as:**
    a) Apoptosis
    b) Atrophy
    c) Necrosis
    d) Autophagy
    e) Senescence

26. **Which of the following terms indicates a malignant neoplasm originating within striated muscle tissue?**
    a) Leiomyosarcoma
    b) Rhabdomyosarcoma
    c) Malignant teratoma
    d) Carcinosarcoma
    e) Sternocleidomastoid tumour

27. **In the absence of excess fluid losses, in order to meet maintenance requirements, adult patients should receive which of the following by the enteral or parenteral route?**
    a) 20–50mmol sodium, 20–40mmol potassium, and 1–1.5L water
    b) 50–100mmol sodium, 40–80mmol potassium, and 1.5–2.5L water
    c) 100–150mmol sodium, 80–120mmol potassium, and 1.5–2.5L water
    d) 50–100mmol sodium, 40–80mmol potassium, and 3–4L water
    e) 100–150mmol sodium, 40–80mmol potassium, and 2–3L water

28. **In biostatistics the proportion of positive tests that are indeed true positives is considered the:**
    a) Sensitivity
    b) Specificity
    c) Negative predictive value
    d) Positive predictive value
    e) Prevalence value

29. **In a patient undergoing elective GI cancer surgery, which of the following agents, when taken in close proximity to surgery, would have the highest risk of impaired wound healing?**
    a) Rapamycin
    b) Cyclophosphamide
    c) Azathioprine
    d) Cetuximab
    e) Neomycin

30. **The medial border of the femoral triangle is bound by:**
    a) The pectineal ligament
    b) The femoral vein
    c) The inguinal ligament
    d) The lacunar ligament
    e) Cloquet's node

31. **In the first 48 hours following major GI surgery which of the following hormonal fluxes is not anticipated:**
    a) Cortisol release increases
    b) Aldosterone release increases
    c) Insulin release increases
    d) Anti-diuretic hormone release increases
    e) Glucagon increases

32. **A 62 year old female is seen with multiple painful subcutaneous lumps over her arms, legs, chest, and abdomen. The lesions have grown slowly over the past 18 months and several now cause severe pain. Her BMI is 38. Which of the following conditions represents the most likely diagnosis?**
    a) Dermatofibrosarcoma protuberens
    b) Pyoderma gangrenosum
    c) Neurofibromatosis type 1
    d) Simple lipomata
    e) Dercum's disease

33. **A 40 year old male has an excision biopsy of an abnormal skin lesion on his back. He weighs 60kg. The procedure is performed under local anaesthesia and he receives 12ml of 1% lidocaine. The maximum safe dose of the drug is 3mg/kg. What dose in milligrams has been administered here?**
    a) 12mg
    b) 18mg
    c) 72mg
    d) 120mg
    e) 180mg

34. **Regarding the recurrent laryngeal nerve (RLN), which of the following statements are false?**
    a) The RLN innervates the intrinsic muscles of the larynx except the cricothyroid.
    b) Both the right and left RLNs emerge at the level of the aortic arch.
    c) The left RLN passes under the arch of the aorta then cranially.
    d) The right RLN passes anterior to the right subclavian artery.
    e) The right RLN lies posterior to the carotid in the trachea–oesophageal groove.

Extended Matching Items

Nutrition

A. Elemental diet
B. Fish oil-based total parenteral nutrition
C. High fibre enteral feed
D. Modular
E. Normal diet
F. Oral nutritional supplements
G. Polymeric enteral feed
H. Puréed/sloppy diet
I. Semi-elemental enteral feed
J. Standard lipid emulsion total parenteral nutrition

For each of the following scenarios, choose the single most appropriate type of feed from the list. Each option may be used once, more than once or not at all.

1. A patient with intestinal failure-associated liver disease.

2. A 78 year old man who has just undergone oesophageal stenting.

3. A 15 year old boy with recently diagnosed severe Crohn's disease.

Nutritional deficiencies

A. Fluorene
B. Iron
C. Magnesium
D. Manganese
E. Molybdenum
F. Selenium
G. Vitamin B1 (Thiamine)
H. Vitamin B12 (hydroxycobalamin)
I. Vitamin D
J. Zinc

In type 3 intestinal failure patients, choose the most likely vitamin deficiency from the list for each of the following scenarios. Each option may be used once, more than once, or not at all.

4. A patient with extreme fatigue, hair loss, and development of a goitre.

5. A patient with numbness and tingling that began in the feet and has progressed proximally with reduced reflexes and impaired proprioception.

6. A patient noted to have a prolonged QT interval on their ECG.

Hernias

A. Bochdalek
B. Femoral
C. Hiatus
D. Incisional
E. Inguinal
F. Lumbar
G. Morgagni
H. Obturator
I. Perineal
J. Spigelian

For each of the following scenarios select the most likely type of hernia for the patient to present with.

7. A 62 year old woman with a swelling in her left groin.

8. A 6 month old boy with progressive dyspnoea.

9. An extremely thin 83 year old woman with chronic obstructive pulmonary disease presenting with small bowel obstruction. There are no external signs of a hernia.

Infection

A. *Bacteroides spp.*
B. *Clostridium difficile*
C. *Escherichia coli*
D. *Proteus spp.*
E. *Staphylococcus aureus*
F. *Staphylococcus epidermidis*
G. *Staphylococcus saphyrophyticus*
H. *Streptococcus bovis*
I. *Streptococcus pyogenes*

For each of the following scenarios select the most likely causative organism.

10. A 32 year old woman presents with a third urinary tract calculus on a background of recurrent urinary tract infection.

11. A 45 year old poorly controlled diabetic presents with a large carbuncle on his upper back.

12. A 63 year old man with bacterial endocarditis who is subsequently found to have colorectal cancer.

Pelvic nerves

A. Genitofemoral nerve
B. Ilioinguinal nerve
C. Iliohypogastric nerve
D. Inferior hypogastric plexus
E. Inferior rectal nerve
F. Perineal nerve
G. Pudendal nerve
H. Sacral sympathetic ganglia
I. Pelvic splanchnic nerves
J. Posterior femoral cutaneous nerve

What is the primary innervation for each of the following structures?

13. External anal sphincter.

14. The male urethra.

15. Uterus.

Statistics

A. ANOVA
B. Bland–Altman
C. Chi square
D. Fisher's exact test
E. Kaplan–Meier
F. Mann–Whitney
G. MANOVA
H. McNemar's test
I. Pearson correlation coefficient
J. Standard deviation

For each of the following descriptions, select the corresponding statistical test.

16. A method of plotting data to analyse the agreement between two different assays or measurement techniques for the same biological variable.

17. A non-parametric statistic estimating the survival function, typically used to estimate mortality or event-free survival.

18. An indicator of variation around the mean for normally distributed data.

Genetic cancer syndromes

A. Fanconi's anaemia
B. Li–Fraumeni syndrome
C. Von Hippel–Lindau disease
D. Lynch syndrome
E. Multiple endocrine neoplasia 1
F. Multiple endocrine neoplasia 2
G. Hereditary breast cancer
H. Hereditary diffuse gastric cancer
I. Familial adenomatous polyposis
J. Von Recklinghausen's disease

From the scenarios, choose the single most appropriate hereditary cancer syndrome from the list. Each option may be used once, more than once, or not at all.

19. Which syndrome is associated with a gain of function mutation in the *RET* proto-oncogene?

20. A loss of function mutation in the *CDH-1* gene is most commonly associated with which hereditary syndrome?

21. Defective DNA mismatch repair due to mutations in genes including *MLH1* and *MSH2* result in which syndrome?

Antibiotics

A. Vancomycin
B. Ciprofloxacin
C. Penicillin
D. Metronidazole
E. Gentamicin
F. Doxycycline
G. Clindamycin
H. Erythromycin
I. Piperacillin
J. Ceftriaxone

From the scenarios, choose the single most appropriate agent from the list. Each option may be used once, more than once, or not at all.

22. Which antibiotic should be considered in severe cases of pseudomembranous colitis?

23. Treatment with which antibiotic can lead to yellow discolouration of the teeth?

24. Which quinolone is commonly used in infections due to gram-negative rods?

Gastrointestinal infection

A. *Shigella*
B. *Cryptosporidium*
C. *Clostridium difficile*
D. *Salmonella*
E. *Pseudomonas aeruginosa*
F. *E. coli* O157
G. *Yersinia enterocolitica*
H. *Giardia lamblia*
I. *Campylobacter jejuni*

For each scenario choose the single most appropriate causative organism from the list. Each option may be used once, more than once, or not at all.

25. A 27 year old female has just returned from India 3 days ago and attends hospital with cramping abdominal pains and bloody diarrhoea.

26. A 43 year old male attends with a 3-day history of cramping abdominal pain and bloody diarrhoea. He has no recent history of foreign travel.

27. A 24 year old homeless male with a history of untreated HIV infection attends with severe watery diarrhoea for the past 2 weeks.

Statistical bias

A. Selection bias
B. Recall bias
C. Lead time bias
D. Classification bias
E. Confounding bias
F. Publication bias
G. Procedure bias
H. Attrition bias
I. Observer-expectancy bias
J. Measurement bias

For each of the following scenarios, choose the single most appropriate type of statistical bias from the list. Each option may be used once, more than once, or not at all.

28. A study aims to evaluate whether treatment with multivitamins may lead to improved five-year survival after oesophagectomy for adenocarcinoma. The study is powered based on a 5-year survival after oesophagectomy of 25%. The study inclusion criteria include absence of residual or recurrent disease. Most patients enter the study at 12–18 months after resection. The study fails to detect a difference in outcome between the treatment groupings.

29. A study evaluates the role of Enhanced Recovery after Surgery (ERAS) pathways during elective colorectal surgery. The primary endpoint is length of hospital stay. The research is undertaken in two centres with similar numbers of surgeons in each hospital. The study aims to recruit 65 patients. Hospital A has seven surgeons who routinely perform laparoscopic surgery and hospital B has two laparoscopic surgeons. Hospital A recruits 33 patients and Hospital B recruits 32 patients. The length of stay is shorter in Hospital A and no clear effect is seen for the role of ERAS.

30. A surgeon decides to evaluate whether single-port laparoscopic cholecystectomy results in a measurable improvement in quality of life after surgery. A small study is designed whereby patients are asked a series of questions at the four-week post-op follow-up appointment. The operating surgeon reads out the questions and documents the answers. In another clinic, patients who undergo standard laparoscopic cholecystectomy are asked the same questions. The study reports improved quality of life measures in the single-port cholecystectomy group with a study size of $n = 40$.

Gastrointestinal polyps

A. Adenomatous polyps
B. Pseudopolyps
C. Hyperplastic polyps
D. Inflammatory polyps
E. Villous polyp
F. Fundic gland polyps
G. Hamartomatous polyps
H. Juvenile polyp
I. Sessile serrated adenoma

For each of the following scenarios choose the single most appropriate diagnosis from the list. Each option may be used once, more than once, or not at all.

31. Often seen in clusters in the upper stomach, usually <1cm in size, smooth, glassy, and sessile.

32. These polyps have a characteristic appearance on microscopy with evidence of dilated crypts which grow laterally along the muscularis propria. They harbour pre-malignant potential.

33. These polyps classically have a core of branching smooth muscle with mucous-filled glands and abundant eosinophils. They are commonly associated with an autosomal dominant condition.

Cancer drugs

A. Gemcitabine
B. Oxaliplatin
C. 5-FU
D. Cyclophosphamide
E. Cisplatin
F. Capecitabine
G. Etoposide
H. Methotrexate
I. Docetaxel
J. Irinotecan

For each of the following scenarios, choose the single most appropriate agent from the list. Each option may be used once, more than once, or not at all.

34. Which alkylating agent has common side effects of marrow suppression, alopecia, and nausea and vomiting?

35. The oral pro-drug of a common direct thymidylate synthase inhibitor, which is preferentially activated in tumour and liver tissue.

36. This anti-metabolite is active in pancreatic, lung, and breast cancer. Toxicities include flu-like syndromes, deranged liver function tests, myelosuppression, and peripheral oedema.

Glasgow Coma Scale

A. 3
B. 4
C. 5
D. 7
E. 8
F. 9
G. 10
H. 12
I. 13
J. 14

For the following scenarios, choose the single most appropriate Glasgow Coma Scale value from the list. Each option may be used once, more than once, or not at all.

37. A man is assessed at the scene of a motor vehicle accident. He was an unrestrained passenger who has been ejected from the vehicle. On assessment he is breathing noisily and is unresponsive. There is a twitching movement in his left arm and leg but this does not appear related to the physician's painful stimulus.

38. A 17 year old female attends the A&E with her friend having fallen on a night out. Her eyes open only after persistent loud questioning and her speech is slurred. She talks as if she is at home in her own bed and wishes to be left alone. When a painful stimulus is applied to her right hand, she uses her left hand to push it away.

39. A 35 year old male has been brought to the A&E. He was found collapsed in a nightclub but on inspection has a laceration over his occiput and bruising on the left side of his face. His eyes are closed throughout the assessment. He is groaning and when a painful stimulus is applied to the right hand, he appears to pull the hand away.

Single Best Answers

1. d) Idarucizumab

Idarucizumab is a monoclonal antibody developed specifically to reverse dabigatran. It is administered as a bolus followed by an infusion. This results in rapid neutralization of dabigatran's anticoagulant effect in the setting of life-threatening haemorrhage or the need for emergency surgery. It is not effective against any of the other novel oral anticoagulants or warfarin (see Figure 1.1).

Veitch AM et al. Endoscopy in patients on antiplatelet or anticoagulant therapy, including direct oral anticoagulants: British Society of Gastroenterology (BSG) and European Society of Gastrointestinal Endoscopy (ESGE) guidelines. *Gut* 2016; 65:374–89.

Pollack Jr CV et al. Idarucizumab for dabigatran reversal. *New England Journal of Medicine* 2015; 373:511–20.

2. c) 48 hours

When discontinuing anticoagulation prior to elective surgery, the nature of the surgery planned and the indication for anticoagulation must be taken into account. In this instance, although the risk of major blood loss is low, the consequences of haematoma at the operation site are severe. The half-life of Apixaban is approximately 12 hours. There should be negligible anticoagulant effect if stopped at least 48 hours prior to surgery. Rivaroxaban and dabigatran have more variable half-lives (5–13 hours for rivaroxaban and 12–17 hours for dabigatran); 48–72 hours should be sufficient for all of these agents. The use of bridging heparin therapy should also be considered. The BRIDGE trial demonstrated no increase in embolic events but less major bleeding in atrial fibrillation patients who were not bridged with heparin perioperatively. The ongoing PERIOP 2 trial aims to answer this question in patients at high thromboembolic risk, including mechanical heart valves.

Douketis JD et al. Perioperative bridging anticoagulants in patients with atrial fibrillation. *New England Journal of Medicine* 2015; 373(9):823–33.

3. d) Lupus anticoagulant

Lupus anticoagulant derives its name from an *in-vitro* anticoagulant effect, which manifests as an isolated prolongation in the activated partial thromboplastin time (APTT). *In-vivo* it is actually prothrombotic and is a significant risk factor for both arterial and venous thrombosis. Lupus anticoagulant is also associated with recurrent miscarriage. Low molecular weight heparin, unlike unfractionated heparin, does not affect APTT. Warfarin therapy will prolong both prothrombin time (PT) and APTT, as will intrinsic liver disease. Factor VII deficiency results in a prolonged PT but normal APTT.

LMWh's do not affect APTT.

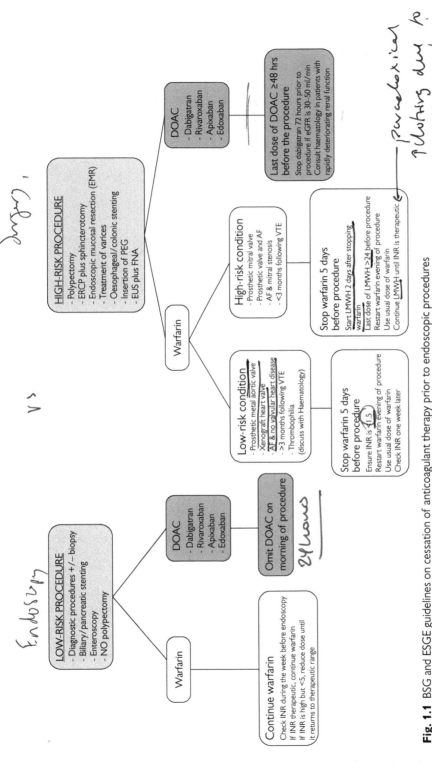

Fig. 1.1 BSG and ESGE guidelines on cessation of anticoagulant therapy prior to endoscopic procedures

[handwritten: LMWn's fondaparunx is 10q]

4. d) Fondaparinux

Heparin induced thrombocytopenia results from antibody formation to the heparin–platelet factor 4 (PF4) complex. It is a prothrombotic state despite the thrombocytopenia and additional anticoagulation should be provided. Fondaparinux is a synthetic factor Xa inhibitor and is suitable for use as it has no affinity for PF4. Dalteparin, enoxaparin, and tinzaparin are all low molecular weight heparins and, although they have a lower incidence of heparin-induced thrombocytopenia, are to be avoided in a patient already sensitized. Clopidogrel is not recommended for VTE prophylaxis and patients taking this for another indication should receive an additional agent.

Kelton JG et al. Nonheparin anticoagulants for heparin-induced thrombocytopenia. *New England Journal of Medicine* 2013; 368:737–44.

5. d) *Streptococcus pneumonia*

Streptococcus pneumoniae is an encapsulated organism. The polysaccharide capsule is resistant to phagocytosis. Opsonization of these organisms is impaired in patients who are either functionally or anatomically asplenic, rendering them more susceptible to these infections. Vaccination against *Strep. pneumoniae*, haemophilus influenza, and Neisseria meningitidis is recommended which should be administered preoperatively in elective splenectomy.

6. b) Lymphoedema praecox

Lymphoedema results from the accumulation of lymph in body tissues. Primary lymphoedema is usually caused by congenital hypoplasia or aplasia of lymphatic vessels or dysfunctional valves within the lymphatic system. Congenital primary lymphoedema is usually present from birth and can be associated with a variety of syndromes such as Turner's syndrome. Primary lymphoedema can also develop in adolescence (lymphoedema praecox) or after the age of 35 (lymphoedema tarda). A female predominance is seen but the mechanism is not understood. Secondary lymphoedema can occur following radiotherapy or nodal dissection, commonly for melanoma or breast cancer. In tropical countries filariasis can cause occlusion of the lymphatic vessels by helminths.

Lymphoedema, <http://emedicine.medscape.com/article/1087313-overview>.

7. b) Third pharyngeal pouch

The thymus gland is formed from portions of the third pharyngeal pouch. The ventral wings of the third pouch fuse to form the cytoreticular cells of the thymus. The dorsal components form the inferior parathyroid glands. The first pharyngeal pouch forms the tubotympanic recess which expands to form the middle ear cavity and auditory tube. The first pharyngeal arch gives rise to Meckel's cartilage which forms the portion of the mandible containing incisor teeth from its ventral end, and the malleus from its dorsal end. The thyroglossal duct is a midline structure at the junction of the anterior two-thirds and posterior one-third of the tongue along which the thyroid gland migrates during development. It normally atrophies as the foramen cecum but may remain patent, potentially forming a thyroglossal duct cyst. Rathke's pouch is a depression in the roof of the mouth, giving rise to the anterior pituitary gland. Benign cysts may develop from Rathke's pouch and craniopharygnioma may develop from the epithelium within the pouch. See Figure 1.2 for overview.

8. a) Human papilloma virus

Approximately 90% of anal cancers are linked to human papilloma virus, most commonly HPV type 16. Epstein–Barr virus was the first human virus to have a proven association with cancer—B-cell lymphoma of various subtypes. Human herpes virus 8, also known as Kaposi sarcoma herpes virus,

[handwritten: post transplant = PTLD]

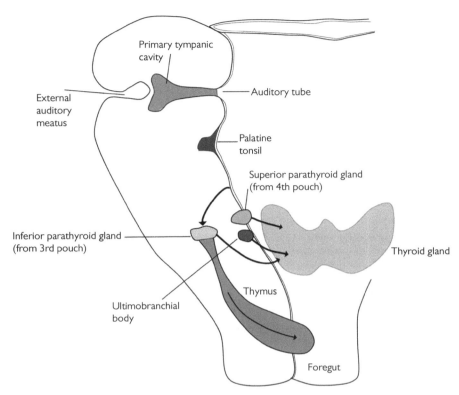

Fig. 1.2 Development of the thymus from the third pharyngeal pouch

is found in almost all cases of Kaposi's sarcoma. Varicella zoster and Coxsackie viruses have not been shown to be carcinogenic. A preparation of Coxsackie virus type A21 is being evaluated as an anti-cancer agent to target and lyse tumour cells.

9. c) *KRAS*

The *KRAS* oncogene is mutated in approximately 40% of colorectal cancers. The 2 most common mutations in codons 12 and 13, which account for 95% of the mutations seen, are negative predictors for response to anti-epidermal growth factor receptor (EGFR) antibodies. Although EGFR is over-expressed in 80% of colorectal cancers, it did not predict clinical outcome with anti-EGFR therapy. HER-2 is an oncogene expressed in 15–20% of breast cancers. BCR–ABL, the Philadelphia chromosome, is a marker for chronic myelogenous leukaemia. Tumour protein p53 is a tumour suppressor. Genetic mutation in p53 can lead to Li–Fraumeni syndrome.

10. e) **Pacemaker reprogramming by cardiology department**

In patients with a cardiac pacemaker, electrical interference from diathermy may be sensed by the pacemaker and wrongly interpreted as intrinsic cardiac activity. This will result in suppression of pacing for the duration of the diathermy burst and, in dependent patients, loss of cardiac output. In the elective setting, the device should be reprogrammed to a non-sensing (asynchronous) mode for the duration of the operation. In an emergency setting, a magnet will usually temporarily produce the same mode. Bipolar diathermy should be used where possible as this produces less electrical interference. Short bursts of monopolar diathermy can be used where this is not available.

Crossley GH et al. The Heart Rhythm Society (HRS)/American Society of Anesthesiologists (ASA) Expert Consensus Statement on the perioperative management of patients with implantable defibrillators, pacemakers and arrhythmia monitors. *Heart Rhythm* 2011; 8:1114–54.

11. b) 2% alcoholic chlorhexidine

There is a growing body of evidence that 2% alcoholic chlorhexidine is superior to all other agents for preoperative skin preparation. It is notable that 2% aqueous chlorhexidine solution has poorer efficacy than its alcoholic counterpart and aqueous povidone-iodine solution.

Sidhwa F and Itani KM. Skin preparation before surgery: options and evidence. *Surgical Infections* 2015; 16(1):14–23.

12. c) 21 days

A muscle at complete rest loses 10–15% of its strength each week. Nearly half of normal strength is lost within three to five weeks of immobilization. Similarly, heart rate increases after immobilization. This is thought to be due to an increase in sympathetic nervous activity. During bed rest the resting pulse rate speeds up by one beat per minute every two days. The consequence of this on diastolic filling means the heart is less able to respond to increased metabolic demand, causing further compromise to a patient who is often already undergoing cardiovascular stress.

Dittmer DK and Teasell R. Complications of immobilization and bed rest. Part 1: Musculoskeletal and cardiovascular complications. *Canadian Family Physician* 1993; 39:1428–32, 1435–7.

13. d) Sodium

After approximately ten days without significant nutritional intake, metabolism adapts to the starvation state. Such patients are at risk of refeeding syndrome. Refeeding syndrome can develop if there is sudden reintroduction of normal caloric intake without anticipation and active replacement of potassium, phosphate, magnesium, and thiamine. Refeeding syndrome occurs when metabolism abruptly shifts from a catabolic to an anabolic state. Carbohydrate intake stimulates insulin release resulting in cellular uptake of potassium, magnesium, and phosphate. Thiamine is not routinely measured but should be assumed to be depleted and should be actively replaced.

Mehanna HM et al. Refeeding syndrome: what it is, and how to prevent and treat it. *British Medical Journal* 2008; 336(7659):1495–8.

14. a) Autosomal dominant

The majority of familial cancer syndromes are inherited in an autosomal dominant fashion. This includes familial adenomatous polyposis, MEN type 1 and 2, and breast cancer related to BRCA1 and BRCA2. Autosomal recessive inherited cancers are often haematological such as Fanconi's anaemia. Epigenetics is the transmission of genetic traits without change in the actual nucleotide sequence and is mediated by DNA methylation and histone modification. It is of relevance in a number of surgical cancers including BRCA1, prostate cancer, and some colon cancers.

15. a) Gastroduodenal artery

The right gastroepiploic artery arises from the gastroduodenal artery, posterior to the duodenum. It runs close to the greater curvature of the stomach supplying it as it passes and anastomoses with the left gastroepiploic artery.

16. b) 10

Number Needed to Treat is calculated as 1/Absolute Risk Reduction (ARR). ARR = (control event rate)—(experimental event rate). Here, control event rate (mortality) is 0.35, experimental event rate 0.25, giving an ARR of 0.1 (10%). 1/0.1 = 10.

17. a) Olfactory

Following minor head trauma where cranial nerve injury is sustained, single nerve palsy has been observed in 77.6% of patients. The most commonly affected nerve in this case is the olfactory nerve, most likely due to shearing of the olfactory fibres as they pass through the cribriform plate. The facial (VII), oculomotor (III), and abducens (VI) nerves are the next most commonly affected. Where multiple cranial nerves are affected, the most frequent combination is the facial (VII) and vestibulocochlear (VIII) nerves.

Coello AF et al. Cranial nerve injury after minor head trauma. *Journal of Neurosurgery* 2010; 113(3):547–55.

18. a) Capacitance coupling

A capacitor is a device that can store charge in which an insulator is sandwiched between two electrode plates. In laparoscopic surgery a capacitor can be constructed by using metallic trochars through which an insulated energy device is passed. The core of the diathermy device acts as one electrode and the trochar as the other with the insulator in between. As a result, despite a well-insulated instrument, it is possible for current to flow into the patient through the trochar. The current flow is relatively small but there is the potential for injury to contacting structures especially if the point of contact is minimal.

19. e) Increasing ventilatory tidal volumes

Adult respiratory distress syndrome is characterized by acute respiratory failure in which an inflammatory process results in non-cardiogenic pulmonary oedema. This in turn results in reduced lung compliance and hypoxia. Numerous local and systemic conditions can result in ARDS. These include, pulmonary contusions, pneumonia, smoke inhalation, aspiration, severe sepsis, massive burns, major trauma, massive transfusion, and pancreatitis. The aim of treatment, in addition to addressing the underlying cause, is to maintain oxygenation, providing supportive care. Airway pressures should be limited to avoid barotrauma and low tidal volumes are used. Modest positive end-expiratory pressure (PEEP) to enhance alveolar recruitment, high-frequency ventilation, prone-position ventilation, and use of fluid restriction/diuresis have all demonstrated benefit.

20. d) *Acanthosis nigricans*

Erythema ab igne is a skin condition due to repeated long-term exposure to heat, for example, the regular use of hot water bottles. This should alert the clinician to the possibility that the heat is being used for analgesic effect and may indicate a painful chronic underlying condition which may include malignancy.

Dermatitis herpetiformis is a blistering skin condition associated with gluten-sensitive enteropathy or coeliac disease. The characteristic itchy blistering erythematous rash is seen on extensor surfaces. Coeliac disease confers an increased risk of small bowel malignancy including lymphoma and adenocarcinoma.

Dermatomysositis is a systemic inflammatory condition characterized by proximal limb weakness and facial erythema with a heliotrope magenta, periorbital, oedematous rash. Nodules and plaques can be seen on the knuckles. Dermatomyositis is an autoimmune condition and in most cases the cause is unknown. However, many cases occur as paraneoplastic syndromes associated with several malignancies including gastrointestinal, pancreatic, breast, cervical, and lung cancer.

Acanthosis nigricans is associated with thickened, dark, velvety patches in flexural areas. The condition is associated with insulin resistance and GI malignancy. Thrombophlebitis migrans is a migratory thrombophlebitis of superficial veins and has been associated with pancreatic malignancy.

21. b) Hypercalcaemia

Massive blood transfusion is defined as replacement of the entire circulatory volume of blood in 24 hours or half of this volume in 3 hours. Other definitions include ongoing blood loss of >150ml/min, the need for 4U of packed red cells in 4 hours or 10U packed red cells in 24 hours. Anticipated effects of massive blood loss and simple RBC transfusion include the development of dilutional coagulopathy which must be prevented using adequate platelets and plasma replacement. RBCs are stored at 4°C and rapid transfusion of volume without blood warmers can result in hypothermia, further impairing metabolic processes in critically ill patients. Red blood cells in cold storage leak intracellular potassium. Upon transfusion, the Na^+–K^+–ATPase pumping mechanism is restored and cellular uptake of potassium usually occurs rapidly. Hyperkalaemia occurs rarely, particularly when the patient is hypothermic and acidotic. Hypocalcaemia (not hypercalcaemia) can occur as a result of chelation of ionized calcium by citrate, which is contained in small concentrations in the additive solution of RBC and FFP transfusions. Transfusion-associated lung injury presents with hypoxia and development of ARDS during or within hours of transfusion.

22. b) L1/2

The spinal cord does not extend the entire length of the spinal column. The distal limit in adults is at the level of the first and second lumbar vertebrae. In neonates the cord can extend to the level of L3/4. Below this level lies the epidural space, a useful landmark as lumbar epidural injections can be targeted here with low risk of cord injury.

23. c) Class III, 1500–2000ml, 30–40% of total volume

Trauma principles are commonly tested in the FRCS examination. This man would be categorized as Class III given he is confused, tachycardic (above 120 but below 140), and hypotensive. The ATLS classification of haemorrhagic shock is as shown in Table 1.1.

Table 1.1 ATLS Classification of haemorrhagic shock

	I	II	III	IV
Blood loss (ml)	<750	750–1500	1500–2000	>2000
Blood loss (% blood volume)	<15	15–30	30-40	>40
Pulse rate (beats/min)	<100	>100	>120	>140
Blood pressure	Normal	Normal	Decreased	Decreased
Respiratory rate (resp/minute)	14–20	20–30	30–40	>35
Urine output (mL/hr)	>30	20–30	5–15	Negligible
CNS symptoms	Normal	Anxious	Confused	Lethargic
Resuscitation fluid	Crystalloid	Crystalloid	Crystalloid + Blood	Crystalloid + Blood

Adapted from *Resuscitation*, 84, 3, Mutschler M, Nienaber U, Brockamp T, et al. A critical reappraisal of the ATLS classification of hypovolaemic shock: does it really reflect clinical reality? pp. 309–13. Copyright (2013) with permission from Elsevier.

Haemorrhagic shock can be divided into four groups using the ATLS classification.

Although this classification is commonly used, a number of recent studies have raised concerns that the classification has substantial deficits. Up to 90% of trauma patients cannot be clearly classified into one of these 4 groups based on heart rate, systolic blood pressure, and Glasgow Coma Scale. In addition, the scale tends to overestimate the degree of tachycardia associated with hypotension and underestimate mental disability in the presence of hypovolaemic shock.

Mutschler M et al. A critical reappraisal of the ATLS classification of hypovolaemic shock: does it really reflect clinical reality? *Resuscitation* 2013; 84(3):309–13.

24. d) Abdominal compartment syndrome is defined as an intra-abdominal pressure >20mmHg with associated organ dysfunction

Normal intra-abdominal pressure (IAP) in critically ill adults is 5–7mmHg. The reference standard for measurement of IAP is via a bladder syringe with a maximum of 25ml sterile saline instilled. Intra-abdominal hypertension (IAH) is classed as Grade 1, IAP 12–15mmHg; Grade II, IAP 16–20mmHg; Grade III, IAP 21–25mmHg; Grade IV, >25mmHg. Abdominal compartment syndrome (ACS) is defined as IAP >20mmHg in the presence of organ dysfunction/failure. Common organ dysfunction associated with ACS includes renal and respiratory impairment and reduced cardiac output. ACS/IAH may be primary (due to intra-abdominal pathology) or secondary (due to conditions not originating in the abdomen or pelvis). Organ function is dependent on abdominal perfusion pressure (APP) calculated by mean arterial pressure minus IAP (APP = MAP - IAP).

25. c) Necrosis

There are two principle forms of cell death: necrosis or apoptosis. Necrosis is a form of cell death due to exogenous injury or hypoxia with resulting enzymatic degradation. Apoptosis implies programmed cell death which usually serves a function for the host organism and unlike necrosis is a clean process without leakage of debris. Atrophy is a term that implies a reduction in size or wasting of a tissue or organ as a result of lack of function or ischaemic changes. Autophagy is the organized destruction and recycling of intra-cellular constituents. Senescence is a state of cell cycle arrest.

26. b) Rhabdomyosarcoma

Sarcomas are malignant neoplasms arising from within mesenchymal tissues and carcinomas arise within epithelial tissues. Liposarcomas originate within adipose tissues, leimyosarcomas originate from smooth muscle, and rhabdomayosarcomas originate from striated muscle. Carcinosarcomas are rare tumours that comprise a mixture of carcinomatous and sarcomatous characteristics. Teratomas are germ cell tumours. A sternocleidomastoid tumour is a benign tumour of infancy that manifests as a firm fibrous growth within the muscle, which can be associated with the presence of torticollis.

27. b) 50–100mmol sodium, 40-80mmol potassium and 1.5–2.5L water

Maintenance requirements for adult patients are 50–100mmol sodium, 40–80mmol potassium, and 1.5–2.5L water (GIFTASUP—British consensus guidelines on intravenous fluid therapy for adult patients <http://www.bapen.org.uk>). If IV fluids are required, then balanced salt solutions such as Hartmann's solution should be administered. One litre of Hartmann's solution contains 131mmol sodium, 5mmol potassium, 111mmol chloride, and 2mmol calcium. Normal saline (0.9%) is not a balanced salt solution and has a higher sodium load with 154mmol sodium and 154mmol chloride. Excess use of normal saline can induce a hyperchloraemic acidosis.

28. d) Positive predictive value

Biostatistical terminology is a common theme of FRCS questions. The terms apply to screening tests and examinees should be familiar with the following definitions shown in Table 1.2.

Table 1.2 Definitions of common statistical terms

Term	Definition
Sensitivity	The probability that the test detects the disease when it is present. Proportion of all patients with the disease who test positive. *TP / TP + FN*
Specificity	Probability that the test indicates absence of disease when negative. Proportion of patients without the disease who test negative. *TN / TN + FP.*
Negative predictive value	Probability that a negative test result is a true negative. Proportion of negative tests that are true negatives. *TN / TN + FN*
Positive predictive value	Probability that a positive test result is a true positive. Proportion of positive tests that are true positives. *TP / TP + FP.*
Prevalence	All current cases of a disease at a given time point.
Incidence	All new cases of a disease in a given time period.

29. a) Rapamycin

Sirolimus like Tacrolimus. IL2 Calcineurin inhibitor. Particularly [illegible]

Rapamycin, or sirolimus, is an mTOR (mammalian target of rapamycin)-inhibiting immunosuppressive agent used clinically to prevent transplant rejection. Wound complications including lymphocoele and wound dehiscence are common in patients taking the drug in close proximity to surgery. Cyclophosphamide can lead to delayed wound healing as well but to a lesser degree. Cetuximab is an anti-EGFR biologic agent used in colorectal cancer. Another monoclonal antibody which has been used in colorectal cancer, bevacuzimab (an anti-VEGF agent), has been reported to increase wound complications. Neomycin is an aminoglycoside antibiotic and is commonly administered as part of oral antibiotic prophylaxis in Europe and North America with no increase in wound complications.

30. d) The lacunar ligament

The femoral canal is a potential hernial orifice through which groin herniae may originate. Femoral hernias make up 5% of male and 20% of female groin herniae. Laterally the femoral vein is a key landmark, which must be appreciated during femoral hernia repair. Anterior to the canal is the inguinal ligament, medially lies the lacunar ligament, and posteriorly lies the pectineal ligament. Cloquet's lymph node is a deep inguinal lymph node that may be present within the femoral canal (see Figure 1.3).

31. c) Insulin release increases

The net effect of the body's response to trauma and surgery is to promote provision of energy substrates including fat, protein, and carbohydrate at the same time as retaining sodium and water. The process is due to systemic neurological, hormonal, and metabolic changes. Sympathetic nervous system activation, an endocrine response involving activation of the hypothalamic pituitary adrenal axis and insulin resistance, in addition to immunological and haematological changes brought about by the systemic inflammatory response are responsible. Table 1.3 details several of the main hormonal changes.

32. e) Dercum's disease

Dercum's disease is a rare condition in which patients develop multiple painful lipomatous lesions in the subcutaneous tissues. Classically, obese, post-menopausal women are affected. The condition is rare but treatment is largely aimed at symptom control. Surgery is reserved for particularly symptomatic lesions given that recurrence is high. Simple lipomata are the other most

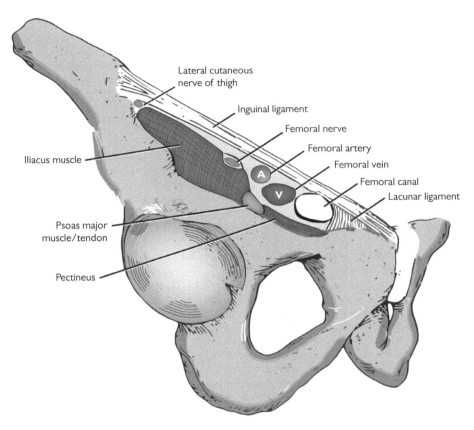

Fig. 1.3 Anatomy of the femoral canal

Table 1.3 Hormonal changes as a response to surgical stress

Endocrine Gland	Hormones	Changes
Anterior pituitary	ACTH	↑ OR ↓
	GH	↑
	TSH	↑ OR ↓
	FSH and LH	↑ OR ↓
Posterior pituitary	ADH	↑
Adrenal cortex	Cortisol	↑↑
	Aldosterone	↑
Pancreas	Insulin	↓
	Glucagon	↑
Thyroid	Thyroxine	↓↓
	Tri-iodothyronine	↓

likely possibility although these lesions are usually painless. Pyoderma gangrenosum is a painful ulcerative skin condition usually affecting the lower limbs and associated with autoimmune diseases (e.g. inflammatory bowel disease and inflammatory arthritides). Neurofibromatosis type 1 or Von Recklinghausen's disease is an autosomal dominant condition characterized by tumours of nerve tissues. Cutaneous neurofibromas develop from the teenage years and can occur anywhere. Dermatofibrosarcoma protuberens (DFSP) is a rare cutaneous malignancy with low-grade malignant potential. DFSP is usually successfully treated by wide local excision.

33. d) **120mg**

Calculating doses of local anaesthesia is another common question. It is important to be familiar with basic percentages and dosing. In a 1% solution there is 10mg of local anaesthesia in 1ml. In a 2% solution there is 20mg of anaesthesia per 1ml. Therefore, in this scenario the patient receives 10mg × 12 = 120mg. If the patient weighs 60kg, then the maximum safe dose is 180mg (3mg × 60kg). The maximum dose of lidocaine is 3mg/kg (5–7mg/kg if administered with adrenaline). For bupivacaine, the maximum dose is 2mg/kg (3mg/kg with adrenaline).

34. d) **The right RLN passes anterior to the right subclavian artery**

The RLNs supply the intrinsic muscles of the larynx, except the cricothyroid muscle. Injury leads to vocal cord paralysis. The nerves arise from the vagus nerve at the level of the aortic arch at T2. The left RLN passes posteriorly under the aorta and the right passes posteriorly under the right subclavian then cranially behind the artery into the neck. The nerves lie posterior to the carotid artery in the trachea–oesophageal groove (see Figure 1.4).

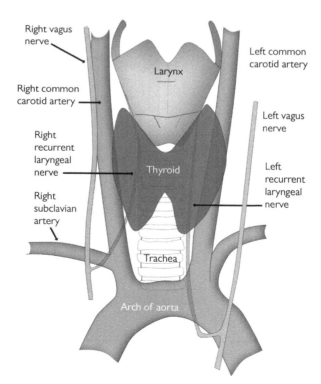

Fig. 1.4 Anatomical relations of the recurrent laryngeal nerve

Extended Matching Items—Answers

Nutrition

1. B. Fish oil-based total parenteral nutrition

Intestinal associated liver disease occurs in 15–40% of adults on home parenteral nutrition (HPN). It is usually related to age, length of time on parenteral nutrition, total caloric intake, and lipid or glucose overload. Its clinical spectrum and progression is similar to that of non-alcoholic fatty liver disease. For patients on HPN, progression can be limited by changing the lipid to omega 3 or fish oil-based lipid emulsion. If progression cannot be halted, visceral transplantation may need to be considered. *small bowel + liver transplant.*

Langnas AN and Tappenden KA. Intestinal failure: current and emerging therapies including transplantation. *Gastroenterology* 2006; 130 (2 suppl 1):S70–7

2. H. Puréed

Patients with oesophageal stents require a diet that will pass easily though the stent without causing occlusion. A puréed or sloppy diet is recommended and, specifically, patients should avoid bread or chunks of meat as these might cause stent occlusion, requiring emergency intervention.

3. A. Elemental   *Crohn's = elemental diet*

Remission in Crohn's disease can be induced in up to 90% of patients using an exclusive elemental enteral diet. This can be achieved without medication such as steroids, which are normally required in adults. Elemental diets contain nitrogen as oligopeptides. Energy is provided as glucose polymers and medium-chain triacylglycerols.

Critch J et al. Use of enteral nutrition for the control of intestinal inflammation in pediatric Crohn disease. *Journal of Pediatric Gastroenterology and Nutrition* 2012; 54(2):298–305.

Nutritional deficiencies

4. F. Selenium   *effectively makes hypothyroidr.*

Selenium is essential for the conversion of thyroxine (T4) to the more active triiodothyronine (T3). The link between selenium deficiency and hypothyroidism was only made in the 1990s. Isoforms of the main selenoproteins glutathione reductase, thioredoxin reductase, and deiodinase are expressed in the thyroid in high quantities.

Contempre B et al. Effect of selenium supplementation in hypothyroid subjects of an iodine and selenium deficient area: the possible danger of indiscriminate supplementation of iodine-deficient subjects with selenium. *Journal of Clinical Endocrinology & Metabolism* 1991; 73:213–5.

5. H. Vitamin B12

Vitamin B12 deficiency can result in sensory and motor deficits, dementia, and other psychiatric symptoms. It may result in sub-acute combined degeneration of the cord (SCD) where there is patchy loss of myelin in the dorsal and lateral columns. This results in progressive weakness of the limbs and trunk with tingling and loss of vibration and touch sense. A similar clinical picture may be seen with copper deficiency. SCD may be precipitated in a patient with both folic acid and vitamin B12 deficiency.

6. C. Magnesium

Acquired prolongation of the QT interval may be caused by many drugs (<http://www.qtdrugs.org>) or by electrolyte deficiencies, principally hypokalaemia, hypomagnesaemia, and hypocalcaemia. This may interact with underlying genetic susceptibility (long QT syndrome) and produce marked prolongation of the QT interval with the risk of arrhythmia (torsades de pointes).

Demling RH and DeBiasse MA. Micronutrients in critical illness. *Critical Care Clinics* 1995; 11:651–73.

Hernias

7. E. Inguinal

Although femoral hernias are three times more common in women than men, a groin hernia in a woman is still three times more likely to be inguinal than femoral.

8. A. Bochdalek

Congenital diaphragmatic hernias occur when there is failure of normal diaphragmatic development. Up to 90% of patients present in the neonatal period or within the first 12 months of life. They are associated with high mortality (up to 50%) and morbidity. Most of this relates to hypoplasia of the lung and pulmonary hypertension on the affected side. Bochdalek hernias account for over 90% of congenital diaphragmatic hernias and caused by a posterolateral defect. Morgagni hernias account for only 5–10% of cases and are anteriorly placed, usually on the right side (Figure 1.5).

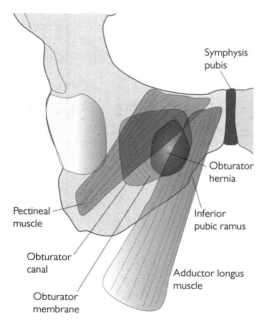

Fig. 1.5 Anatomical relations of the obturator canal

9. H. Obturator

Obturator hernias are rare and typically occur in elderly women or patients with chronically raised intra-abdominal pressure. Pregnancy has been suggested as a cause of the female preponderance, potentially due to a wider and more horizontal obturator canal. In general obturator hernias are asymptomatic unless they compress the obturator nerve or present with bowel compromise. This particular patient is more likely to have an obturator rather than femoral hernia (which would usually be more common) due to there being no palpable hernia despite her low BMI.

Infection

10. D. *Proteus*

Chronic proteus infection can lead to renal tract calculi. Proteus organisms alkalinize the urine by hydrolysing urea to ammonia by means of urease. This can lead to precipitation and struvite calculi (magnesium ammonium phosphate). Proteus infections account for 1–2% of urinary infections in healthy women but a prevalence of 20–45% when associated with catheterization.

11. E. *Staphylococcus aureus*

Coagulases produced by *Staphylococcus aureus* are an essential component in abscess formation, a hallmark of this organism. Patients with diabetes are more prone to skin infections. Tight post-operative glycaemic control is associated with a reduced frequency of wound infections

Cheng AG et al. Genetic requirements for *staphylococcus aureus* abscess formation and persistence in host tissues. *Federation of American Societies for Experimental Biology Journal* (FASEB J) 2009; 23:3393–404.

Sebranek JJ et al. Glycaemic control in the perioperative period. *British Journal of Anaesthesia* 2013; 111(suppl 1):18–34.

12. H. *Streptococcus bovis*

The association between endocarditis and colorectal cancer has been established since 1951 with *Streptococcus bovis* being identified as a causative agent in bacterial endocarditis two decades later. *Strep. bovis* endocarditis is associated with colon cancer in 50–70% of endocarditis cases at presentation and should prompt colonoscopy with surveillance for up to 4 years.

Klein RS et al. Association of *Streptococcus bovis* with carcinoma of the colon. *New England Journal of Medicine* 1977; 297:800–2.

Wentling GK et al. Unusual bacterial infections and colorectal carcinoma—*Streptococcus bovis* and *Clostridium septicum*: report of three cases. *Diseases of the Colon & Rectum* 2006; 49:1477–84.

Pelvic nerves

13. G. Pudendal nerve

The pudendal nerve is the main nerve of the perineum, supplying the motor function to the external anal sphincter, external urethral sphincter, and pelvic muscles. It supplies sensory innervation to the external genitalia and skin around the perineum and anus. Damage during childbirth may lead to faecal incontinence and loss of sensation.

14. F. Perineal nerve

The perineal nerve is the larger inferior branch of the pudendal nerve. It accompanies the perineal artery and further subdivides into superficial and deep branches. It is the deep branch that supplies the male urethra (see Figure 1.6).

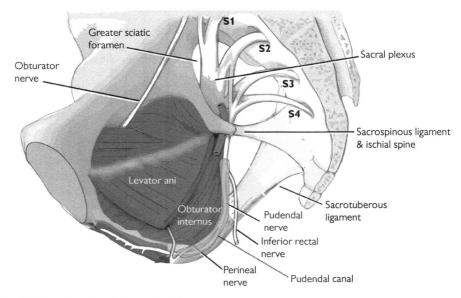

Fig. 1.6 Relationships of the pudendal nerve

15. D. Inferior hypogastric plexus

The nerve supply of the uterus is complex but its sympathetic supply is primarily from the inferior hypogastric plexus.

Statistics

16. B. Bland–Altman

The Bland–Altman is used to compare two clinical measurements, both of which are subject to error. It is designed to go beyond correlation between the two measurements and look at the level of agreement. A high level of correlation between two different measures of the same variable does not guarantee good agreement. The technique allows identification of systematic differences and outliers. 95% limits of agreement are commonly calculated.

17. E. Kaplan–Meier

The Kaplan–Meier estimator is presented as a plot of declining horizontal steps and is one of the most commonly used survival analyses. It is a time-to-event model where the time to a certain level of events can be predicted. It is typically used to present data on mortality, recovery, and event-free survival.

18. J. Standard deviation

Standard deviation is a measure of the variation of a set of data values. A low standard deviation (SD) indicates that the data points lie close to the mean. It assumes that the data are normally distributed. If this is not the case then non-parametric tests are more appropriate, with a box and whisker plot of the five-number summary being useful.

Genetic cancer syndromes

19. F. Multiple endocrine neoplasia 2

MEN 2 is a rare inherited syndrome caused by mutations in the RET proto-oncogene. It is characterized by medullary thyroid cancer and phaeochromocytoma. MEN 2A is distinguished from MEN 2B by the presence of parathyroid hyperplasia and absence of mucosal neuromas and marfanoid habitus. It is inherited as an autosomal dominant condition but up to 50% of cases of MEN 2B result from *de novo* mutations. MEN 1 syndrome includes pituitary and pancreatic islet tumours in addition to parathyroid hyperplasia.

20. H. Hereditary diffuse gastric cancer

E-cadherin (*CDH1*) mutations predispose to hereditary diffuse gastric cancer. Loss of E-cadherin expression or function is implicated in a variety of tumour types and it is intimately related to the process of epithelial–mesenchymal transition. Loss of E-cadherin is also a characteristic of the process of adenomatous transformation in familial adenomatous polyposis (FAP); however, this condition is characterized by a loss of function mutation in the tumour-suppressor APC gene.

21. D. Lynch syndrome

Lynch syndrome (hereditary non-polyposis colorectal cancer, HNPCC) is a cancer syndrome which results from defective DNA mismatch repair. Mutations in the *MSH2, MLH1, MSH6, PMS2,* and *PMS1* are implicated giving rise to HNPCC (2–4% of colorectal cancers) and resulting in the microsatellite instability phenotype (right-sided predominance, poor tumour differentiation, higher mucin content, and pronounced lymphocytic infiltrate). Most cancers arise from *MLH1* and *MSH2* mutations. Predisposed individuals are thought to have one inactivated copy of the mismatch repair gene and the second is lost as a somatic mutation. In sporadic microsatellite unstable colorectal cancer (15% of all CRCs), most cases arise via an epigenetic phenomenon with hypermethylation of the *MLH1* gene promoter region.

Antibiotics

22. A. Vancomycin

Treatment of mild to moderate *Clostridium difficile* colitis is with oral metronidazole (400–500mg TDS for 10–14 days), which has been shown to be as effective as vancomycin. Severe *C. difficile* infection (CDI) is considered in the presence of a rising leukocyte count (WCC >15 × 10^9), acute rise in creatinine (>50% over baseline), temperature (>38.5°C), and evidence of severe colitis based on abdominal signs or radiological findings. CDI is best treated with oral vancomycin (125mg QDS for 10–14 days), which is preferred to oral metronidazole because of lower failure rates. Fidaxomicin could be considered in severe *C. difficile* infection with a high risk of recurrence (Public Health England Guidance on the Management and Treatment of *Clostridium Difficile* infection 2013).

23. F. Doxycycline

Doxycycline is a tetracycline antibiotic commonly used in the treatment of lower respiratory tract infections, rickettsial diseases, acne, and chlamydia. Side effects include gastrointestinal upset, photosensitivity, and, more rarely, permanent discolouration of dentition, which is reported in young children and during pregnancy.

24. B. Ciprofloxacin

Quinolones include ciprofloxacin, ofloxacin, and levofloxacin. Ciprofloxacin is effective against gram-negative bacteria, including those that cause gastrointestinal and urinary tract infections such as *E. coli, Klebsiella, salmonella, Shigella,* and *campylobacter*, as well as *pseudomonas*.

Gastrointestinal infection

25. A. *Shigella*

Shigella is a non-flagellated organism spread by the faecal–oral route. It is a common cause of travellers' diarrhoea in addition to *salmonella* and enterotoxigenic *E. coli* (ETEC). Unlike *salmonella* and *giardiasis*, *shigella* commonly causes bloody diarrhoea. It usually follows a self-limiting course but antibiotics (e.g. ciprofloxacin) can be used in severe cases.

26. I. *Campylobacter jejuni*

Campylobacter jejuni and *campylobacter coli* are common causes of food poisoning and can result in bloody diarrheoa. It is transmitted via the faecal–oral route through uncooked foods such as poultry, meat, and unpasteurized milk. This patient's short-lived history and lack of travel make *campylobacter* the most likely cause. *E. coli* O157 is a toxin-producing enterohaemorrhagic strain of *E. coli* (EHEC) capable of life-threatening haemorrhagic syndromes. This bacterium can also be spread via contaminated meats in the United Kingdom; however, cases are relatively rare and therefore this answer is less likely.

27. B. *Cryptosporidium*

This protozoal infection is seen in immunocompromised patients but can also present with milder diarrhoea in non-immunocompromised hosts. It is spread through contaminated water. *Cryptosporidium* oocysts are seen in stool cultures.

Statistical bias

28. A. Selection bias

Selection bias occurs when a study selects patients that are not truly representative of the target population. This can be due to non-randomization or a small study population. In the example a power calculation is based on all patients after oesophagectomy. By recruiting at 12–18 months they have already biased the population by excluding early recurrences. The population is no longer representative of the target population and therefore selection bias is present.

29. G. Procedure bias

Procedure bias occurs where subjects in different groups receive different treatment, which is a confounding factor in the analysis. Here, clearly different treatments that may confound the primary outcome measure (length of stay) are employed. The study should stratify appropriately for the use of laparoscopic surgery.

30. I. Observer-expectancy bias

This occurs where the researcher has a strong belief in the efficacy of a given treatment. Consciously or unconsciously this may interfere with the documentation of results. It is minimized by allocation concealment (blinding). In this case the operating surgeon is asking subjective research questions and documenting the answers, which is not appropriate.

Other types of statistical bias:

Recall bias—This occurs when study subjects are asked to recall events, as occurs in retrospective research. An awareness of a disorder can alter the recall by study subjects, as can the passage of time, with recent events more clearly recalled than older events.

Lead time bias—This occurs when cases are not detected at the same stage of the disease. Follow-up starts from the time of detection. The disease course may not be altered and this 'lead time' may result in a systemic error in results.

Classification bias—This occurs where ambiguity in the definition of included patients leads to less sharply defined groupings for analysis.

Confounding bias—This occurs where multiple factors could influence the outcome. Such factors may be inextricably linked and can confuse the analysis. For example, colorectal cancer risk is greater in obese people but it is also higher in those with a sedentary lifestyle and those who have a high dietary fat intake. It requires validation studies, case controls, and matching study design to reduce bias.

Publication bias—This occurs where journals preferentially publish positive results compared with negative trial results.

Attrition bias—This occurs where there is a differential drop-out rate between the study groups.

Measurement bias—This occurs when groups under study may behave differently than they would otherwise. This is known as the Hawthorne effect.

Gastrointestinal polyps

31. F. Fundic gland polyps

These are the most commonly seen polyps on upper GI endoscopy and are characteristically 1–5mm transparent lesions occurring in clusters in the gastric body or fundus. They may be sporadic (as in the vast majority) or can be associated with familial adenomatous polyposis. This diagnosis should be considered in young patients (i.e. consider colonoscopy). In the absence of a genetic basis they harbour little malignant potential (dysplasia in <1%). Spontaneous regression is reported and regular observation is usually not required after a biopsy to exclude dysplasia.

32. I. Sessile serrated polyps

These polyps have only recently been recognized as a variant of the hyperplastic polyp. They have pre-malignant potential and may account for 15–33% of colorectal cancers. Tumours developing via this pathway have several characteristics including a right-sided predominance, sporadic microsatellite instability, BRAF mutations, and CpG island methylator phenotype. Simple hyperplastic polyps have limited malignant potential and are characteristically <5mm in size and located in the region of the distal colon and rectum.

33. H. Hamartomatous polyps

Peutz–Jeghers syndrome is an autosomal dominant condition associated with multiple hamartomatous polyps of the GI tract and mucocutaneous pigmentation. The polyps are characterized by a connective tissue core. The condition is associated with gastro-oesophageal, pancreatic, colorectal, and breast cancers. Colonoscopy is recommended 2–yearly from the age of 25 years (BSG Guidelines on Colorectal Cancer Surveillance 2010).

Cancer drugs

34. D. Cyclophosphamide

Alkylating agents are anti-proliferative drugs and include Melphalan, Chlorambucil, Ifosfamide, and Cyclophosphamide. They bind via alkyl groups to DNA. Crosslinking leads to arrest in G1–S transition. They are commonly used in haematological malignancies and solid cancers including ovarian and breast cancer.

35. F. Capecitabine

This is an oral pro-drug of 5-FU, a pyrimidine analogue that inhibits thymidilate synthase and RNA synthesis. It is used in a variety of tumour types, particularly gastrointestinal malignancies. Side effects include myelosuppression, gastrointestinal upset, and cardiotoxicity.

36. A. Gemcitabine

Anti-metabolites include anti-folates (methotrexate and thymidilate synthase inhibitors), anti-purines (azathioprine), cytosine analogues (gemcitabine), and adnenosine analogues (fludarabine). The active metabolite of gemcitabine (df-CTP) is incorporated into DNA during replication resulting in growth arrest and apoptosis. It is commonly used in pancreatic cancer, bladder cancer, lung cancer, and breast cancer.

Glasgow Coma Scale

37. A. 3

This man is unconscious (E1, M1, V1, GCS = 3) and makes no movements or sounds in response to stimulus. He requires urgent airway management.

38. H. 12

This patient opens her eyes to voice (E3), is confused (V4), and localizes to a painful stimulus with her other hand (M5)

U = (N) / confused = IV / inapropriate words = 3 grunts = 2 (= Ji le

39. D. 7

This patient has no eye opening (E1), makes incomprehensible sounds (V2), and withdraws from pain (M4)

Calculating the GCS is a common scenario in the exam and therefore candidates should ensure they are well prepared for these questions (See Table 1.4).

Teasdale G and Jennett B. Assessment of coma and impaired consciousness. A practical scale. *The Lancet* 1974; 13(2):81–4.

Table 1.4 Glasgow Coma Scale

Behaviour	Response	Score
Eye opening response	Spontaneously	4
	To speech	3
	To pain	2
	No response	1
Best verbal response	Orientated, normal conversation	5
	Confused, disorientated	4
	Inappropriate words	3
	Incomprehensible sounds	2
	Makes no sounds	1
Best motor response	Obeys commands	6
	Localizes to pain	5
	Flexion/withdrawal from pain	4
	Abnormal flexion to painful stimulus (decorticate response)	3
	Abnormal extension to painful stimulus (decerebrate response)	2
	No movements	1

Reprinted from *The Lancet*, 13, 2, Teasdale G and Jennett B. Assessment of coma and impaired consciousness. A practical scale, pp. 81–4. Copyright (1974), with permission from Elsevier.

PERIOPERATIVE AND CRITICAL CARE

QUESTIONS

Single Best Answers

1. **Which of the following is required to undertake testing for diagnosis of death using neurological criteria (DNC)?**
   a) Evidence for irreversible brain damage
   b) Normothermia
   c) Consent from the patient's family or Power of Attorney
   d) Two medical practitioners
   e) Glasgow Coma Score of 3 or mechanical ventilation with apnoea

2. **Which of the following should be present when undertaking testing for the diagnosis of death using neurological criteria?**
   a) Normal serum creatinine
   b) Cardiovascularly stable without the use of vasoactive agents
   c) Normal arterial blood gases
   d) Patient should be well sedated
   e) Apnoea

3. **Which of the followings statements is correct when considering the provision of enteral nutrition in the acute phase of a critical illness?**
   a) Nutrition be commenced within 24 hours of admission to the intensive care unit (ICU)
   b) Should be supplemented with parenteral nutrition to match the measured caloric requirements
   c) Should contain supplemental glutamine
   d) Can be delayed for up to seven days
   e) Reduces the risk of nosocomial infection in comparison to parenteral nutrition

4. **When considering the micronutrient requirements of critically ill patients, which of the following statements is correct?**
   a) Replacement of selenium in severely septic patients improves survival
   b) Administration of vitamin C to alcoholics with a critical illness is beneficial
   c) Vitamin B_6 replacement should be considered in in-patients who have undergone a gastrectomy or ileal resection
   d) Additional calcium may be required to replace losses from pancreatic fistulae
   e) Phosphate, magnesium, and potassium deficiencies should be considered upon refeeding a malnourished patient

5. **Which of the following statements is correct when comparing parenteral nutrition to the use of enteral nutrition in critically ill patients?**
   a) Parenteral nutrition is associated with an increased incidence of acquired infections
   b) Enteral nutrition is associated with a reduction in mortality rates
   c) The use of parenteral nutrition shortens the length of stay
   d) Parenteral nutrition is associated with a shortened duration of mechanical ventilation
   e) Parenteral nutrition is more expensive

6. **Critically ill patients in the ICU are subject to invasive procedures and multiple direct contacts with staff and the environment. Which of the following interventions has been shown to reduce the risk of acquired infection in critically ill patients?**
   a) Hand-washing with alcohol rub before and after patient contact
   b) Whole-patient bathing with Chlorhexidine
   c) Application of intra-oral Chlorhexidine gel
   d) The liberal use of antibiotics
   e) Five days of prophylactic intravenous antibiotics

7. **Which of the following has been shown to reduce the incidence of acquired central venous line sepsis?**
   a) Administration of intravenous (IV) vancomycin prophylaxis at the time of line insertion
   b) Utilizing the femoral vein site of insertion
   c) Using a multiple lumen catheter
   d) Daily review and removal of the catheter at the earliest opportunity
   e) Changing the lines every seven days

8. **When considering the APACHE II scoring system, which of the following statements are correct?**
   a) It can be used to predict functional recovery and quality of life following ICU
   b) It can predict a patient's risk of death in ICU
   c) It can be recalculated at any time during their admission in ICU
   d) It can be used to calculate a standardized mortality ratio for an ICU allowing benchmarking between units
   e) It is no longer regarded as a valid assessment of the severity of disease

9. **A Quality Indicator helps in understanding a health care system, the ability to compare it with others and then to improve it. Which of the following is the most commonly used Quality Indicator when evaluating critical care?**
   a) Length of stay
   b) Mortality rate
   c) APACHE II scores
   d) Re-admission rates
   e) Overnight admission rates

10. **A 68-year-old man remains sedated and requiring mechanical ventilation 6 days following surgery. He has a measured haemoglobin level of 86g/L. The critical care team have decided not to transfuse him. What is the most likely reason for this decision?**
    a) There is a high risk of transfusion-associated lung injury
    b) The currently recommended transfusion trigger is 70 g/L
    c) The patient is unable to provide consent
    d) It may increase his risk of developing a deep venous thrombosis
    e) The patient does not have a central venous catheter

11. **Anaemia is common in critically ill patients, affecting around 70% of patients in the ICU. This is multifactorial in aetiology. Which of the following is the most effective strategy to prevent this type of anaemia?**
    a) The administration of erythropoietin
    b) Prompt red cell transfusion to maintain a haemoglobin level above 100g/L
    c) Routine iron supplementation
    d) Avoiding fluid overload
    e) The use of blood-conservation sampling devices to reduce phlebotomy-associated blood loss

12. **A 73 year old woman undergoes drainage of an empyema of her gallbladder. On the second post-operative day her platelet count is 55 × 10^9/L. What is the most likely cause?**
    a) Hypersplenism
    b) Heparin-induced thrombocytopenia (HIT)
    c) Haemolytic uraemic syndrome (HUS)
    d) Antibiotic administration
    e) Septic response

13. **A 65 year old man is admitted to the ICU following a Hartmann's procedure for perforated diverticular disease. Bloods taken 6 hours after his admission show a rise in lactate to 4.1nmol/l. He requires ongoing mechanical ventilation, inotropes, and intravenous fluids. What is the most likely cause for the rising lactate?**
    a) The patient's deteriorating renal function
    b) The patient's ongoing septic response
    c) Mesenteric ischaemia
    d) Impaired hepatic function
    e) The norepinephrine infusion

14. **Venous thromboembolism (VTE) is common in hospitalized patients and those with critical illness are at particular risk. When considering prophylactic measures, which of the following statements is correct?**
    a) Inferior vena cava (IVC) filters are used routinely with pharmacological prophylaxis or in individuals where pharmacological prophylaxis is contraindicated
    b) The use of low molecular weight Heparin (LMWH) is reserved for use in patients with a history of heparin-induced thrombocytopenia (HIT)
    c) Prophylaxis should be commenced within 24 hours of admission to the ICU
    d) Mechanical thromboprophylaxis is used in critically ill patients when pharmacological prophylaxis is contraindicated. In this setting, intermittent pneumatic compression is superior to graduated compression stockings
    e) Patients with stable or improving traumatic brain injury should be considered for pharmacological prophylaxis within 24 hours of injury

15. **A 62 year old man has had a particularly stormy post-operative course following a return to theatre and a prolonged stay on the Intensive Care Unit. He has now developed a sustained pyrexia, high white cell count and some new changes on his chest X-ray. The diagnosis is ventilator-associated pneumonia (VAP). Which of the following interventions has been shown to reduce the risk of ventilator-associated pneumonia?**
    a) Early initiation of enteral nutrition
    b) Intravenous ranitidine or omeprazole
    c) Early establishment of tracheostomy
    d) Nebulized antibiotics
    e) Nursing the patient in a 30–45° head-up position

16. **Tracheostomy is among the most common procedures undertaken in patients in the Intensive Care Unit. Which of the following statements is correct when considering the benefits of tracheostomy in this setting?**
    a) Reduced incidence of ventilator-associated pneumonia
    b) Reduced mortality rate
    c) Reduced rate of sub-glottic stenosis
    d) Improved patient psychological well-being
    e) Earlier discharge to a non-critical care ward

17. **The nursing staff are concerned regarding the behaviour of 78 year old man recovering from a ruptured aortic aneurysm. He was extubated earlier in the day but he has now become very aggressive and difficult to manage. What is the most likely cause for his deterioration?**
    a) Mesenteric ischaemia
    b) Delirium
    c) Myocardial infarction
    d) Untreated anaemia
    e) Alcohol withdrawal

18. **According to the Frank–Starling law of the heart, stroke volume is related to which of the following?**
    a) Central venous pressure
    b) Coronary perfusion pressure
    c) Heart rate
    d) Left ventricular afterload
    e) Left ventricular end diastolic volume

19. **Which of the following hormones mediates positive inotropy independent of adrenoceptors?**
    a) Adrenaline
    b) Dopamine
    c) Noradrenaline
    d) Glucagon
    e) Vasopressin

20. **A 71 year old man with chronic obstructive pulmonary disease and mild left ventricular systolic dysfunction is listed for a right hemicolectomy for cancer. He undergoes cardiopulmonary exercise testing as part of his preoperative assessment. Which of the following parameters has been shown to predict mortality after intra-abdominal surgery?**
    a) Anaerobic threshold
    b) Peak heart rate
    c) Peak minute ventilation
    d) Peak oxygen consumption
    e) Ventilatory equivalent for carbon dioxide

21. **A 65 year old man is referred with mild discomfort from a reducible inguinal hernia. He had a drug-eluting coronary stent inserted three months ago and remains on dual antiplatelet therapy following this. Which of the following is the most appropriate course of action?**
    a) Advise against an operation
    b) Continue both antiplatelet agents, avoid spinal anaesthesia, and operate
    c) Defer the operation until six months after coronary stenting
    d) Stop both antiplatelet agents and operate
    e) Stop one antiplatelet agent and operate

22. **A 72 year old man is listed for an anterior resection. He has had a mechanical aortic valve replacement and takes warfarin. How should his anticoagulation be managed perioperatively?**
    a) Continue warfarin throughout the perioperative period
    b) Omit warfarin on the day of surgery only
    c) Stop warfarin three days before surgery and commence aspirin
    d) Stop warfarin five days before surgery and commence prophylactic enoxaparin
    e) Stop warfarin three days before surgery and commence unfractionated heparin

23. **A 52 year old woman with well-controlled type 2 diabetes, hypertension, and hypercholesterolaemia is scheduled for an incisional hernia repair as a day case procedure under general anaesthesia. Her current medications are metformin, gliclazide, atenolol, and simvastatin. Which of these should she omit preoperatively?**
    a) Atenolol
    b) Gliclazide
    c) Metformin
    d) None
    e) Simvastatin

24. **A 70 year old man with a past medical history of chronic obstructive pulmonary disease undergoes a laparoscopic right hemicolectomy. Which of the following approaches to intra-operative ventilation is shown to improve outcomes?**
    a) Avoidance of recruitment manoeuvres
    b) High inspired oxygen concentration
    c) Permissive hypercapnia
    d) Positive end expiratory pressure
    e) Tidal volume 6–8 ml/kg actual body weight

25. Which of the following are effective in reducing the incidence of delirium?

a) The use of benzodiazepines
b) Early mobilization
c) Regularly administered anti-psychotics, for example Haloperidol
d) Effective night sedation
e) The provision of written and verbal information about delirium to patient's relatives

26. Which of the following does not predict post-operative pneumonia?

a) Advancing age
b) Chronic obstructive pulmonary disease
c) Ischaemic heart disease
d) Previous cerebrovascular accident
e) Weight loss

27. A 68 year old man undergoes serial intra-abdominal pressure monitoring following repair of a ruptured abdominal aortic aneurysm. A diagnosis of abdominal compartment syndrome is made after sustained intra-abdominal pressure reaches what level?

a) 5mmHg
b) 12mmHg
c) 15mmHg
d) 20mmHg
e) 25mmHg

28. A 75 year old woman with faecal peritonitis due to a diverticular perforation undergoes serial intra-abdominal pressure monitoring. Where are standard intra-abdominal pressure measurements made?

a) Bladder
b) Inferior vena cava
c) Portal vein
d) Rectum
e) Stomach

29. A 23 year old man with polytrauma is found to have raised intra-abdominal pressure. Which of the following treatments does not reduce intra-abdominal pressure?

a) Neuromuscular blockade
b) Nasogastric decompression
c) Percutaneous drainage of intra-abdominal collections
d) Liberal fluid resuscitation
e) Surgical decompression

30. **A 75 year old male with a past history of COPD falls at home, injuring his right chest wall. He is admitted through A&E with tachypnoea, hypoxaemia, and pain. A chest X-ray (CXR) shows a moderate right-sided pneumothorax with multiple fractured ribs and raises the potential diagnosis of a flail segment. He is transferred to Critical Care for ongoing monitoring, with an intercostal drain *in situ*, but he develops an ongoing and rising oxygen demand. His SpO$_2$ is 93% on a FiO$_2$ of 0.8 via facemask and a respiratory rate (RR) of 28.**

    What is the best approach in this patient?
    a) Continuous positive airway pressure (CPAP)
    b) High-flow nasal oxygen
    c) High thoracic epidural analgesia
    d) Invasive ventilation
    e) Patient-controlled analgesia (PCA) with opioids

31. **An elderly gentleman undergoes an emergency colonic resection for large bowel obstruction with local contamination found at laparotomy and he returns ventilated to Critical Care. He is rapidly weaned from vasopressor support but encounters great difficulty when sedation is reduced as he becomes very agitated. He has one attempted extubation that fails within four hours due to delirium and sputum retention.**

    What is the most appropriate management strategy?
    a) Benzodiazepine sedation
    b) Non-invasive ventilation via face-mask
    c) Palliation with end-of-life care
    d) Reintubation
    e) Reintubation with a view to tracheostomy

32. **An elderly gentleman with a history including an MI (myocardial infarction), heart failure, and stroke presents in septic shock with a marked area of cellulitis extending from his scrotum to the anterior abdominal wall. On examination this appears to demonstrate crepitus and he has hypotension and biochemical evidence of acute kidney injury. A diagnosis of Fournier's gangrene is made.**

    What is the most appropriate management strategy?
    a) Antibiotics
    b) Debridement and extubation
    c) Debridement and Critical Care admission
    d) End-of-life care
    e) ICU admission alone

33. **A 36 year old is admitted with moderate pancreatitis but no CT evidence of necrosis. She develops type 1 respiratory failure due to a combination of abdominal distension and bilateral pleural effusions. She is ventilated for several days with failure of nasogastric (NG) feeding due to high volume aspirates. She then passes small amounts of melaena and altered blood on NG suction. There is no haemodynamic compromise and no significant haemoglobin drop.**

    What is the most appropriate management strategy?
    a) Continue with nasogastric feeding
    b) Continuous PPI infusion—'Hong Kong' regime
    c) Histamine receptor blockade
    d) Upper GI endoscopy
    e) Proton pump inhibitor

34. **A 24 year old is a victim of an assault with multiple contusions across his abdomen, allegedly due to being struck with a baseball bat. He presents to A&E with signs of peritonism and a FAST (Focused Assessment with Sonography for Trauma) scan suggests free fluid. He is anxious but alert with a heart rate of 130bpm and a non-invasive blood pressure of 90/50mmHg. A venous lactate is 3.8. You are informed that it will be 45 minutes until a theatre slot is available.**

    What is the most appropriate management strategy?
    a) Blood resuscitation
    b) Crystalloid resuscitation
    c) Deployment of aortic occlusion device
    d) Permissive hypotension
    e) Vasopressors to an MAP >65mmHg

35. **A young man is admitted following an assault with multiple stab wounds to his abdomen, shocked and acidotic with evidence of marked haemorrhage. He is rapidly taken to theatre where multiple enterotomies and vascular injuries are found. His vascular injuries are repaired and his bowel injuries begin to be addressed. After a period of time closing enterotomies the anaesthetist raises concerns that his acidosis and hypothermia are worsening despite optimum treatment.**

    What is the most appropriate management strategy?
    a) Cessation of surgery for a period to allow on-table warming
    b) Closure of abdomen and palliation
    c) Formal bowel resection with stoma formation
    d) Temporary bowel stapling, abdomen left open, transfer to ICU
    e) Temporary bowel stapling, closure of abdomen, transfer to ICU

36. **A 65 year old patient undergoes a Hartmann's procedure for a perforated sigmoid volvulus with faecal peritonitis. She is admitted to Critical Care for ongoing care but despite optimization with fluids and vasopressors her renal function deteriorates. On the third post-operative day she is passing 10ml/hr of urine with a potassium of 6.1mmol/L, a bicarbonate of 9mmol/L, and a creatinine of 430micromol/L. Her initial CT scan ruled out obstructive uropathy.**

    What is the most appropriate management strategy?
    a) Aminophylline
    b) Further fluid resuscitation
    c) Intravenous diuretic infusion
    d) Renal replacement therapy
    e) Terlipressin

37. **A middle-aged alcoholic is admitted with haematemesis and melaena. After a period of observation haemodynamic instability supervenes and the case progresses to endoscopy. At endoscopy a number of large oesophageal varices are encountered and banded. During the procedure a 7-unit transfusion of packed red cells occurs. The patient returns to Critical Care where they continue to have small volume melaena and some oozing around invasive lines. Laboratory tests return showing a haemoglobin of 88g/L, a platelet count of 40 × 10^9, a PT ratio of 2.2, and an APTT ratio of 2.0.**

    What is the most appropriate management strategy?
    a) Activation of major haemorrhage protocol
    b) Administration of calcium chloride
    c) Correction of haemoglobin to >100g/dL
    d) Correction of coagulation abnormalities
    e) Vitamin K

38. **A 72 year old man is operated on for an incarcerated and obstructed inguinal hernia. At the end of the procedure he is extubated and immediately vomits copiously, desaturating, and becoming tachypnoeic. He is reintubated and endobronchial toilet is carried out. He is subsequently referred to ICU.**

    What is the most appropriate management strategy?
    a) Antibiotics with anaerobic coverage
    b) Bronchoscopy
    c) Corticosteroids
    d) CT scanning
    e) Expectant monitoring

Extended Matching Items

Physiological response to haemorrhage

A. Adrenaline
B. Aldosterone
C. Angiotensin II
D. Antidiuretic hormone
E. Aortic arch baroreceptor
F. Atrial volume receptor
G. Carotid sinus baroreceptor
H. Erythropoietin
I. Noradrenaline
J. Renin

For each statement select the most appropriate mediator from the list of options.

1. Reduces signalling via the glossopharyngeal nerve in response to hypotension.

2. Increases heart rate, contractility, and systemic vascular resistance when secreted from post-ganglionic sympathetic nerve fibres.

3. Promotes water reabsorption by translocation of aquaporin channels in the epithelial cells of the distal convoluted tubule and collecting duct.

Partial pressure of oxygen

A. 0kPa
B. 2kPa
C. 3.5kPa
D. 5.3kPa
E. 10kPa
F. 13kPa
G. 21kPa
H. 75kPa
I. 100kPa
J. 101kPa

For each scenario select the most appropriate partial pressure from the list of options.

4. A fit 23 year old man is brought to theatre for an appendicectomy. Prior to induction of anaesthesia, effective pre-oxygenation with 100% oxygen is achieved. What is the approximate arterial partial pressure of oxygen at this time?

5. The alveolar–arterial gradient may be calculated when severity scoring surgical patients admitted to intensive care. What is a normal value for the alveolar–arterial pressure gradient?

6. A 59 year old with septic shock secondary to cholangitis has her central venous oxygen saturation measured as 75%. Assuming she is currently afebrile and has a normally positioned oxyhaemoglobin dissociation curve, what is the corresponding venous partial pressure of oxygen?

Lung volumes

A. Closing volume
B. Forced expiratory volume in one second
C. Functional residual capacity
D. Inspiratory reserve volume
E. Ratio of forced expiratory volume in one second to forced vital capacity
F. Residual volume
G. Tidal volume
H. Total lung capacity
I. Vital capacity

For each scenario select the most appropriate lung volume from the list of options.

7. A 69 year old woman with chronic obstructive pulmonary disease presents for a mastectomy. Which of the following is used to gauge the severity of her lung disease?

8. A 42 year old man with a suspected duodenal ulcer undergoes rapid sequence induction of general anaesthesia. Which of the following acts as an oxygen reservoir until the trachea is intubated and ventilation resumed?

9. A 38 year old man develops acute respiratory distress syndrome secondary to pancreatitis and requires invasive ventilation. Which of the following should be carefully controlled to avoid further lung injury?

Bleeding and shock

A. Acute coagulopathy of trauma
B. Acute hepatic failure
C. Disseminated intravascular coagulation
D. Haemolytic uraemic syndrome
E. Heparin-induced thrombocytopenia
F. Hypersplenism
G. Immune thrombocytopenic purpura
H. Myelodysplasia
I. Sepsis-induced thrombocytopenia
J. Thrombotic thrombocytopenic purpura

For each of the following scenarios, select the most likely diagnosis from the list of options.

10. A 45 year old woman is involved in a multi-vehicle accident and is transferred to the ICU after fixation of multiple long-bone fractures and intra-abdominal injuries. On day 2 she develops marked bleeding from all wounds and catheter sites with prolonged PT (prothrombin time), APTT (activated partial thromboplastin time), and reduced platelet counts.

11. A 79 year old man is admitted to the ICU with acute cholecystitis, sepsis, and renal failure. He is ventilated, on vasopressors and renal replacement therapy, and develops marked thrombocytopenia after six days. He has a prolonged PT and obstructive pattern of liver function tests. His APTT indicates therapeutic anticoagulation with heparin. On a sedation hold he is found to have a right-sided hemiparesis.

12. A 42 year old woman is admitted to Critical Care after a sudden deceleration injury while wearing a seatbelt. She has had a CT scan confirming free intra-abdominal air and fluid and is taken for a laparotomy. She undergoes a prolonged procedure and returns to Critical Care hypothermic and acidotic with bleeding from her laparotomy wound and several line sites.

Bleeding and shock

A. Acute adrenal insufficiency
B. Cardiogenic shock
C. Fat embolism
D. Haemorrhagic shock
E. Neurogenic shock
F. Pulmonary embolism
G. Relative adrenal insufficiency
H. Septic shock
I. Spinal shock
J. Thyroid storm

For each of the following scenarios, select the most likely diagnosis from the list of options.

13. A 32 year old suffers a femoral fracture in a motor accident. Following a prolonged operation he is admitted to Critical Care for prolonged recovery. On the third day he is mobilizing with physiotherapy when he collapses, with hypotension, distended neck veins, and hypoxaemia.

14. A 74 year old man is found at the bottom of a stairwell with an occipital laceration and an open ankle fracture. He has diaphragmatic breathing, no motor response to painful stimulus, and hypotension refractory to 20ml/kg of IV fluid resuscitation.

15. A 65 year old attends A&E after worsening of her Crohn's disease. She has a tachycardia of 150bpm and an invasive BP of 80/40mmHg. She has cool peripheries and prolonged capillary refill time despite 3L of crystalloid resuscitation. She has a prolonged PT and mildly deranged LFTs (liver function tests), with a lactate of 3.2mmol/L. A CT scan shows inflammation of the terminal ileum with a large retroperitoneal collection.

Respiratory dysfunction

A. Adult respiratory distress syndrome
B. Atelectasis
C. Bronchopneumonia
D. Bronchopulmonary fistula
E. Bronchospasm
F. Fibrosing alveolitis
G. Negative pressure pulmonary oedema
H. Pulmonary embolism
I. Pulmonary vasculitis
J. Sarcoidosis

For each of the following scenarios, select the most likely diagnosis from the list of options.

16. A 23 year old man is admitted to ICU following repair of a perforated duodenal ulcer. He self-extubates the next morning and is acutely stridulous leading to an emergency reintubation. His oxygen saturations remain at 88% on an FiO_2 of 1.0. On examination he has bilateral inspiratory crepitations.

17. A 46 year old is admitted to Critical Care with acute severe pancreatitis. A CT scan shows marked necrosis of the pancreatic tail and bilateral small pleural effusions. He is given fluid resuscitation, vasopressors, and post-pyloric feeding. On day 6 he develops tachypnoea, a rising oxygen demand, and a portable CXR shows florid bilateral pulmonary infiltrates.

18. A 62 year old is admitted to hospital for a laparoscopic left hemicolectomy for colonic carcinoma that proceeds uneventfully. On the fifth post-operative day he is mobilizing to the shower when he collapses with cyanosis, hypotension, and a sinus tachycardia. An ABG (arterial blood gas) on high-flow oxygen shows a PaO_2 of 6.3kPa and a $PaCO_2$ of 3.2kPa with a metabolic acidosis. A focused echocardiogram reveals a dilated right ventricle with septal bulging into the left ventricle.

Renal dysfunction

A. Acute interstitial nephritis
B. Cardiorenal syndrome
C. Cerebral salt wasting
D. Goodpasture's syndrome
E. Hepatorenal syndrome
F. Nephrogenic diabetes insipidus
G. Neurogenic diabetes insipidus
H. Polyuric renal failure
I. Pre-renal failure
J. Rhabdomyolysis

For each of the following scenarios, choose the most likely diagnosis from the list of options.

19. A 49 year old with a history of bipolar disease is admitted following a negative laparotomy for suspected large bowel obstruction. A presumptive diagnosis of Ogilvie's syndrome secondary to her psychiatric medications has been made. She is intubated and ventilated with low-dose vasopressor support. It is noted during the first day of admission that her sodium is climbing and marked polyuria is recorded.

20. A 45 years old is involved in a road traffic accident (RTA) where he is trapped and requires extrication from his car. He is hypothermic and hypotensive with profound and tense lower limb compartments. He is transferred to hospital, where he is given fluid resuscitation, vasopressors, and intubated for airway protection. He produces small amounts of reddish-brown urine for the first six hours in Critical Care before this reduces to virtual anuria. Investigations reveal a potassium of 7mmol/L and a creatinine of 300micromol/L.

Anti-microbials

A. Ciprofloxacin
B. Clindamycin
C. Cefotaxime
D. Vancomycin
E. Co-amoxiclav
F. Amphotericin
G. Fluconazole
H. Posaconazole
I. Caspofungin

For each of these clinical scenarios select the most appropriate anti-microbial.

21. Following a 2-week stay in Critical Care and a re-laparotomy, a 41 year old man with Crohn's disease has a swinging pyrexia, raised inflammatory markers and cardiovascular instability. A Candida has been isolated in a blood culture. Which anti-microbial should be commenced?

22. A 79 year old gentleman remains septic following his fall and subsequent orthopaedic injuries. A septic screen was undertaken at the time of admission. The likely infecting organism is a *Staph. aureus*. Which anti-microbial should be commenced?

23. Which of these antibiotics can be used to treat *Clostridium difficile* infection?

Single Best Answers

1. b) Normothermia

The criteria and process for the diagnosis of death using neurological criteria in the United Kingdom are clearly defined. There must be evidence of irreversible cessation of brainstem function of known aetiology. The patient should be normothermic with a temperature of at least 34⁰C. They should also have a GCS of 3 and be mechanically ventilated with apnoea. The diagnosis requires the presence of two senior medical practitioners, often consultants, and does not require the consent of family or power of attorney to be undertaken.

Academy of Medical Royal Colleges (2008). *A Code of Practice for the Diagnosis and Confirmation of Death.* <http://www.aomrc.org.uk>.

2. e) Apnoea — *Inotropes are allowed*

For diagnosis of death by neurological criteria it is important that the electrolytes, sodium and potassium, are within normal limits.

In addition, the patient is haemodynamically stable. This may require the administration of vasoactive agents to maintain an effective perfusion pressure and that any sedative agents or neuromuscular blockers received by the patient are no longer active.

Arterial blood gases should be taken before and during the apnoeic test to ensure that the CO_2 levels have risen to at least 6kPa.

3. d) Can be delayed for up to seven days

A number of recent trials have demonstrated that full caloric replacement feeding early in critical illness does not provide benefit and may cause harm in some populations or settings. The Early Parenteral Nutrition and Supplemental Parenteral Nutrition trials suggest that the use of parenteral nutrition in itself may not increase the risk of infectious complications. Therefore, current recommendations for clinical practice include allowing hypocaloric enteral feeding in the acute phase of critical illness for up to seven days in previously well-nourished patients. Current evidence does not support glutamine supplementation early in critical illness.

Casaer MP and Van den Berghe G. Nutrition in the acute phase of critical illness. *New England Journal of Medicine* 2014; 370:1227–3.

4. e) Phosphate, magnesium, and potassium deficiencies should be considered upon refeeding a malnourished patient

There is no evidence that selenium replacement significantly improves outcomes in the severely septic patient. Thiamine deficiency is well described in alcoholics and replacement is recommended. Vitamin B12 replacement may be required in patients following gastrectomy or ileal resection. Zinc losses can occur from pancreatic fistulae. Calcium levels may fall in acute pancreatitis. Precipitous falls in magnesium, phosphate, and potassium can occur in previously malnourished patients on the commencement of nutrition. Micronutrient supplementation in critically ill patients should be monitored carefully, particularly in patients with renal failure.

5. e) Parenteral nutrition is more expensive

Recent methodologically sound and adequately powered randomized, controlled trials have failed to provide unequivocal evidence that feeding protocols targeting full-replacement nutrition early in the course of critical illness result in clinical benefits such a reduction in mortality, shorter length of stay in ICU, or reduced requirement for mechanical ventilation. The findings of the EPaNIC and EDEN trials raise concern that targeting full-replacement feeding early in critical illness does not provide benefit and may cause harm in some populations or settings. These trials suggest that parenteral nutrition in itself may not increase the risk of infectious complications.

Casaer MP et al. Early versus late parenteral nutrition in critically ill adults. *New England Journal of Medicine* 2011; 365:506–17.

The National Heart, Lung, and Blood Institute Acute Respiratory Distress Syndrome (ARDS) Clinical Trials Network. Initial trophic vs full enteral feeding in patients with acute lung injury: the EDEN randomized trial. *Journal of the American Medical Association* 2012; 307:795–803.

6. a) Hand washing with alcohol rub before and after patient contact

Hand washing has repeatedly been demonstrated to be the most effective method of reducing spread of infection. Alcohol hand rub is ineffective against *Clostridium difficile* or norovirus, in which case soap and water is required.

Shedding of MRSA should be reduced by the use of topical suppression such as nasal mupirocin and topical chlorhexidine washes during ICU stay. However, evidence from well-conducted studies suggests oral chlorhexidine gel and chlorhexidine washes are not effective.

Antibiotic treatment should be used only when clearly indicated, reviewed daily, and discontinued as soon as it is no longer needed. In most cases five days of treatment is sufficient. Intravenous antibiotics as a component of selective decontamination of the digestive tract (SDD) has been demonstrated to reduce hospital-acquired infections.

7. d) Daily review and removal of the catheter at the earliest opportunity

The use of central venous lines has become a fundamental part of management of critically ill patients. Uses include haemodynamic monitoring and the delivery of intravenous fluids, blood products, antibiotics, chemotherapy, haemodialysis, and total parenteral nutrition (TPN). Despite preventative measures, central venous catheter-related infections are common, with rates of 0.5–2.8/1000 catheter days.

There is no evidence that intravenous Vancomycin prophylaxis at the time of insertion or weekly changing of central venous lines reduces the incidence of line sepsis. There is an increased incidence of infection when utilizing the femoral vein and an increased number of lumens in the catheter.

Length of time in situ - key determinant.

Prevention is paramount, using a variety of measures including tunnelling of long-term devices, chlorhexidine antisepsis, maximum sterile barriers, aseptic non-touch insertion technique, minimal line accessing, and evidence-based care bundles reduces line sepsis rates. This includes removal of the line at the earliest opportunity.

Marschall J et al. Strategies to Prevent Central Line–Associated Bloodstream Infections in Acute Care Hospitals: 2014 Update. *Infection Control & Hospital Epidemiology* 2014; 35 (7):753–71.

8. d) Be used to calculate a standardized mortality ratio for an ICU allowing benchmarking between units

There are a number of scoring systems used in critical care. Physiology-based scoring systems are applied to critically ill patients and have a number of advantages over diagnosis-based systems that may be used in other patient groups. Patients admitted to ICU can have single or multiple organ failure and therefore will not fit a clearly defined diagnostic group. Sometimes, no diagnosis can be made, either on admission or retrospectively. Diagnosis-based scoring systems would therefore be inapplicable.

One of the more commonly used physiology-based scoring systems is the APACHE II system. The APACHE scoring system is a combination of an acute physiology severity score (which is a number—the higher the number the more severe the derangement in physiology), a further score for the patient's age, and an additional score if the patient has a significant chronic morbidity. The acute physiology score is calculated using the physiological parameters recorded in the initial 24 hours in the ICU.

The APACHE II score can be used to calculate the probability of mortality of a patient. Over a period of time this can be used to calculate a standardized mortality ratio for an individual ICU and allows benchmarking of units.

Scoring systems for use in ICU patients have been introduced and developed over the last 30 years. They allow an assessment of the severity of disease and provide an estimate of in-hospital mortality, not ICU mortality. Despite initial development of APACHE II occurring over 30 years ago it remains valid in current UK ICU practice.

9. d) Re-admission rates

Although Quality Indicators help in understanding a healthcare system, all have their limitations. They can only serve as flags or pointers which summarize and prompt questions about complex systems of clinical care and so they must be understood in that context.

The length of stay, mortality rate, and APACHE II score are dependent on many variables, in particular the characteristic of the patient population. For example, the length of stay and mortality rate of a critical care unit admitting a large proportion of post-operative elective surgery will be very different from a neuro-critical care unit. Discharge of patients out of hours has been associated with poorer outcomes and is normally avoided. The rate of re-admission to ICU is a widely utilized measure of quality of care.

10. b) The currently recommended transfusion trigger is 70g/L

Clinicians need to assess the relative risk-to-benefit balance of transfusing stored allogeneic red blood cells (RBCs) to critically ill patients because it is recognized that stored RBCs have potential adverse effects. These can include transfusion-associated lung injury. However, it is unlikely that this would be an issue in this patient due to the small quantity of red cells to be transfused. There is strong evidence to support a generally restrictive approach to RBC transfusion in the critically ill.

This patient does not have capacity to provide consent for transfusion. However, if there was an appropriate indication for transfusion this can be documented in the notes. Red cell transfusion is not particularly associated with an increased risk of DVT. It is preferable to administer red cells through a peripheral venous line.

Carson JL et al. Outcomes using lower vs higher hemoglobin thresholds for red blood cell transfusion. *Journal of the American Medical Association* 2013; 309:83–4.

11. e) The use of blood-conservation sampling devices to reduce phlebotomy-associated blood loss

Multiple factors contribute to the development of anaemia in critically ill patients, including haemodilution, bleeding, and blood sampling. Strategies to decrease blood sampling frequency and volume can decrease anaemia and RBC transfusions. ICU patients do not display increased erythropoietin concentrations or reticulocytosis in response to anaemia as they exhibit an acute inflammatory anaemia with impaired erythropoiesis. However, the administration of exogenous erythropoietin treatment generates modest increments in haemoglobin therefore it is not an effective transfusion-sparing therapy in critically ill patients. In trials it was also associated with increased thromboembolic events.

Retter A et al. British Committee for Standards in Haematology. Guidelines on the management of anaemia and red cell transfusion in adult critically ill patients. *British Journal of Haematology* 2013; 160: 445–64.

12. e) Septic response

Thrombocytopenia is the most common haemostatic disorder in critically ill patients. Up to 40% of these patients develop thrombocytopenia during their ICU stay. The cause of thrombocytopenia is often multifactorial and may be attributed to enhanced platelet consumption as a component of the septic/inflammatory response, reduced platelet production, or haemodilution. *concern for DIC.*

Most patients are exposed to heparin during their ICU stay, and heparin-induced thrombocytopenia (HIT) is often suspected, although rarely proven. It is very early in this patient's illness to have developed HIT. Critically ill patients receive other drugs such as antibiotics, histamine receptor-2 antagonists, and antiplatelet agents, which have also occasionally been associated with thrombocytopenia.

HUS and hypersplenism are also causes of thrombocytopenia but are unlikely in this patient.

13. b) The patient's ongoing septic response

Glycolysis – Clot prese of sepsis.

Increased blood lactate levels are common in critically ill patients. Although frequently used to diagnose inadequate tissue oxygenation, other processes unrelated to tissue oxygenation may increase lactate levels. Especially in critically ill septic patients, increased glycolysis may be an important cause of hyperlactataemia and the presence of mitochondrial dysfunction in septic patients can limit pyruvate metabolism (and thus increase lactate levels) in the absence of limited oxygen availability. This is the likely situation in this patient.

Other notable causes of hyperlactataemia include the administration of epinephrine which results in a dose-dependent increase in lactate levels due to increased production of energy by glycolysis. Liver dysfunction impairs lactate clearance and the substantial tissue hypoxia resulting from mesenteric ischaemia.

14. c) Prophylaxis should be commenced within 24 hours of admission to the ICU

Where a DVT is present and a contraindication exists to anticoagulation, an IVC filter may be considered. In these exceptional circumstances, a temporary IVC filter could be used although early retrieval and anticoagulation should be initiated once the contraindication has resolved. There is no evidence to support their routine use.

Low molecular weight Heparin can induce HIT.

DVT prophylaxis should be commenced within 24 hours of ICU admission but is contraindicated within the first 72 hours after a traumatic brain injury.

In patients with a contraindication to pharmacological prophylaxis mechanical thromboprophylaxis should be used. Intermittent pneumatic compression is of equal efficacy to graduated compression stockings.

Even with appropriate preventative intervention the risk of PE (pulmonary embolism) in intensive care remains significant.

Agu O et al. Graduated compression stockings in the prevention of venous thromboembolism. *British Journal of Surgery* 1999; 86:992–1004.

National Institute of Health and Clinical Excellence. Venous thromboembolism: reducing the risk for patient in hospital. London: NICE, June 2015. <https://www.nice.org.uk/guidance/cg92>.

15. e) Nursing the patient in a 30–45° head-up position

Some studies have shown that VAP occurs in 10–20% of ICU patients. Preventing VAP should be part of an overall strategy to reduce healthcare-acquired infections. The best definition of VAP and the optimal criteria for diagnosis remain controversial, and studies in VAP prevention are limited by inconsistent definitions. Furthermore, although many interventions have reduced rates of VAP, few have had an impact on length of stay or mortality.

The pathogenesis of VAP is micro-aspiration of potential pathogens into the respiratory tract. Therefore, nursing mechanically ventilated patients in a semi-recumbent rather than a supine position reduces the rate of VAP. Micro-aspiration can be reduced further by maintaining an endotracheal tube (ETT) cuff pressure greater than 20cmH$_2$O. The use of an ETT with a subglottic drainage port has been associated with a reduction in VAP and length of ICU stay. However, the use of a tracheostomy has not been demonstrated to be a factor, nor has the use of nebulized antibiotics. Topical intra-oral antimicrobials have been demonstrated to be effective.

The prevention of stress ulcers must be weighed up against the increased risk of VAP as raising the pH of the stomach contents promotes colonization with potentially pathogenic organisms. Therefore, the use of ranitidine and omeprazole is associated with increased rates of VAP.

16. d) Improved patient psychological well-being

There are a number of potential benefits of using a tracheostomy over translaryngeal intubation. These include the protection from laryngeal injury caused by a translaryngeal tube, decreased airway resistance, and hence decreased work of breathing, which may allow early extubation. They may provide a more secure airway particularly in patients with a difficult airway. They allow patients to eat and speak which is the likely reason for improvements seen in patients' psychological well-being. However, they are associated with tracheal issues, particularly stenosis. They have not been proven to reduce mortality or ventilator-associated pneumonia rates.

Non-critical care ward staff require ongoing training on the management of tracheostomy patients and in many hospitals it is not possible to discharge these patients before tracheostomy de-cannulation.

17. b) Delirium

It is possible that any of these conditions could complicate a recovery from aneurysm repair. All should be considered and investigated. However, delirium is common. It is a manifestation of acute brain dysfunction, with altered wakefulness and cognition resulting in a confused patient.

It has a rapid onset and fluctuates in severity. The incidence of delirium in critically ill patients is around 30% overall. Patients who develop delirium have increased risk of dying and long-term cognitive problems, equivalent to moderate traumatic brain injury or mild Alzheimer's disease, regardless of age. The longer the delirium is maintained the worse the outcome.

Delirious patients can be hyperactive (agitated, combative, insomniac), hypoactive (immobile, compliant, drowsy), or a mixture of these.

18. e) Left ventricular end diastolic volume

Landmark studies by Otto Frank and Ernest Starling identified an intrinsic regulatory mechanism of the heart, whereby the initial length of cardiac muscle (preload) governs its contraction. This is typically expressed as left ventricular end-diastolic volume determining stroke volume. Initially, stroke volume will increase with the volume of blood in the left ventricle at end-diastole. At a molecular level, this reflects closer proximity of actin and myosin at longer sarcomere lengths (due to length-dependent reductions in lateral spacing) resulting in more cross-bridges being formed and greater contraction ensuing. However, beyond a certain point further increases in left ventricular end-diastolic volume lead to a reduction in stroke volume. This is due to diminishing overlap between the actin and myosin filaments impeding contraction. The left ventricle normally functions on the ascending limb of this length–force relationship but volume overload causes contractility to fall. See Figure 2.1.

Starling EH. *The Linacre Lecture on the Law of the Heart.* London: Longmans, Green and Co, 1918.

19. d) Glucagon

Endogenous catecholamines (dopamine, adrenaline, and noradrenaline) enhance myocardial contractility via β_1-adrenoceptors. These receptors are coupled to stimulatory G-proteins that activate adenylate cyclase thereby increasing cyclic adenosine monophosphate (cAMP). This leads to a rise in cytosolic calcium concentration that facilitates the actin-myosin interactions that bring about contraction. Glucagon also confers positive inotropy by stimulating adenylate cyclase to produce cAMP. However, this effect is mediated by glucagon G-protein coupled receptors and so bypasses β_1-adrenoceptors. Vasopressin has a neutral or negative impact on contractility, attributable to the rise in systemic vascular resistance and reflex increase in vagal tone.

20. a) Anaerobic threshold

Cardiopulmonary exercise testing quantifies a patient's functional capacity to respond to the increased metabolic demands of major surgery. The test involves cycling at a constant speed against controlled changes in resistance while connected to an ECG, blood pressure cuff, pulse oximeter, and gas analyser that measures oxygen consumption and carbon dioxide production. Different patterns of test results are characteristic of specific disease states. Moreover, certain parameters have been found to predict post-operative morbidity and mortality. The most useful in this regard are the peak oxygen consumption and anaerobic threshold (defined as the oxygen consumption above which muscle cells generate ATP (adenosine triphosphate) anaerobically producing lactic acid). A low anaerobic threshold reflects little cardiorespiratory reserve and predicts morbidity and mortality in various types of intra-abdominal surgery. Cardiopulmonary

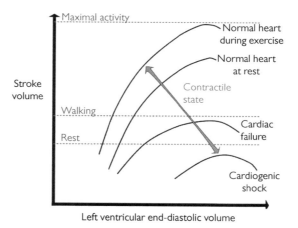

Fig. 2.1 Frank–Starling Law of the Heart

exercise testing therefore permits individualized risk assessment, preoperative optimization, and allocation of critical care resources.

Moran J et al. Role of cardiopulmonary exercise testing as a risk-assessment method in patients undergoing intra-abdominal surgery: a systematic review. *British Journal of Anaesthesia* 2016; 116:177–91.

21. c) Defer the operation until <u>six months after coronary stenting</u>

Dual antiplatelet therapy should be administered for one month with bare metal stents and six months with drug-eluting stents in stable coronary disease. In acute coronary syndromes, this should be extended to one year. When possible, elective non-cardiac surgery should be deferred until completion of the course of dual antiplatelet therapy. If surgery has to proceed, single anti-platelet therapy (preferably with aspirin) should be continued. Clopidogrel and ticagrelor should be withheld for five days and prasugrel for seven days prior to surgery unless there is a high risk of stent thrombosis. For patients in the latter group, bridging therapy with intravenous, reversible glycoprotein inhibitors should be considered. Dual anti-platelet therapy should be resumed as soon as possible after surgery and, preferably, within 48 hours.

Kristensen SD et al. ESC/ESA Guidelines on non-cardiac surgery: cardiovascular assessment and management. *European Heart Journal* 2014; 35:2383–431.

22. e) Stop warfarin three days before surgery and commence unfractionated heparin

Patients with mechanical heart valves undergoing major intra-abdominal surgery need bridging therapy with unfractionated heparin (UFH) or therapeutic-dose low molecular weight heparin (LMWH) in the perioperative period. Warfarin is generally discontinued three days before surgery and daily INR (international normalized ratio) measurements performed. UFH or LMWH should be started when the INR falls below 2 and continued until no less than 12 hours before surgery in the case of LMWH and 4 hours before surgery for UFH. Consideration should be given to postponing the procedure if the INR remains above 1.5. Post-operatively, LMWH or UFH is recommended at the same dose 12–48 hours after surgery, depending on the patient's haemostatic status. Warfarin should be resumed at 24–48 hours with 1.5 times the preoperative maintenance dose given for 2 consecutive days and the usual maintenance dose thereafter. LMWH or UFH should be continued until the INR returns to therapeutic levels.

Kristensen SD et al. ESC/ESA Guidelines on non-cardiac surgery: cardiovascular assessment and management. *European Heart Journal* 2014; 35:2383–431.

23. b) Gliclazide

In well-controlled type 2 diabetics undergoing non-emergency surgery and likely to miss only one meal, safe perioperative glycaemic control can be achieved by manipulating the patient's normal medication. Drugs that act by lowering blood glucose concentrations (e.g. sulphonylureas, meglitinides) should be omitted when fasting, whereas those that prevent glucose levels rising (e.g. metformin) may be continued without the risk of hypoglycaemia. Observational studies have consistently shown increased mortality following preoperative beta-blocker withdrawal so current guidelines advocate perioperative maintenance of beta blockade. Continuation of statin therapy is likewise advocated.

Barker PE et al. Peri-operative management of the surgical patient with diabetes. Association of Anaesthetists of Great Britain and Ireland. *Anaesthesia* 2015; 70:1427–40.

24. d) Positive end expiratory pressure

A recent multicentre trial randomized 400 adults at intermediate to high risk of respiratory complications after major abdominal surgery to conventional or lung-protective ventilation intraoperatively. The latter comprised target tidal volumes 6–8 ml/kg predicted body weight, positive end expiratory pressure 6–8cmH$_2$O, and recruitment manoeuvres. Both the intervention and control groups had less than 50% oxygen applied and normocapnia maintained. This study found that use of lung-protective ventilation reduced complications and need for ventilation within seven days of surgery and shortened hospital stay.

Futler et al. A trial of intraoperative low-tidal-volume ventilation in abdominal surgery. *New England Journal of Medicine* 2013; 369:428–37.

25. b) Early mobilization

The incidence of delirium is high in critically ill patients and often goes unrecognized. It is a predictor of worse outcomes for patients, including death and long-term cognitive impairment. It is important to prevent in ICU patients.

All critically ill patients are at risk of delirium due to a combination of risk factors, in particular infection and coma from any cause including sedation. Efforts should be made to mobilize patients early and minimize sedation, particularly avoiding the use of long-acting drugs. Sleep/wake disturbances are common in delirium, and sleep deprivation is probably an aggravating factor. Good sleep needs to be promoted through measures including a reduction in noise, light, and interventions at night but not by pharmacological measures.

There is currently no evidence to support the use of antipsychotics in critically ill patients, either to prevent or treat delirium. Currently, antipsychotics should be reserved for the management of acute agitation. In general benzodiazepines should be avoided but again may be required to manage an acutely agitated patient.

Barr J et al. Clinical practice guidelines for the management of pain, agitation, and delirium in adult patients in the intensive care unit. *Critical Care Medicine* 2013; 41(1):263–306.

26. c) Ischaemic heart disease

Arozullah and colleagues devised a risk index for predicting post-operative pneumonia. This takes account of the type and urgency of surgery, and the age and functional status of the patient. Comorbidities such as previous cerebrovascular disease, chronic obstructive pulmonary disease, weight loss, and impaired sensorium (but not ischaemic heart disease) are also factored in. General anaesthesia, transfusion, abnormal urea levels, steroid use, smoking and alcohol excess further elevate the risk of post-operative pneumonia. Besides identifying patients at increased likelihood of complications, this risk prediction equation may have a role in guiding perioperative respiratory support.

Arozullah AM et al. Development and validation of a multifactorial risk index for predicting postoperative pneumonia after major non-cardiac surgery. *Annals of Internal Medicine* 2001; 135:847–57.

27. d) 20mmHg

Normal intra-abdominal pressure in critically ill adults is 5–7mmHg. It rises when fluid accumulates in the abdomen and compliance falls. Intra-abdominal hypertension is defined by sustained or repeated elevation in intra-abdominal pressure greater than or equal to 12mmHg. It is graded I to IV using ranges of 12–15, 16–20, 21–25, and >25mmHg, respectively. Abdominal compartment syndrome is diagnosed when intra-abdominal pressure is sustained above 20mmHg and accompanied by new organ dysfunction. Common organ dysfunction associated with ACS includes renal and respiratory impairment and reduced cardiac output. ACS/IAH may be primary (due to intra-abdominal pathology) or secondary (due to conditions not originating in the abdomen or pelvis). Organ function is dependent on abdominal perfusion pressure (APP) calculated by mean arterial pressure minus IAP (APP = MAP − IAP).

Kirkpatrick A et al. Intra-abdominal hypertension and the abdominal compartment syndrome: updated consensus definitions and clinical practice guidelines from the World Society of the Abdominal Compartment Syndrome. *Intensive Care Medicine* 2013; 39:1190–206.

28. a) Bladder

Standard intra-abdominal pressure measurement uses the transbladder technique. This requires an indwelling urinary catheter connected to a pressure transducer. According to the World Society of the Abdominal Compartment Syndrome, the transducer is zeroed at the iliac crest in the mid-axillary line (although other sources suggest using the pubic symphysis). Intra-abdominal pressure is the bladder pressure 60 seconds after instillation of 25ml saline in the supine position at end expiration and in the absence of active abdominal muscle contraction. It is usually measured every four hours if normal or more frequently if raised. Falsely high readings are seen with a non-compliant bladder (e.g. secondary to chronic or radiation cystitis) and falsely low readings occur if there is a leak in the system.

Kirkpatrick A et al. Intra-abdominal hypertension and the abdominal compartment syndrome: updated consensus definitions and clinical practice guidelines from the World Society of the Abdominal Compartment Syndrome. *Intensive Care Medicine*; 39:1190–206.

29. d) Liberal fluid resuscitation

Raised intra-abdominal pressure may result from a variety of pathologies, so no one management strategy can be uniformly applied to every patient with the condition. However, interventions that may be of value in reducing intra-abdominal pressure include sedation/analgesia with or without neuromuscular blockade (to improve abdominal wall compliance) and drainage of intra-luminal contents and peritoneal collections. While correction of hypovolaemia is important to maintain mean arterial pressure (and hence abdominal perfusion pressure), indiscriminate fluid administration is implicated in causation and should be avoided. Surgical decompression is recommended in abdominal compartment syndrome refractory to other treatment. The open abdomen must be covered by some form of protective dressing. A variety of techniques (e.g. Bogota bag, Wittmann patch, and vacuum-assisted closure) has been proposed but none are shown superior. Recurrent abdominal compartment syndrome is possible with any of these techniques and should be addressed by removal and reapplication of the dressing.

30. c) High thoracic epidural analgesia

This patient has had significant pulmonary trauma with a high-impact injury leading to a flail segment and undoubtedly pulmonary contusions. Respiratory dysfunction following this type of injury is multifactorial including hypoventilation, VQ (ventilation/perfusion) mismatch, collapse, and regional oedema. The timeframe of injury is such that contusions worsen over the first few days following injury and the trajectory is important to observe and react to. While the other options are all valid, the most important point to address with chest trauma is analgesia. PCA analgesia and single-shot intercostal or paravertebral blocks are all effective but are limited by side-effects and temporal duration. Thoracic epidural analgesia remains the gold standard, minimizing the hypoventilation seen with opioids, and allowing for effective interaction with physiotherapists, mobilization, and enabling patient-delivered recruitment manoeuvres and coughing. Using a mixture of local anaesthetic and low-dose opioid for epidural infusion gives optimal analgesia while avoiding motor-blockade and cardiovascular sequelae. A suitably high level of insertion needs to be achieved to allow full dermatomal coverage.

31. e) Reintubation with a view to tracheostomy

Delirium is a particularly difficult issue in the elderly undergoing surgery and critical care. It is independently linked with prolonged ventilation, increased mortality, and long-term cognitive dysfunction. Predisposing factors include age, sepsis, pre-existing cognitive issues, alcohol excess, and benzodiazepine use. No reliable treatment exists with a variety of different sedatives being in common use including atypical antipsychotics. Tracheostomy insertion allows for marked reduction in sedation need due to placement below the glottis and therefore allows for more accurate assessment of neurological function. Assessing who will benefit from tracheostomy is difficult and studies of the optimum time for tracheostomy insertion have failed to show a benefit from early (<D4) versus late (>D10) tracheostomy, with no difference in mortality. Most clinicians would aim for a trial of extubation on the first occasion but insertion of a tracheostomy in the case of failure allows for reduction in sedation as well as more gradual weaning from mechanical ventilation in difficult cases.

32. d) End-of-life care

It can be difficult when operative and supportive options exist to realize that non-treatment is the better option. In high-pressure situations, the ability to de-escalate is crucial. The treatment for Fournier's with established organ dysfunction would be debridement followed by prolonged critical care and multi-organ support prior to attempting to rehabilitate to fitness before proceeding to further skin-grafting operations. Embarking upon a line of treatment requires the attending doctor to assess how likely it is that the patient will be able to reach the end of the therapeutic path, and whether the risks of the treatment outweigh the benefits. Providing high-quality end-of-life care is as much a part of modern critical care as multi-organ support and many departments have links with palliative care. Other presentations to Critical Care may need end-of-life care to include support to the point of organ donation, with organ support ongoing at the same time as comfort measures. End-of-life care needs to be tailored to patients with family considerations and prior wishes taken into account.

33. c) Histamine receptor blockade

Stress ulcers in the critically ill occur in 6–8% of the whole cohort, rising up to 15–20% if no prophylaxis is used. Classically, bleeding with stress ulcers occurs in the absence of abdominal pain, in contrast with peptic ulceration. On endoscopy the ulcers are usually erosions found in the corpus or fundus (rather than antrum or duodenum), and are often asymptomatic. Continuous PPI infusion only has an evidence base in patients who have undergone endoscopic intervention and endoscopy is usually reserved for patients with high-volume blood loss or haemodynamic compromise. The choice between H2RA (H2 receptor antagonist) and PPI (proton pump inhibitor) is often made on institutional or clinician driven favour but large-scale cohort studies would suggest that no significant difference is seen in GI bleeding between the two classes but side-effect profile is significantly higher with PPIs. Gastric bacterial colonization is clearly linked to the development of nosocomial or ventilator-associated pneumonia with the risk higher in the PPI group, and similar increased risk of *C. difficile* infection.

MacLaren R et al. Histamine-2 receptor antagonists vs proton pump inhibitors on gastrointestinal tract haemorrhage and infectious complications in the intensive care unit. *JAMA Internal Medicine* 2014; 174(4):64–574.

34. d) Permissive hypotension

In a patient with a traumatic injury and no signs of vital organ hypo-perfusion, use of permissive hypotension is a viable option. This approach is largely based on extending the evidence base from penetrating trauma to blunt injuries. The theoretical basis is that avoidance of large volume fluid resuscitation will avoid cyclical blood and pressure changes that lead to continual disruption of clot formation, dilution of coagulation factors, and worsening of hypothermia from infusate. Much of the evidence is from animal models and human evidence is limited to mainly non-blinded or semi-randomized trials. Limitations of this approach include time to theatre, definitions of hypo-perfusion and what approach should be used in the trauma patient with intracranial injuries. A general approach would be, for a time-limited period, of limiting resuscitative efforts to maintaining a radial pulse (commensurate with a systolic pressure of 70mmHg) in the absence of confusion or symptomatic cardiac ischaemia, with targeted low-volume boluses if this occurs. If time to definitive management is likely to be ≥90 minutes, then this approach should be stopped.

35. d) Temporary bowel stapling, abdomen left open, transfer to ICU

In a cohort of patients with multiple serious injuries, or victims of trauma, the concept of damage control resuscitation and damage control laparotomy is gaining acceptance. The initial focus is on rapid diagnosis and appropriate imaging that does not delay access to theatre. From theatre onwards the approach can be split into three phases. Phase 1 is focused on restoring physiology and controlling haemorrhage and contamination. Prolonged resections should be avoided and anatomical continuity is not expected. Simple drainage procedures are favoured and re-operation is expected from the start. The abdomen is left relatively open to guard against intra-abdominal hypertension. Phase 2 is based on critical care with restoration of physiological 'normality' while dealing with the neuro-hormonal consequences of trauma and surgery. Coagulopathy and acidosis are corrected and if they are slow to improve or worsen then return to theatre is mandated. Phase 3 is the return to theatre for definitive management and should occur in a semi-elective fashion with meticulous planning performed, on the backdrop of normalized physiology.

36. d) Renal replacement therapy (RRT)

Acute kidney injury (AKI) requiring RRT still carries a significant mortality despite improvements in technology. Traditional indications for instituting RRT include acidosis, hyperkalaemia, fluid overload, and uraemia. Modern critical care practice tends towards earlier utilization with oliguria being the most common precipitant. RRT can be instituted intermittently using haemodialysis-based techniques, or continually with haemofiltration. Most UK critical care units use predominantly continuous techniques, using dedicated dual lumen venous access devices. Historical use of 'renal rescue' medications including aminophylline and diuretic infusions have categorically been shown to either have no benefit or to cause harm. Once pre-renal fluid replacement has occurred and euvolaemia achieved, further fluid boluses cease to be useful, increasing renal parenchymal oedema and venous engorgement, and should be avoided. Terlipressin has been shown to be of some utility in hepatorenal syndrome but not in other aetiologies of renal dysfunction.

37. d) Correction of coagulation abnormalities

This is a difficult situation with the most likely diagnosis being a multifactorial coagulopathy secondary to consumption, alcoholic liver disease, massive transfusion, and an element of DIC (disseminated intravascular coagulation). While many of the options are probably correct, this will require multiple different clotting products and close liaison with Haematology. Both nutritional and disease pathways will have led to extrinsic pathway defects and consumption of platelets with ongoing bleeding to be expected. Over-transfusion during active bleeding is common and leads to dilution of coagulation factors as well as potentially causing hypocalcaemia, volume overload, hyperkalaemia, and hypothermia. Studies of restrictive versus liberal transfusion in variceal bleeding support a restrictive transfusion trigger in the absence of other indicators or comorbidities, which mirrors findings in the critically ill where a trigger of 70g/L appears to be safe and well tolerated.

38. e) Expectant monitoring

Aspiration pneumonitis and aspiration pneumonia are two overlapping but different conditions. Aspiration of gastrointestinal contents, such as occurs occasionally in peri-anaesthetic practice, largely cause a chemical pneumonitis dependent upon volume and acidity of fluid aspirated. The pneumonitis causes bronchospasm, VQ mismatch, and localized pulmonary oedema that is acute in onset but is usually sterile in nature. Over time, secondary bacterial infection can occur with formation of erosive abscesses and associated parenchymal destruction. Corticosteroids have been used historically but have little firm supportive evidence and can potentially worsen outcomes. Endobronchial toilet should be carried out after reintubation and ideally before application of positive pressure ventilation. Formal bronchoscopy is only indicated for lobar collapse or in the presence of larger particulate matter in vomitus. A reasonable approach would be to provide lung protective ventilation for a period of time to assess resolution of gas exchange abnormality whilst providing surveillance for secondary infection.

Extended Matching Items

Physiological response to haemorrhage

1. G. Carotid sinus baroreceptor

Baroreceptors are stretch receptors located in the tunica adventitia of the aortic arch and carotid sinus. They reduce their rate of firing via the vagus and glossopharyngeal nerves respectively when blood pressure falls. This is conveyed to brainstem nuclei resulting in sympathetic stimulation (and parasympathetic inhibition). The consequent increase in heart rate, contractility, and systemic vascular resistance restores arterial blood pressure, which in turn increases baroreceptor signalling, and so achieves negative feedback control.

2. I. Noradrenaline

Sympathetic preganglionic neurons originate in the lateral horn of the spinal cord from the first thoracic segment down to the second lumbar segment. They are short myelinated fibres that leave the spinal nerves as white rami communicantes and release acetylcholine at synapses with postganglionic neurons in the sympathetic chain. The postganglionic neurons are longer unmyelinated fibres that leave the sympathetic chain as grey rami communicantes and join the spinal or visceral nerves to the target organ, whereupon they release noradrenaline. In the heart and vasculature, this acts on adrenoceptors to exert positive inotropic, chronotropic, and pressor effects that ultimately raise blood pressure. *Norad - post-synaptic*

3. D. Antidiuretic hormone

Antidiuretic hormone is a nonapeptide produced by the hypothalamus but secreted from the posterior pituitary gland in response to hyperosmolarity or hypovolaemia. It acts on V1 receptors in vascular smooth muscle to cause vasoconstriction and V2 receptors in the distal convoluted tubules and collecting ducts of the kidney to promote water reabsorption. This antidiuresis is mediated by translocation of aquaporin channels that increase the water permeability of tubular cells. Aldosterone also promotes water reabsorption by the distal nephron in the context of hypovolaemia but this effect is secondary to increased sodium reabsorption mediated by synthesis of apical sodium channels and enhanced basolateral Na+/K+–ATPase pump activity.

Partial pressure of oxygen

4. H. 75kPa   *e.g ↑ functional residual capacity.*

The purpose of pre-oxygenation is to increase physiological stores of oxygen in order to prolong the time to desaturation during a period of apnoea, such as frequently happens with induction of anaesthesia. This is particularly the case during a rapid sequence induction when positive pressure ventilation is avoided prior to intubation of the trachea. Theoretically, when an FiO_2 of 1.0 is applied via a tight-fitting face mask (to prevent entrainment of room air), perfect pre-oxygenation will raise the alveolar partial pressure of oxygen to 88kPa in accordance with the alveolar gas equation. In reality, tidal breathing over 3 minutes or 8 vital capacity breaths over 1 minute will raise the alveolar (and arterial) partial pressures of oxygen to 70–80kPa. This provides around 1500ml of oxygen in the functional residual capacity of the lungs. Assuming standard oxygen consumption of 250ml/min, this reservoir will prevent desaturation for up to 6 minutes following the onset of apnoea, allowing time for an airway to be secured.

5. B. 2kPa

The alveolar–arterial gradient ($A–aO_2$) is the difference between partial pressures of oxygen in the pulmonary alveoli and systemic arteries. The former is calculated from the alveolar gas equation and the latter measured in blood. $A–aO_2$ is a measure of the integrity of the alveolar–capillary unit. In diffusion disorders, ventilation–perfusion mismatch, and right-to-left shunts, oxygen is not effectively transferred from the alveoli to the blood and $A–aO_2$ rises. In contrast, at high altitude, both pressures will be low and the difference normal. A–aO2 forms part of the APACHE II severity score commonly used in Intensive Care.

Knaus WA et al. APACHE II: a severity of disease classification system. *Critical Care Medicine* 1985; 13:818–29.

6. D. 5.3kPa

The oxyhaemoglobin dissociation curve relates the proportion of haemoglobin in its saturated form (y axis) to the partial pressure of oxygen in the blood (x axis). This relationship takes the form of a sigmoid curve because binding of the first oxygen molecule induces a conformational change in the haemoglobin molecule that facilitates binding of subsequent molecules. The partial pressure of oxygen at which haemoglobin is 50% saturated is known as the P50 and has a normal value of 3.5kPa. Venous blood is usually about 75% saturated, which corresponds to a partial pressure of oxygen of 5kPa. If more oxygen is extracted in the tissues because of decreased oxygen delivery or increased tissue oxygen consumption, venous saturations will fall. This has been used to direct therapy in septic shock. At partial pressures of oxygen above about 8kPa, the oxyhaemoglobin dissociation curve flattens out as it approaches maximum oxygen saturation.

Dellinger RP et al. Surviving Sepsis Campaign: international guidelines for management of severe sepsis and septic shock. *Critical Care Medicine* 2013; 41:580–637.

Lung volumes

7. B. Forced expiratory volume in one second

According to the GOLD guidelines, chronic obstructive pulmonary disease (COPD) is diagnosed when chronic dyspnoea or cough is accompanied by risk factors for the disease and the ratio of forced vital capacity (FVC) to forced expiratory volume in one second (FEV1) is <0.7 post-bronchodilator. Thereafter, the severity of COPD is given by the FEV1 measurement. An FEV1 ≥80% predicted indicates mild disease, 50–79% predicted moderate disease, 30–49% predicted severe disease, and <30% predicted very severe disease. Spirometric criteria are used for simplicity. However, there is poor correlation between FEV1, symptoms, and impaired health-related quality of life. For this reason, symptoms and exacerbations should also be acknowledged when assessing the severity of COPD.

Global Strategy for the Diagnosis, Management and Prevention of COPD, Global Initiative for Chronic Obstructive Lung Disease (GOLD) 2016. Available from: <http://www.goldcopd.org/>.

8. C. Functional residual capacity $FRC = ERV + residual volume.$

Functional residual capacity (FRC) is the volume of air present in the lungs at the end of tidal exhalation. It is the sum of the residual volume and the expiratory reserve volume. At FRC, the elastic recoil of the lungs is balanced by the opposing tendency of the chest wall to spring outwards. FRC measures approximately 2500ml in the average adult male but varies with age, sex, height, and weight. It also changes with posture, respiratory disease, anaesthesia, pneumoperitoneum, and other causes of abdominal distension. The FRC maintains oxygenation of blood passing through the lungs during exhalation and breath-holding. It is also important to anaesthetists as the oxygen reservoir that postpones desaturation when apnoea occurs and ventilation is deferred (as in a rapid sequence induction) or proves difficult (see Figure 2.2).

9. G. Tidal volume

The goals of invasive ventilation in acute respiratory distress syndrome are to maintain acceptable gas exchange and prevent further lung injury while the underlying cause is addressed. Inappropriate ventilation may actually compound the problem by causing overdistension (volutrauma) or collapse (atelectatrauma) of alveoli and consequent release of inflammatory mediators. The seminal ARDSNet trial showed improved mortality when patients were ventilated with a tidal volume of 6ml/kg predicted body weight (compared to the traditional 12ml/kg). Targeting lower tidal volumes may lead to hypercapnia, which in most patients will be tolerated as the lesser insult (permissive hypercapnia).

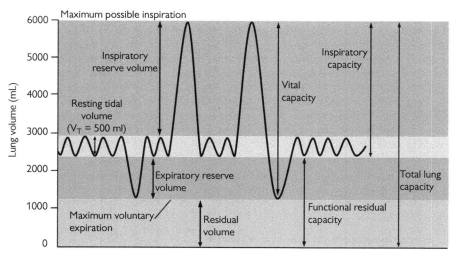

Fig 2.2 Diagram of lung volumes

Acute Respiratory Distress Syndrome Network. Ventilation with lower tidal volumes as compared with traditional tidal volumes for acute lung injury and the acute respiratory distress syndrome. *New England Journal of Medicine* 2000; 342:1301–8.

Bleeding and shock

10. C. Disseminated intravascular coagulation (DIC)

DIC is a final common pathway of a number of wide-ranging systemic pathologies, most likely mediated by excessive release of tissue factor (TF) within small-calibre blood vessels. This exaggerated response to local factors leads to widespread thrombosis within small vessels as well as accelerated conversion of plasmin to plasminogen and attendant thrombolysis. Coagulopathy is produced by consumption of circulating clotting factors and this is exacerbated by the local vascular damage caused by deposition of unregulated thrombus. Products of clot breakdown, including D-dimers, activate complement and kinase systems leading to clinical features of hypotension, capillary leak, and shock. Laboratory studies confirm coagulopathy (prolonged PT, APTT, hypofibrinogenaemia, and thrombocytopenia) as well as thrombosis (increased D-dimers, FDPs (fibrin/fibrinogen degradation products)). Treatment is focused on addressing the underlying cause with replacement of clotting factors guided by Haematology. Blood products should be used to address bleeding or in cases of high risk of haemorrhage rather than solely abnormal laboratory values. Occasionally anticoagulation is required, despite the presence of coagulopathy, to limit the extent of microvascular thrombosis or significant peripheral ischaemia.

11. E. Heparin-induced thrombocytopenia.

HIT is a rare prothrombotic complication of the use of heparin associated with thrombocytopenia. It is mediated by an interaction between heparin and platelet factor 4 (PF4) that leads to a hapten that is targeted by IgG antibodies. This complex then binds to the platelet surface causing platelet activation and aggregation, which in turn leads to thrombosis and thrombocytopenia. Patients who have previously been exposed to heparin may develop systemic signs of a drug reaction but most will be asymptomatic. Diagnosis is complicated by the fact that many patients receiving heparins will develop heparin-PF4 complexes but most will not progress to HIT. The current approach is to assess patients using the Warkentin or '4T' score that assesses the severity of thrombocytopenia, the timing of thrombocytopenia, the presence of thrombosis, and the presence of alternative diagnoses. This score guides further investigations that include functional assays of platelet activation. If diagnosed with HIT, the heparin should be stopped and an alternative anticoagulant used given the high risk of thrombosis. Suitable alternatives include danaparoid, argobatran, and fondaparinux.

12. A. Acute coagulopathy of trauma

The Acute Coagulopathy of Trauma (ACOT) appears to be a separate entity from simple dilutional or consumptive coagulopathy with emerging evidence that it represents an imbalance between procoagulant, anticoagulant, and endothelial factors. There are animal and human data supporting impaired fibrinogen activity in trauma patients. Additional evidence from thromboelastography shows that hyperfibrinolysis can be seen with early clot breakdown, even in the presence of normal traditional laboratory coagulation values. Traditional management of trauma patients with large volumes of cold crystalloid fluid exacerbates ACOT, producing additional damage through inducing hypothermia and further dilution of procoagulants. Much has been written about the 'lethal triad' of coagulopathy, hypothermia, and acidosis. A major aim of damage control surgery is to perform timeous and limited operations that avoid the development of this triad. The use of <u>tranexamic</u> acid, as evidenced by the CRASH2 trial, aims to reduce fibrinolysis while the early use of plasma and other coagulation products has been shown to be of benefit in normalizing point-of-care coagulation studies in a wide range of traumatic presentations.

Bleeding and shock

13. C. Fat embolism

Fat embolism is common following trauma or orthopaedic surgery. Fat embolism occurs when fat globules enter the circulation and obstruct capillaries in the lung and other sites. Fat embolism syndrome (FES) is a distinct entity representing a severe manifestation of fat embolism characterized by the triad of respiratory insufficiency, neurological abnormalities, and a petechial rash. The mechanical theory of FES is based upon emboli passing through the right heart, impacting in the pulmonary circulation causing large rises in right-sided pressures and opening the foramen ovale to allow paradoxical embolization to occur. Echogenic material can be seen first in the right ventricle, then the left when myocardial dysfunction occurs. Treatment of developed FES is supportive with the key step being consideration of the diagnosis. There exists no specific pharmacotherapy and the observed mortality rate of 5–10% is lower than that previously reported, probably due to improvement in general critical care. With the lack of therapeutic options comes the interest in preventing FES. Early fixation of fractures reduces the incidence of FES with one study showing a 70% reduction in all pulmonary complications.

14. E. Neurogenic shock

This man has evidence of a high spinal cord injury with refractory hypotension suggestive of neurogenic shock. This is caused by unopposed <u>parasympathetic activity leading to bradycardia and profound vasodilation</u>, both of which lead to hypotension that is not fully reversed by fluid resuscitation. Around <u>50%</u> of high cord injuries will result in neurogenic shock which takes between 1 and 3 weeks to resolve. Spinal shock is the description given to the flaccid areflexia below the level of a spinal cord injury and not a description of hypotension. Treatment involves close monitoring and the consideration of vasopressors, either noradrenaline or phenylephrine, to counteract vasodilation. Historical papers suggest a benefit in function if high (>85mmHg) MAP targets are used but this should be addressed on an individual patient basis. Vagolytics, such as atropine, rarely resolve the bradycardia seen but can be useful prophylactically in avoiding asystole in response to vagal stimulation if oropharyngeal suction or laryngoscopy is to be conducted. Bladder catheterization should be undertaken to avoid distension and vagal stimulation.

15. B. Septic shock

Sepsis is now defined as 'life-threatening organ dysfunction due to a dysregulated host response to infection', with septic shock being defined as hypotension requiring vasopressors AND a lactate of >2mmol/L after adequate fluid resuscitation. The hallmark of sepsis is macro- and microvascular derangement of vasomotor tone in response to infection. This leads to organ dysfunction, despite often cardiac output being raised. Treatment focuses on early diagnosis, administration of broad-spectrum appropriate antibiotics and source control guided by investigations and imaging. Hypotension and hypo-perfusion is treated with fluid resuscitation, and vasopressors titrated to MAP and organ function. In septic shock, targeting a higher MAP (>75mmHg) was no better than a lower MAP (>65mmHg) in terms of mortality but the higher group had lower rates of AKI and renal replacement. Source control has to find the balance between invasiveness and efficacy: radiological control has established itself, but loculated or multiple collections may be better addressed by surgery dependent upon patient condition. Organ failure that initially improves then deteriorates should prompt the surgical team to consider repeating source control as appropriate.

Shankar-Hari M et al. Developing a new definition and assessing new clinical criteria for septic shock: For the third international consensus definitions for sepsis and septic shock (Sepsis-3). *Journal of the American Medical Association* 2016; 315(8):775–87.

Respiratory dysfunction

16. G. Negative pressure pulmonary oedema   *bronchospasm / laryngospasm*

This case features a period of upper airway obstruction, most likely from a combination of laryngospasm and glottic swelling that is followed by pulmonary oedema that markedly impairs gas exchange despite resolution of the obstruction. The pulmonary oedema that ensues is felt to be due to a combination of different factors and can take up to 24 hours to be resorbed. Development of profoundly negative intrathoracic pressures leads to both increased afterload and preload, resulting in elevated end-diastolic and end-systolic pressures. Allied with low alveolar pressures, this preferentially leads to formation of alveolar oedema. Oxygen consumption increases in the pulmonary cells and, augmented by the hypoxaemia caused by airway obstruction, leads to disruption of cellular junctions and endothelial competence, further favouring oedema formation. Treatment focuses on resolution of airway obstruction normally with induction of anaesthesia and/or neuromuscular relaxation. Most patients will require a period of positive pressure ventilation such as CPAP, while up to one-third will need formal invasive ventilation until intrathoracic pressures are normalized and oedema resorbed.

17. A. Adult respiratory distress syndrome (ARDS)

ARDS is a common final pathway for many critical illnesses, characterized by bilateral non-cardiogenic pulmonary oedema, impaired gas exchange, and progressive pathological destruction of the alveolar architecture. The Berlin criteria classifies ARDS as lung injury of acute onset (<1 week after insult), bilateral changes on CXR not explained by other disease, no signs of cardiac dysfunction, and change in oxygenation as explained by a PaO_2/FiO_2 ratio of <39.9kPa for mild, <26.6kPa for moderate, and <13.3kPa for severe. The majority of patients with ARDS will be mechanically ventilated where there is evidence for mortality benefit with lung-protective ventilation (low tidal volumes and low airway pressures), prone position ventilation, and early use of neuromuscular blockade to reduce airway stress. There is a growing acceptance that mechanical support in the form of extracorporeal membrane oxygenation (ECMO) may improve survival in severe ARDS by allowing reduction in ventilatory support. Treatment of the precipitating cause (in this case, pancreatitis) is key. All-cause mortality in recent RCTs is around 35–40%.

18. H. Pulmonary embolism

Pulmonary embolism (PE) is a difficult diagnosis to make but is still felt to account for around 15% of all sudden cardiac deaths. The incidence increases in the perioperative period, especially with risk factors such as active malignancy and immobilization. Classically small PEs cause more symptoms, such as pain, while large central PEs cause more signs, such as haemodynamic instability. This case would be classified as a massive PE with haemodynamic instability caused by obstructive shock and the resulting right ventricular dysfunction leading to low left-sided pressures and output. Treatment should focus on confirmation of diagnosis and, in massive pulmonary embolism, consideration should be given to systemic thrombolysis with tissue plasminogen activator. This treatment appears to convey a mortality benefit in this subgroup of PEs that is not so convincingly seen in less severe subgroups. The major side effect seen is haemorrhage, with intra-cerebral haemorrhage having a tenfold higher incidence in thrombolysed patients. Anticoagulation should continue acutely with unfractionated heparin while cardiovascular support is often needed to a 'stunned' right ventricle, either with noradrenaline or dobutamine.

Renal dysfunction

19. F. Nephrogenic diabetes insipidus

This patient is demonstrating an inability to concentrate urine which may be polyfactorial. Diagnosing the cause can be done by a water suppression test (polyuria will cease in polydipsia) and an antidiuretic hormone test (polyuria will cease with neurogenic DI but continue with nephrogenic DI). Nephrogenic DI is largely drug-induced with the two most common culprits being lithium and tetracyclines. The exact molecular mechanism is unknown but tubular response to ADH (antidiuretic hormone) is impaired with resulting loss of urinary concentration. DI can occur at therapeutic levels of lithium but is more likely in toxicity. In health, the physiological response is that of polydipsia to maintain normal electrolyte levels. If polydipsia ceases, then water excretion is in excess of sodium excretion and hypernatraemia intervenes. Therefore, water intake has to be maintained in the form of hypotonic dextrose until extubation occurs. For chronic treatment there has been demonstrated benefit from thiazide diuretics, as these increase natriuresis which reduces the degree of water loss by increasing urinary osmolarity.

20. J. Rhabdomyolysis

Crush injuries to musculature can be caused by immobilization if comatose or incapacitated, similar to those seen in trauma. Damaged musculature swells with restoration of blood flow and many inflammatory mediators and breakdown products are released into the bloodstream. Several of these, including myoglobin and creatine kinase, are directly nephrotoxic with myoglobin accumulating in the renal tubules alone, and in combination with Tamm–Horsfall protein, to form casts that obstruct ultrafiltrate flow. Levels of uric acid and hypotension both lead to acidification of the ultrafiltrate that affect ion channel function. This all combines to effect a reduced glomerular filtration rate. Treatment is based on intravenous fluid resuscitation, aiming to restore circulating volume and clear tubules of obstructing casts. The choice of fluid has little evidence to support choice. Urinary alkalinization has been used to try and reduce cast formation. A significant number of patients with rhabdomyolysis will need renal replacement therapy to deal with complications including hyperkalaemia and fluid overload. Muscle compartments should be examined for evidence of swelling and consideration given to fasciotomy.

Anti-microbials

21. I. Caspofungin

Candidaemia is a life-threatening illness and prompt initiation of therapy is important. An understanding of the local epidemiology of Candida species is helpful. Although the majority of Candida infections are caused by Candida albicans there has been an increase in the isolation of Candida glabrata that are less sensitive to Fluconazole. Therefore, echinocandins including Caspofungin is the initial drug of choice, with de-escalation possible when sensitivities become available. Amphotericin is often avoided due to toxicity. Posaconazole is not licensed for this indication. It is important that any central venous catheters are changed as this may be the source of the Candida infection.

Kollef M et al. Septic shock attributed to Candida infection: importance of empiric therapy and source control. *Clinical Infectious Diseases* 2012; 54:1739.

22. D. Vancomycin

It is important to discuss the case with a microbiologist familiar with the current epidemiology. Factors within this patient's recent clinical history are relevant as recent antibiotic therapy or healthcare exposure increase the likelihood that the *Staph. aureus* may be methicillin resistant. Vancomycin is the most appropriate empirical therapy. This can be adjusted following antibiotic susceptibility testing.

There is some evidence that continuous infusion of some antibiotics in critically ill patients may provide a survival benefit and this should be considered in this patient.

23. D. Vancomycin

Diarrheoa is a common problem in critically ill patients regardless of the disease process that necessitated admission to the intensive care unit. Overall, up to 40% of patients will develop diarrheoa after admission to the ICU. Furthermore, patients that develop diarrheoa are at risk of other complications such as dehydration, hemodynamic instability, malnutrition, electrolyte imbalances, and skin breakdown. Enteral feeding is the most common cause of diarrheoa in the intensive care setting. *Clostridium difficile* infection (CDI) is the most common cause of infectious diarrheoa in the ICU. Oral vancomycin can used to treat CDI. Intravenous vancomycin is not effective for CDI since there is minimal bowel excretion meaning faecal drug concentration is low. Avoiding the use of the so-called four C antibiotics listed (clindamycin, cephalosporins, co-amoxiclav, and ciprofloxacin) is associated with reducing the incidence of CDI.

GENERAL SURGERY

Single Best Answers

1. **An 81 year old woman develops a chest infection following a total hip replacement. On the fifth post-operative day she is noted to have painless abdominal distension. An abdominal film demonstrates gaseous distension of the whole colon with a caecal diameter of 12cm. What is the most appropriate next step in her management?**
   a) Caecostomy using local anaesthetic
   b) Tube caecostomy using radiological guidance
   c) Conservative treatment with IV fluids and observation
   d) Laparotomy and colectomy
   e) Colonoscopic decompression

2. **Which of the following statements is not correct in relation to venous thromboembolism prophylaxis?**
   a) Knee-length and thigh-length anti-embolic stockings have similar efficacy
   b) Pneumatic compression devices are superior to anti-embolic stockings for patients at significant risk of VTE
   c) Unfractionated heparin has a similar efficacy to low molecular weight heparin
   d) Pulmonary oedema is a contraindication to anti-embolism stockings
   e) Anti-platelet agents should not be considered as prophylaxis

3. **Which of the following is not associated with stercoral perforation?**
   a) Long-term use of opiates
   b) Tricyclic antidepressants
   c) Neostigmine
   d) Hypothyroidism
   e) Diabetic enteropathy

4. **A 68 year old man attends the A&E with acute onset of severe right loin pain. He is normotensive but is sweating and his heart rate is 110bpm. There is no preceding history of trauma. He had an uncomplicated appendicectomy as a teenager. He has hypertension controlled by an ACE (angiotensin-converting enzyme) inhibitor. What is the most likely cause of his pain?**
    a) Ascending urinary tract infection
    b) Ruptured abdominal aortic aneurysm
    c) Perforated intra-abdominal organ
    d) Ureteric colic
    e) Adhesional small bowel obstruction

5. **A 42 year old lady with a BMI of 42 is admitted with upper abdominal pain and deranged liver function tests. A US is reported as showing cholelithiasis with a dilated CBD (8mm). The ultrasonographer who performed the scan also thought she could see a stone in the distal CBD (common bile duct). What is the most appropriate next step in her management?**
    a) MRCP
    b) Repeat US by a consultant radiologist
    c) Discharge with elective laparoscopic cholecystectomy planned
    d) ERCP +/− sphincterotomy
    e) Endoscopic ultrasound

6. **Which of the following conditions is most commonly associated with the development of an intussusception in adults?**
    a) Inflammatory bowel disease
    b) Villous adenoma
    c) Large intramural lipoma
    d) Inflamed Peyer's patch
    e) Meckel's diverticulum

7. **Which of the following statements is true regarding intestinal malrotation?**
    a) Corrected by a Pringle's procedure
    b) May be associated with volvulus around a narrow-based mesentery
    c) Diagnosed if the duodenojejunal flexure lies to the left of the midline on a contrast study
    d) Can involve the entire hindgut
    e) Most commonly presents in the second to third year of life

8. **A 55 year old man is admitted with a 10-day history of right iliac fossa (RIF) pain. He has a tender mass in his RIF. Urinalysis is unremarkable. A CT shows an appendix mass centred on a 3cm abscess at the tip of the appendix. His symptoms settle with conservative measures. What should the next step in his management be?**
    a) Percutaneous drainage of the abscess
    b) Appendicectomy on this admission
    c) Discharge with elective colonoscopy
    d) Discharge with elective interval appendicectomy
    e) Follow up with family doctor

9. **An 85 year old man with peritonitis is found at laparotomy to have a perforated gastric ulcer high on the lesser curve. His past medical history includes COPD and angina. What is the most appropriate treatment?**
    a) Excision of the ulcer
    b) Oesophago–gastrectomy
    c) Partial gastrectomy
    d) Total gastrectomy
    e) Patch repair of the ulcer

10. **Which of the following responses typically occurs during the ebb phase of the body's response to injury and trauma?**
    a) Increased metabolic rate
    b) Decreased sympathetic nervous system activity
    c) Increased fat breakdown
    d) Increased glycogenolysis
    e) Pyrexia

11. **What is the most common management strategy in patients who present with neutropenic enterocolitis?**
    a) Right hemicolectomy with hand-sewn anastomosis
    b) Non-operative management
    c) Granulocyte colony-stimulating factor (GCSF)
    d) Subtotal colectomy
    e) Right hemicolectomy and stapled anastomosis

12. **A surgical trainee is involved in undertaking a national multicentre randomized controlled trial of a new technique to close abdominal wounds. When writing the final manuscript for submission to a journal, which is the most appropriate reporting guideline statement to follow?**
    a) PRISMA
    b) STROBE
    c) CONSORT
    d) TRIPOD
    e) SQUIRE

13. **In statistical terms, how would you define specificity?**
    a) The false-positive rate
    b) The true-negative rate
    c) The false-negative rate
    d) The true-positive rate
    e) P<0.05

14. **A 35 year old male presents to A&E with a 5-hour history of severe upper abdominal pain of sudden onset. He is lying still and is distressed. His heart rate is 120bpm, blood pressure is 90/40mmHg, and he has a prolonged capillary return (4 seconds). The only abnormalities in his bloods are a WCC of 21.2×10^9/L and an amylase of 269U/L. What is the next most appropriate intervention?**
    a) Transfer immediately to theatre to repair the perforated duodenal ulcer
    b) Transfer immediately to the high-dependency unit for resuscitation prior to laparotomy
    c) CT abdomen/pelvis
    d) Insertion of NG tube
    e) Administration of oxygen and IV fluids

15. **A 56 year old female with no significant past medical history is referred to hospital with an acute onset of severe upper abdominal pain radiating to her back. This is associated with vomiting of undigested food mixed with bile. She is tender in the upper abdomen. Her amylase is 1568U/L with a bilirubin of 96μmol/L. An erect CXR is unremarkable. What is the most appropriate imaging modality in this patient?**
    a) CT abdomen
    b) Upper abdominal ultrasound
    c) CT abdomen/pelvis
    d) MRCP
    e) FAST scan in A&E

16. **A 25 year old female is re-admitted 5 days following a laparoscopic appendicectomy for acute appendicitis with colicky central abdominal pain associated with profuse bile-stained vomiting. The operation note records a 'difficult dissection'. Her abdomen is distended but not peritonitic. Her BMI is 36. Plain AXR (abdominal X-ray) shows laddering of distended small bowel loops with a featureless colon. Her WCC (white cell count) is 13.5 × 10⁹/L and CRP (C-reactive protein measurement) is 35mg/L. Bloods are otherwise unremarkable. Her heart rate is 110bpm. What is the next appropriate step in her management?**

    a) Diagnostic laparoscopy
    b) Abdominal ultrasound
    c) Emergency laparotomy
    d) Low-dose CT abdomen/pelvis
    e) CT abdomen/pelvis with IV contrast

17. **A 34 year old male presents with a short history of colicky central and lower abdominal pain associated with nausea and abdominal distension. Abdominal CT shows signs of two concentric rings of enhancing bowel, involving the distal ileum and proximal colon in the right upper quadrant causing proximal small bowel obstruction. What is the optimal strategy to treat this patient's condition?**

    a) Right hemicolectomy
    b) Open reduction and four point caecopexy
    c) Colonoscopic reduction and biopsy
    d) Therapeutic air enemata
    e) Conservative management with 'drip and suck' with regular clinical review

18. **A 56 year old male presents 4 weeks following an open appendicectomy for perforated appendicitis. He has a swinging pyrexia and a tender fullness in the right iliac fossa. The wound is indurated and discharging pus. Preliminary microbiology report of a wound pus swab shows the presence of filamentous Gram-positive rod-shaped bacteria with sulphur granules. What is the likely causative organism?**

    a) *Staphlyococcus aureus*
    b) *Actinomyces israelii*
    c) *Streptococcus faecalis*
    d) *Clostridium spp.*
    e) *Proteobacteria spp.*

19. **A 34 year old female presents with sudden onset of constant severe lower abdominal pain. On examination she has tenderness and guarding across the lower abdomen. Her last period was two weeks ago. A pelvic ultrasound shows a trace of free fluid at the pouch of Douglas. A diagnostic laparoscopy reveals brown fluid and altered clot coming from a large cyst of the left ovary. What is the most likely diagnosis?**
    a) Pelvic inflammatory disease
    b) Ruptured corpus luteum cyst
    c) Ruptured ectopic pregnancy
    d) Krukenberg tumour of the ovary
    e) Ruptured ovarian endometrial cyst

20. **An 83 year old female presents with a large bowel obstruction and right iliac fossa tenderness. CT images suggest an obstructing tumour of the distal sigmoid colon with intramural gas affecting the grossly distended caecum and ascending colon. There is no evidence of metastatic disease. Her past medical history includes COPD, ischaemic heart disease, and non-insulin dependent diabetes (well controlled) but she is fully independent with a reasonable exercise tolerance. What is the optimal treatment for her obstruction?**
    a) Hartmann's procedure
    b) Total colectomy and ileorectal anastomosis
    c) Total colectomy and end ileostomy
    d) Sigmoid colectomy with primary anastomosis
    e) Insertion of a colonic stent

21. **A 45 year old obese male presents with left iliac fossa pain, mild localized tenderness and elevated inflammatory markers (WCC 16 ×10⁹/L; CRP 124mg/L). A CT scan shows a 3.8cm paracolic collection surrounding an area of inflamed diverticular disease in the sigmoid colon. What is the best initial treatment for this patient?**
    a) IV antibiotics
    b) Laparoscopic washout and drainage
    c) Radiologically guided percutaneous drainage
    d) Sigmoid colectomy with primary anastomosis
    e) Laparoscopic washout without drainage

22. ***Clostridium difficile* is a**
    a) Gram-positive anaerobic spore-forming bacillus
    b) Gram-positive aerobic spore-forming bacillus
    c) Gram-negative anaerobic spore-forming bacillus
    d) Gram-negative aerobic spore-forming bacillus
    e) Gram-positive anaerobic non-spore-forming bacillus

23. **A 44 year old insulin-dependent diabetic male presents to the clinic with a troubling pilonidal sinus causing repeated bouts of localized sepsis. There are three midline pits in the natal cleft and one just above the anal margin. There is also a lateral tract that extends 8cms superiorly and 6cms to the right of the most superior of the pits. He has previously undergone excision and primary closure of a pilonidal sinus and scarring can be seen in the surrounding skin. The patient is keen for further intervention. What would be the most appropriate next step?**
    a) Conservative management with analgesia advice
    b) CT natal cleft
    c) MRI natal cleft
    d) Primary excision and reconstruction with Karydakis flap
    e) Primary excision and reconstruction with Limberg flap

24. **A 6 week old male infant is brought to hospital by his mother who reports a short history of bilious vomiting. The child is inconsolable and pulling his legs up. An upper GI contrast study is performed which shows the duodenojejunal flexure to the right of the midline. What is the correct surgical management option?**
    a) Reduction, Ladd's procedure, and appendicectomy
    b) Ramstedt's pyloromyotomy
    c) Air enemata
    d) Resection of Meckel's diverticulum
    e) Duodeno-duodenostomy

25. **An elderly female patient presents with generalized peritonitis due to perforated diverticular disease. She is scheduled to go to theatre for a Hartmann's procedure. Her family want to know about the anticipated risks of surgery. Which scoring system would provide an estimate of post-operative morbidity and mortality?**
    a) mGPS
    b) APACHE II
    c) Mannheim Peritonitis Index
    d) ASA grade
    e) P-POSSUM

26. **A 58 year old lady presents as an emergency admission to the surgical unit with an episode of mild pancreatitis. She is on steroids for polymyalgia rheumatica and her LFTs demonstrate mildly raised transaminases with a bilirubin of 52μmol/L. A US shows biliary sludge. She denies any alcohol intake. What is the next most appropriate step in her management?**
    a) Repeat US
    b) No further investigations as the diagnosis is steroid-induced pancreatitis
    c) MRCP (magnetic resonance cholangiopancreatography)
    d) ERCP and sphincterotomy
    e) Laparoscopic cholecystectomy

27. **A 22 year old pregnant lady (28 weeks, para 1+0), presents with a 2-day history of right iliac fossa pain. She has a fever but looks well. Her abdomen is soft but tender down the right side. Her WCC is 13.5 × 10^9 and the CRP is 41mg/L. Her urinalysis is negative. What would you do next?**
    a) Start IV antibiotics and observe
    b) Diagnostic laparoscopy
    c) US abdomen/pelvis
    d) MRI abdomen
    e) Open appendicectomy

28. **A 39 year old male presents with a 12-hour history of abdominal pain. On examination, he looks well but has a heart rate of 120bpm and his blood pressure (BP) is 100/55mmHg. His abdomen is soft but he is tender across his lower abdomen. There are no external findings. He admits to placing a penknife per rectum three days ago. You cannot feel the object on digital examination. What is the next most appropriate step in the management of this patient?**
    a) Rigid sigmoidoscopy at the bedside and remove the object if identified
    b) Perform an examination under anaesthesia in theatre
    c) Erect CXR
    d) CT scan
    e) Laparotomy

29. **Which of the following chest-wall injuries is not associated with an increased risk of intrathoracic or intra-abdominal injury?**
    a) Scapula fracture
    b) Flail segment
    c) Multiple rib fractures
    d) Anterior sternoclavicular dislocation
    e) Sternal fracture

30. **A 21 year old male is admitted with a single stab wound to his right anterior chest wall. Clinically there is a haemothorax and a chest drain is inserted. There is a significant amount of blood in the drain. Which of the following is an indication for an emergency room thoracotomy?**
    a) 500ml of immediate chest tube drainage
    b) Ongoing bleeding at a rate of 100ml/hr
    c) 1500ml of immediate chest tube drainage
    d) Ongoing bleeding at a rate of 150ml/hr
    e) 1000ml of immediate chest tube drainage

31. **A 76 year old lady is admitted after a collapse and fresh rectal bleeding is noted. Her medications include apixaban for atrial fibrillation. An endoscopy reveals an actively bleeding ulcer in the first part of the duodenum. The most appropriate immediate management option is:**
    a) Inject the ulcer base with adrenaline
    b) Apply hemoclips
    c) Spray with haemostatic powder
    d) Inject adrenaline and apply hemoclips
    e) Transfer to theatre for laparotomy

32. **Endoscopic signs or stigmata of recent haemorrhage are of prognostic value in the management of duodenal ulcers. Which of the following endoscopic signs carries the highest risk of further bleeding?**
    a) Clean ulcer base
    b) Adherent clot
    c) Spurting vessel
    d) Non-bleeding visible vessel
    e) Pigmented spot

33. **A 75 year old man presents after a collapse at home. On arrival to hospital, he is noted to have fresh rectal bleeding. He looks well. His heart rate is 105bpm and the BP is 100/50mmHg. He responds to an initial fluid bolus but on transfer to the ward there is a further collapse with rectal bleeding. He again responds to resuscitation. He is unable to give any past history but you note a previous midline laparotomy scar and his wife said he was under the care of the vascular surgeons in the past. What is the next best course of action?**
    a) Urgent CT angiogram
    b) Laparotomy
    c) Transfer to the high dependence unit (HDU) for further resuscitation before CT
    d) Upper GI endoscopy
    e) Call a vascular surgeon

34. **A 66 year old lady presents two weeks following a laparoscopic anterior resection for a colovaginal fistula. She is clinically well but has a fever, a raised WCC, and CRP. A CT scan confirms a 6 × 5cm pelvic collection. What is the next most appropriate step in her management?**
    a) Antibiotic therapy alone
    b) EUA and drain collection per rectum
    c) CT-guided percutaneous drainage of collection
    d) Laparotomy and lavage
    e) Laparotomy and formation of stoma

35. **A 32 year old male presents with a 1-day history of a tender lump at his perineum. On examination there is a tender, tense bluish lump at the anal margin. The best course of action would be:**
    a) Bed rest and topical anaesthesia
    b) Incision and drainage of the clot under local anaesthesia
    c) Proctoscopy and banding
    d) Excision of haemorrhoid under general anaesthesia
    e) Haemorrhoidal artery ligation

36. **You have been asked to review a 76 year old man with a past history of paroxysmal atrial fibrillation (AF). He underwent a right hemicolectomy for cancer 3 days previously and his heart rate is 130bpm. An ECG confirms AF. On examination he looks unwell with a mildly distended abdomen. An NG tube is placed and 1100mls of bile is aspirated with some resolution of his symptoms. Blood tests reveal a mild acute kidney injury. What is the most appropriate management?**
    a) Continue with IV fluid therapy and await cardiology opinion
    b) Obtain an abdominal film
    c) Contrast CT abdomen and pelvis
    d) Non-contrast CT abdomen and pelvis
    e) Transfer to theatre for laparotomy

37. **A 66 year old lady presents with abdominal pain and distension. She has a past history of cervical cancer and was treated with pelvic radiotherapy two years previously. On examination, her abdomen is distended and an erect chest film confirms free intraperitoneal gas. What is the most likely structure to have perforated?**
    a) Duodenum
    b) Ileum
    c) Stomach
    d) Colon
    e) Rectum

38. **A 35 year old presents to the clinic with a symptomatic incisional hernia. He is keen for surgical repair. He had a laparostomy performed three years previously for abdominal compartment syndrome following a critical illness. On examination he is noted to have a 20 × 15 cm defect between the edges of his rectus muscle. What is the most appropriate operation to fix his hernia?**

a) Mesh implantation as inlay repair

b) Suture repair with monofilament continuous suture

c) Mesh implantation as onlay repair

d) Mesh implantation as sublay repair

e) Laparoscopic (intraperitoneal) repair with mesh

39. **A 27 year old male falls from the top of a stepladder onto a concrete floor. On arrival in hospital he is noted to be hypotensive with distended neck veins. Which of the following is unlikely to be a possible diagnosis?**

a) Tension pneumothorax

b) Open pneumothorax

c) Pericardial tamponade

d) Myocardial contusion

e) Air embolism

Extended Matching Items

Evidence-based medicine

A. Chi-squared test

B. Chi-squared trend test

C. Fisher's exact test

D. Kruskal–Wallis test

E. McNemar's test

F. One-way ANOVA

G. Paired t-test

H. Unpaired t-test

I. Wilcoxon rank sum test

J. Wilcoxon signed rank test

Choose the most appropriate statistical test for each of the following scenarios from the preceding list. Each option may be used once, more than once, or not at all.

1. A research nurse wants to use a visual analogue scale to compare pain scores before and after a new technique to treat haemorrhoids. The study has recruited more than 350 patients. The pain score data from each group are normally distributed.

2. A clinical research fellow wishes to know whether patients are more likely to develop post-operative pelvic collections whether undergoing open or laparoscopic appendicectomy. To date, he has collected data on 136 patients, of which 43 have developed a collection.

3. A core surgical trainee is involved in analysing data from a pilot study of 14 patients that examined the CRP level on day 2 following elective ($n = 7$) versus emergency ($n = 7$) laparoscopic surgery for ulcerative colitis. Analysis of the raw CRP data suggests that it is not normally distributed in either group.

The acute abdomen

A. 1
B. 2
C. 3
D. 4
E. 5
F. 6
G. 7
H. 8
I. 9
J. 10
K. 11
L. 12

For each of the following clinical scenarios, please select the correct score. Each option may be used once, more than once, or not at all.

4. A 36 year old male patient presents with acute severe upper abdominal pain and vomiting after a weekend of binge drinking. His amylase is 1678. He is treated for acute pancreatitis. On day 2 of his admission, his results are as follows:

- WBC 25.4×10^9/L
- PaO$_2$ 7.9kPa on air
- Random blood glucose 9.7mmol/L
- Urea 15.4mmol/L
- Corrected calcium 2.45mmol/L
- Albumin 34g/L
- AST 34 iu/l
- ALT 43 iu/l
- LDH 150 iu/l

What is his modified Glasgow–Imrie criteria score?

5. A 23 year old male presents with a short history of central abdominal pain localizing to his right lower abdomen associated with nausea, vomiting, and anorexia. On examination he has tenderness in the right iliac fossa with rebound signs. His temperature is 37.8°C and his WCC is 16.5×10^9/L with a left shift. What is his Alvarado score?

Bowel obstruction

A. Adhesions
B. Caecal volvulus
C. Colon cancer
D. Faecal impaction
E. Femoral hernia
F. Gallstone ileus
G. Ileocolic intussusception
H. Inguinal hernia
I. Obturator hernia
J. Sigmoid volvulus
K. Small bowel lymphoma
L. Terminal ileal Crohn's disease

For each of the following clinical scenarios, please select the most likely cause of bowel obstruction from the preceding list. Each option may be used once, more than once, or not at all.

6. A 78 year old female patient presents with a small bowel obstruction. She previously had an open appendicectomy as a teenager via a large gridiron incision. There are no hernias on examination. Plain AXR shows multiple dilated small bowel loops and an unusual gas pattern in the right upper quadrant.

7. A 64 year old male from a long-stay mental health unit presents with an acute large bowel obstruction. The mental health nurse who accompanies him informs you that he has been more introvert than usual and has not opened his bowels in five days. His bloods are as follows: Hb 94g/L, MCV 67fl, CRP 34mg/L, Albumin 22g/L. Plain abdominal X-ray shows a large bowel obstruction with dilated colon from the caecum to the mid-descending colon.

8. A 67 year old female presents with small bowel obstruction. She has lost more than 12kg in weight over recent months and her BMI is 15. She is currently under investigation by the respiratory team for an abnormality in her right lung. She has a distended abdomen with a tender mass in her right groin.

Post-operative complications

A. Abdominal compartment syndrome
B. Acute adrenal insufficiency
C. Acute pancreatitis
D. Adult respiratory distress syndrome
E. Alcohol withdrawal
F. Anastomotic leak
G. Cystic duct stump leak
H. Duodenal perforation
I. Intra-abdominal collection
J. Peripancreatic fluid collection
K. Unrecognized injury to small bowel or colon

From the preceding list, please select the most likely post-operative complication for each of the following clinical scenarios. Each option may be used once, more than once, or not at all.

9. A 56 year old male develops sepsis and respiratory failure 4 days after an uncomplicated laparoscopic high anterior resection for a diverticular stricture. His CXR shows patchy infiltration in both lungs and no pneumoperitoneum. He has a past medical history of heavy alcohol use, COPD, and he has recently been given prednisolone to treat a flare of polymyalgia rheumatica.

10. An obese 74 year old male undergoes an emergency laparotomy for an incarcerated upper abdominal midline incisional hernia containing a loop of perforated transverse colon. The emergency general surgeon struggled to obtain fascial apposition and closed the abdominal wall using an absorbable inlay mesh. Post-operatively he develops worsening respiratory failure with rising peak airways pressures, hypotension, and acute renal failure.

11. A 52 year old female undergoes an urgent and technically difficult laparoscopic cholecystectomy for acute calculous cholecystitis. On the second post-operative evening she develops right upper quadrant pain with nausea and vomiting. A CT of abdomen and pelvis suggests a large fluid collection in the right upper quadrant.

Trauma scoring systems

A. 1
B. 2
C. 3
D. 4
E. 5
F. 6
G. 7
H. 8
I. 9
J. 10
K. 11
L. 12
M. 13
N. 14
O. 15

For each of the following scenarios, select the correct score from the preceding list. Each option may be used once, more than once, or not at all.

12. A 16 year old motorcyclist is involved in a high speed RTA and sustains a significant head injury. He is intubated and ventilated on ICU. Two independent assessments in ICU confirm brainstem death and his family give consent for organ donation. What should the anaesthetist record the ASA score as during the organ retrieval?

13. A 74 year old male from a nursing home falls out of bed, striking his head on a wooden table, and sustains a blunt head injury. His carer informs you that he had a stroke three years previously and has a dense right-sided weakness. On examination his eyes open on command. His speech is slurred and difficult to understand but he can say his name. He is unable to move his right arm or leg but can localize to pain with his left arm. What is his GCS?

14. A 24 year old female is the restrained driver involved in a head-on RTA. A CT shows a 6cm-long superficial liver laceration (maximum 2.4cm deep) of the lateral aspect of the right lobe. What is the grade of this liver injury?

Wound management

A. Debridement
B. Conservative management with dressings
C. Primary intention
D. Secondary intention
E. Negative pressure wound therapy
F. Free flap
G. Amputation
H. Larval therapy
I. Rotational flap
J. Vascular reconstruction

For each of the following scenarios, select the most appropriate treatment from the preceding list. Each option may be used once, more than once, or not at all.

15. A patient presents with a non-healing ulcer over the first metatarso-phalangeal joint. Preoperative investigations have revealed a long stenotic lesion of the superficial femoral artery on the ipsilateral side.

16. An intravenous drug user presents to the A&E in septic shock with purulent discharge from an injection sinus and rapidly spreading cellulitis around a small area of bruising.

17. A 55 year old diabetic previously underwent removal of a 20 × 10cm area of skin necrosis on the thigh. This was thought to be secondary infection at an insulin injection site. There is an exudate from the wound that is requiring a twice-daily dressing change.

18. A 60 year old male nursing home resident with dementia was initially referred up with a deep pressure sore on the right buttock and thigh. He is known to have an occlusion of the superficial femoral artery on the same side. The wound was initially debrided and now looks reasonably clean although a deep 15 × 20cm cavity remains.

Microbiology

A. *Clostridium difficile*
B. *Staphylococcus aureus*
C. *Yersinia enterocolitica*
D. *Mycobacterium tuberculosis*
E. *Chlamydia trachomatis*
F. *Campylobacter*
G. *Neisseria gonorrhoea*
H. *Salmonella*
I. *Candida albicans*
J. *Pseudomonas aeruginosa*
K. *Escherichia coli*

For each of the following scenarios, select the most likely causative organism from the preceding list. Each option may be used once, more than once, or not at all.

19. A 25 year old female patient presents to her GP with a short history of new-onset vaginal discharge and lower abdominal pain.

20. A 37 year old male patient presents to the A&E with a 3-day history of diarrhoea and abdominal pain. He gives a history of eating a meat dish at a restaurant which he felt was not cooked properly.

21. Which organism can cause an infection that mimics appendicitis by causing localized right iliac fossa tenderness and low-grade pyrexia?

22. Secondary infection with which organism results in poorer outcome in patients with complicated severe acute pancreatitis.

Major trauma

A. Mattox manoeuvre
B. Left antero-lateral thoracotomy and clamping of the descending aorta
C. Extra-peritoneal packing
D. Pringle manoeuvre
E. Cattall–Brasch manoeuvre
F. Clamshell thoracotomy
G. Damage control laparotomy
H. Angio-embolization
I. Extended Kocher procedure

For each of the following questions, please select the most appropriate answer from the preceding list. Each option may be used once, more than once, or not at all.

23. What intervention might be considered to access/control bleeding from a stab injury involving the aorta and left renal pedicle?

24. A 36 year old man is crushed by a forklift truck at work. On arrival to hospital he is hypotensive and has a tachycardia. Examination reveals contusions over the upper abdomen and abdominal distension. He is taken straight to theatre and undergoes immediate four-quadrant packing. Despite this he continues to bleed from between the packs in the right upper quadrant. What is the most appropriate next step in his management?

25. A 25 year old man sustains a shotgun injury to the chest and abdomen. On arrival to A&E he is hypotensive and has a tachycardia. He has an open sucking chest wound on the left thorax and an intercostal drain has been inserted prior to your assessment. This drained 250mls of blood when first inserted but there has been little ongoing drainage of blood since. What is the most next most appropriate intervention?

26. Which technique should be considered first in a physiologically normal patient with pelvic haemorrhage related to pelvic fractures not controlled with pelvic binding/fixation?

Hernias

A. Indirect inguinal hernia
B. Amyand's hernia
C. Richter's hernia
D. Littre's hernia
E. Maydl's hernia
F. Petit's hernia
G. Pantaloon hernia
H. Spigelian hernia

For each of the following scenarios, please select the most appropriate answer from the preceding list. Each option may be used once, more than once, or not at all.

27. An elderly patient presents with an incarcerated right inguinal hernia. A CT scan suggests the caecum descends into the hernia sac with surrounding inflammatory change. What is the name of the eponymous hernia described on the scan?

28. A patient is referred to the outpatient clinic with a left flank swelling. What is the name of the hernia which describes this presentation?

29. You perform a laparotomy for small bowel obstruction secondary to an incarcerated umbilical hernia. Intra-operatively you find the hernia sac contains small bowel with what appears to be a diverticulum approximately 60cm from the ileo-caecal valve. What is the name of this eponymous hernia?

Thoracic trauma

A. Median sternotomy
B. Left anterolateral thoracotomy
C. Clamshell thoracotomy
D. Midline laparotomy
E. Trapdoor thoracotomy
F. Left posterior thoracotomy

For each of the following clinical scenarios, please select the most appropriate operative approach from the preceding list. Each option may be used once, more than once, or not at all.

30. A 31 year old male presents with a single penetrating wound to his left anterior chest wall, medial to the left nipple. He is haemodynamically unstable and requires intervention. Which would be the most appropriate incision?

31. A 45 year old presents with a gunshot to his right upper quadrant (RUQ). The exit wound is below his left scapula. At this time, he has no abdominal signs. Which incision would you perform initially?

32. A 21 year old man presents with a stab wound to his posterior left chest. He is in extremis. A left anterolateral thoracotomy is performed but no bleeding is identified. What would you do now?

33. An 18 year old girl is admitted after a fall onto a metal fence. She has sustained a single penetrating injury just above her right clavicle. She in unstable and requires urgent surgical intervention. What incision would you begin with?

Biologic agents

A. Bevacizumab
B. Adalimumab
C. Infliximab
D. Vedolizumab
E. Basiliximab
F. Trastuzumab
G. Golimumab
H. Cetuximab
I. Imatinib

Please select the biological agent from the preceding list that is most accurately described by each of the following statements. Each answer may be used once, more than once, or not at all.

34. This agent blocks the action of vascular endothelial growth factor A (VEGF-A)

35. Used in combination with other immunosuppressive drugs to prevent acute organ rejection

36. A monoclonal antibody that interferes with the HER2/neu receptor

37. A 'gut-selective' monoclonal antibody used to treat inflammatory bowel disease

38. An epidermal growth factor receptor inhibitor used in the treatment of metastatic colorectal cancer, metastatic lung cancer, and head and neck cancer

Single Best Answers

1. e) Colonoscopic decompression

Acute colonic pseudo-obstruction (ACPO), also known as Ogilvie's syndrome, is a condition which clinically presents like a mechanical obstruction but with no demonstrable occlusive lesion. It is characterized by abdominal distension, nausea, and/or vomiting, with a failure to pass flatus. If the condition progresses, massive colonic dilatation can cause ischaemia and perforation, with subsequent peritonitis. Such complications affect up to 15% of patients with ACPO. Despite best care, the mortality associated with these complications is approximately 50%.

ACPO is most commonly seen in association with orthopaedic, spinal, or pelvic surgery, trauma, burns, and caesarean section. It occurs predominantly in elderly or institutionalized patients with other comorbidities. Chronic intestinal pseudo-obstruction (CIPO), by contrast, is usually idiopathic and much rarer, affecting the paediatric population. It can lead to malnutrition and intestinal failure.

Conservative management, with IV fluid and electrolyte replacement, nil by mouth, and NG drainage, should not normally exceed 72 hours. Reversible causes should be treated, medications with an anti-motility effect should be stopped/avoided, and Lactulose is also contraindicated. Patients should be carefully monitored with serial X-rays and examination and urgent surgery should be considered for cases of suspected ischaemia or perforation.

Pharmacological treatment (IV/SC Neostigmine) or colonoscopic decompression should be considered for patients who fail to respond to conservative management. In the current scenario, a caecum of 12cm is a cause for concern and merits colonoscopic decompression. The success rates of colonoscopic decompression are high (>80%) and may be further improved by placement of a flatus tube. Recurrence can also be reduced by prescribing oral polyethylene glycol (PEG) solution.

De Giorgio R and Knowles CH. Acute colonic pseudo-obstruction. *British Journal of Surgery* 2009; 96:229–39.

Ponec RJ et al. Neostigmine for the treatment of acute colonic pseudo-obstruction. *New England Journal of Medicine* 1999; 341:137–41.

Committee ASoP et al. The role of endoscopy in the management of patients with known and suspected colonic obstruction and pseudo-obstruction. *Gastrointestinal Endoscopy* 2010; 71:669–79.

2. b) Pneumatic compression devices are superior to anti-embolic stockings for patients at significant risk of VTE

All patients undergoing a surgical procedure should be fully assessed for their risk of venous thromboembolism with consideration given to the most appropriate method of prophylaxis.

Knee-length and thigh-length anti-embolism stockings have not been shown to have any significant difference in efficacy. Both lengths of stocking are seen as appropriate prophylaxis in surgical patients providing there are no contraindications to their use.

There is little evidence available to suggest superiority for either intermittent pneumatic compression devices or anti-embolism stocking providing neither are contraindicated

Both unfractionated heparin and low-molecular weight heparin (LMWH) significantly reduce the risk of symptomatic DVT, PE, and fatal PE in surgical patients deemed at risk. Both agents are licenced for this indication and unfractionated heparin is as effective as LMWH. Anti-embolism stocking have an additive benefit to pharmacological agents in high-risk patients.

Contraindications to anti-embolism stockings include massive leg oedema, pulmonary oedema, severe peripheral vascular disease, peripheral neuropathy, leg deformity, and dermatitis.

Meta-analysis suggests that anti-platelet agents may reduce the risk of VTE. However, use of anti-platelet agents as the sole agent for VTE prophylaxis is not recommended by either NICE or SIGN guidelines due to a lack of evidence compared to the effect of heparin and fondaparinux.

Scottish Intercollegiate Guidelines Network. Prevention and management of venous thromboembolism: A national clinical guideline. SIGN Guideline 122. October 2014. <http://www.sign.ac.uk/sign-122-prevention-and-management-of-venous-thromboembolism.html>.

National Institute for Health and Care Excellence. Venous thromboembolism: reducing the risk for patients in hospital. NICE Clinical Guideline [CG92]. June 2015. <https://www.nice.org.uk/guidance/cg92>.

3. c) Neostigmine

Stercoral perforation is a relatively rare condition which presents as a perforation of the bowel secondary to pressure necrosis from hard luminal faeces. It occurs most commonly in elderly patients and is associated with long-term constipation. It has also been noted to occur in association with megacolon, scleroderma, hypercalcaemia, renal failure, and renal transplantation. Any conditions or medication which predispose to chronic constipation may be a factor in its aetiology. In this regard, stercoral perforation has also been recorded in patients on long-term opiates, tricyclic antidepressants, and in those suffering from hypothyroidism, diabetic enteropathy, and hemiparesis. Neostigmine has not been associated with the development of stercoral perforation and indeed is sometimes used to treat colonic pseudo-obstruction.

CT is helpful in establishing the diagnosis. The commonest findings seen on CT are a combination of faecal impaction (84%) and subphrenic (90%) or extra-luminal air (61%). The sigmoid colon is the commonest site of perforation (50%) followed by perforation of the rectosigmoid junction (24%). The stercoral perforation is often large, circular and located on the anti-mesenteric border of the bowel with minimal surrounding inflammation. This is often found in association with formed stool contaminating the peritoneal cavity which can be identified on CT in 10–15% of patients.

Overall mortality in a recent systematic review was 34%. The authors concluded that the condition should be suspected in elderly and chronically constipated patients who present with unexplained abdominal pain.

Chakravarty S et al. A systematic review of stercoral perforation. *Colorectal Disease* 2013; 15:930–5.

4. b) Ruptured abdominal aortic aneurysm

Given the patient's age, it is more likely that the patient is suffering from a ruptured aortic aneurysm than a first presentation of ureteric colic. Considering that he has a tachycardia and is sweating, he should be moved into the resuscitation area and the on-call vascular team should be alerted. Initial management should include administration of oxygen and large-bore IV access should be established. Bloods should be taken for FBC (full blood count), U&Es (urea and electrolytes), amylase, and crossmatch as well as arterial blood gases and an arterial line catheter if possible. A strategy of permissive hypotension should be adopted with the aim of maintaining a systolic pressure of >70mmHg. Referral to a specialist vascular unit offers the chance for optimum outcome but in many hospitals this will require off-site transfer. Initial investigations should not be allowed to delay specialist referral in patients with a suspected rAAA (ruptured abdominal aortic aneurysm). A FAST scan may be undertaken in the Emergency Department to confirm the presence of an abdominal aortic aneurysm (AAA). CT scanning has a higher sensitivity for rAAA and may be considered in stable patients but should not delay appropriate transfer. Patients who are intubated or have had a cardiac arrest should not be considered for transfer. Very elderly or frail patients with comorbidities should be discussed by senior clinicians before deciding whether they are suitable for surgical intervention. Overall mortality in rAAA is 90% but mortality in those who undergo surgery is 50%.

Royal College of Radiologists: Best practice guidelines for the management and transfer of patients with a diagnosis of ruptured abdominal aortic aneurysm to a specialist vascular centre. London: Royal College of Radiologists, September 2012.

5. d) ERCP +/– sphincterotomy

There are a number of specific trans-abdominal US and clinical findings which are helpful in identifying patients who are likely to have stones in the CBD. However, the sensitivity of these findings is limited; that is, the absence of such a finding does not infer the absence of CBD calculi. No single US, biochemical, or clinical finding can therefore be used in isolation as a predictive test for ductal stones. Rather, clinicians should consider such variables in combination when deciding on whether a patient needs further investigation. It is useful to have an algorithm in mind for dealing with common presentations during an emergency surgical take. These should take into consideration the local availability of imaging and interventional services, as well as the skillset of the various surgeons in the department (see Figure 3.1).

Williams EJ et al. Guidelines on the management of common bile duct stones. *Gut* 2008; 57:1004–21.

National Institute for Health and Care Excellence. Gallstone disease: diagnosis and initial management. NICE clinical guideline published October 2014. <http://www.nice.org.uk/guidance/cg188>.

6. b) Villous adenoma

Intussusception occurs when a segment of bowel (the intussusceptum) becomes invaginated into another segment of bowel just distal to it (the intussuscipiens). Although the condition is a common cause of intestinal obstruction in children aged 6–18 months, it may also occur in adults. Whereas intussusception in children commonly occurs because of enlarged Peyer's patches within the terminal ileum, in adults bulky polyps or tumours frequently act as the lead point of the intussusception. They tend to develop in the right and transverse colon.

In addition to villous adenomas and polypoid tumours acting as the lead for the intussusception, other risk factors include a history of inflammatory bowel disease, Meckel's diverticulum, metastatic neoplasms or the presence of intestinal tubes, jejunostomy feeding tubes, or a history of previous intussusception.

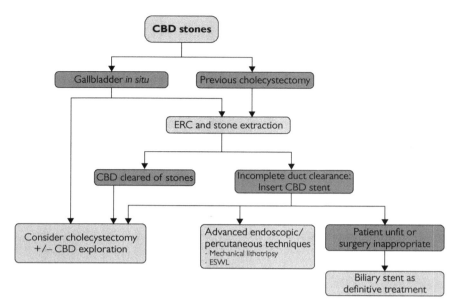

Fig 3.1 Suggested guidelines on the management of CBD stones. NICE.

Adapted by permission from BMJ Publishing Group Limited, *Gut*, 57, Williams EJ, Green J, Beckingham I et al., Guidelines on the management of common bile duct stones, pp. 1004–21, 2008.

The condition is relatively rare in adults and accounts for only 1–5% of cases of bowel obstruction. The classic triad of crampy abdominal pain, bloody diarrhoea, and a tender palpable mass, seen in paediatric patients, is rarely present in adults. Adults tend to present with a more chronic, non-specific history suggestive of partial obstruction. The diagnosis of intussusception is becoming more common due to the use of CT scanning which is highly sensitive both for the diagnosis and the cause of the condition. The characteristic appearances on CT include a 'doughnut' or 'target' sign and mesenteric fat within the mass is also a supportive feature. The most common locations for intussusception are entero-enteric and ileocaecal-colic.

In children the condition is usually a primary benign intussusception and can be treated with pneumatic or hydrostatic reduction. This is successful in up to 80% of patients. In contrast, however, the vast majority of adults who present with intussusception have significant underlying pathology. Up to 65% of adult cases are secondary to a benign or malignant tumour therefore, surgical resection is usually the treatment of choice in adults. With the increased sensitivity of CT it is now possible to differentiate between benign and malignant causes preoperatively meaning that a conservative or non-resectional approach can be considered in some patients. This is particularly true in entero-enteric intussusceptions which have a much lower risk of malignancy compared to colonic types.

Marinis A et al. Intussusception of the bowel in adults: A review. *World Journal of Gastroenterology* 2009; 15(4):407–11.

7. b) May be associated with volvulus around a narrow-based mesentery

During normal abdominal development the foregut, midgut, and hindgut herniate out of the abdominal cavity through the anterior abdominal wall, where they undergo a 270° counterclockwise rotation around the superior mesenteric vessels. The GI tract then returns to the abdominal cavity where the duodenal/jejunal loop becomes fixed to the left of midline and the caecum becomes fixed in the right lower quadrant. Intestinal malrotation (also referred to as incomplete rotation) refers to any condition where this complete 270° rotation and fixation does not occur. The rotation may be interrupted during foetal development, which may result in a wide range of acute and chronic conditions. The most common presentation in paediatric patients is incomplete rotation, predisposing to midgut volvulus.   ← Commoner then conceived

Intestinal malrotation occurs in between <u>1 in 200</u> and <u>1 in 500</u> live births; however, the vast majority of cases of are asymptomatic. Malrotation may be an isolated abnormality although many children with malrotation are affected by another congenital abnormality including diaphragmatic hernia, gastroschisis, and omphalocele. Patients with malrotation may also have evidence of either duodenal atresia or jejuno-ileal atresia or congenital cardiovascular disease.

Volvulus describes the torsion of the bowel around the narrow-based mesentery. This involves the sigmoid colon, caecum, and transverse colon in 76%, 22%, and 2% of cases respectively. Approximately 50% of patients will have had previous episodes of obstruction. Midgut volvulus is a serious condition that requires emergency surgery and can be associated with mortality rates of up to <u>20%</u>. This is particularly the case if the diagnosis is delayed or there is evidence for intestinal necrosis. Children undergoing surgery for midgut volvulus have an even higher overall mortality because of other associated anomalies.

Paediatric patients typically present with bilious vomiting. Contrast imaging may show the duodenojejunal flexure lies to the right of the midline. The treatment is de-rotation and, if the bowel is viable, the condition is corrected by Ladd's procedure which broadens the base of the mesentery and places the bowel in a non-rotated state. Necrotic bowel must be resected. On occasion, a near total enterectomy may be necessary.

Adults may present with chronic midgut volvulus due to intermittent or partial twisting which gives rise to recurrent abdominal pain. Other clinical features include recurrent bouts of diarrhoea, constipation, intolerance of solid food, jaundice, and gastro-oesophageal reflux. In adults there are a number of treatment options depending on the acuteness of presentation and severity of the obstruction. Simple decompression, resection, or a range of procedures to stabilize the small bowel and colon can be performed.

Lee HC et al. Intestinal malrotation and catastrophic volvulus in infancy. *Journal of Emergency Medicine* 2012; 43(1):e49–51.

Durkin ET et al. Age-related difference in diagnosis and morbidity of intestinal malrotation. *Journal of the American College of Surgeons* 2008; 206:658–63.

8. c) Discharge with elective colonoscopy

Appendicitis can evolve in three ways: it can resolve; become gangrenous and perforate; or become walled off by a mass of omentum and small bowel. In the latter situation, patients present with lower abdominal pain which may be of several days' duration. They are usually systemically well. At this stage, and once the diagnosis is confirmed, the risk of perforation has passed. Initial management remains controversial. Surgery to remove the appendix can be technically difficult and has been shown to be associated with an increased risk of morbidity, although most of the evidence is largely historical. The traditional conservative approach has more recently been challenged, with some believing equivalent results can be achieved by urgent appendicectomy.

In the scenario presented it is likely that a 3cm abscess will resolve with conservative management, which remains the most common approach. A percutaneous drain should not be required unless there is a clinical deterioration. Given this man's age, elective colonoscopy should be performed at around six to eight weeks to exclude either an alternative diagnosis or malignancy as a cause of the appendicitis. Elective interval appendicectomy remains a controversial management option. The majority of patients will not experience recurrent symptoms and therefore a policy of routine interval appendicectomy does not seem warranted. Patients who experience recurrent symptoms will usually present within the first six months after the initial episode and should proceed to appendicectomy. There has been no apparent increase in morbidity or mortality with such an approach.

Simillis C et al. A meta-analysis comparing conservative treatment versus acute appendectomy for complicated appendicitis (abscess or phlegmon). *Surgery* 2010; 147(6):818–29.

9. a) Excision of ulcer

Statistically, gastric ulcer perforation tends to occur in the elderly. It is more likely in those taking non-steroidal anti-inflammatory drugs (NSAIDs). Other aetiologies include carcinoma, lymphoma, and gastrointestinal stromal tumours. Omental patch closure and ulcer excision are as effective as gastrectomy in the management of perforated gastric ulcer and merit consideration as first-line therapy in technically applicable cases. However, patch repair with biopsies of the ulcer edge can lead to missed cancer diagnoses and so ulcer excision and closure is the preferred technique.

In the scenario presented, the patient has a high risk of mortality due to the presence of medical comorbidities and therefore a stomach-sparing technique should be preferred to a resectional approach. Several scoring systems exist to predict the risk of mortality related to perforated peptic ulcer disease including the Boey score. Medical comorbidity, delay in presentation, and haemodynamic compromise are all known to significantly increase the risk of mortality.

Boey J et al. Risk stratification in perforated duodenal ulcers. A prospective validation of predictive factors. *Annals of Surgery* 1987; 205(1):22–6.

10. d) Increased glycogenolysis

Sir David Cuthbertson described the loss of nitrogen from skeletal muscle that occurred from trauma and concluded the response to injury could be considered in two phases: ebb and flow.

The ebb phase is a short-lived response to injury, associated with hypovolaemic shock, increased sympathetic nervous system activity, and reduced metabolic rate. This results in increased glycogenolysis and a decrease in resting energy expenditure. The predominant hormones regulating this phase are catecholamines, cortisol, and aldosterone. The main role is to conserve circulating volume and energy stores.

The flow phase begins 24–48 hours after injury and mobilizes body stores for repair and recovery. It is characterized by:

- Increased heat production, leading to pyrexia
- Increased muscle catabolism and breakdown
- Increased breakdown of fat and reduced fat synthesis
- Increased gluconeogenesis

Desborough JP. The stress response to trauma and surgery. *British Journal of Anaesthesia* 2000; 85(1):109–17.

11. b) Non-operative management

Also known as typhlitis, neutropenic enterocolitis is a potentially life-threatening condition characterized by a pronounced inflammatory process of the terminal ileum, caecum, or ascending colon. It occurs most often as a consequence of chemotherapy for haematological malignancies but is also seen with other high-dose chemotherapy regimens, in transplant patients and in patients with AIDS. Progression to transmural necrosis and perforation is possible but the majority of patients recover with non-operative management.

Patients may present with diarrhoea, abdominal pain, distension, right iliac fossa tenderness, and pyrexia. Other modes of presentation include GI bleeding, obstruction, or perforation. When surgery is required the mortality rates are high and immediate anastomosis should be avoided.

Colonic emergencies. In: Paterson-Brown S (ed.). *Core Topics in General and Emergency Surgery*, 5th edn. Philadelphia, PA: Saunders Ltd, 2014, pp. 179–203.

Cunningham SC et al. Neutropenic enterocolitis in adults: case series and review of the literature. *Digestive Diseases and Sciences* 2005 February 50(2):215–20.

12. c) CONSORT

Various reporting guideline statements are commonly used in medical literature worldwide to improve the quality of reporting of all levels of evidence. The CONSORT (CONsolidated Standards Of Reporting Trials <http://www.consort-statement.org>) statement is an evidence-based checklist of recommendations used when reporting randomized trials to facilitate transparency of methodology and aid critical appraisal and interpretation of results. The following guideline statements are commonly used when reporting other levels of evidence:

- PRISMA-Preferred Reporting Items for Systematic Reviews and Meta-Analyses <http://www.prisma-guidelines.org>
- STROBE-STrengthening the Reporting of OBservational studies in Epidemiology <http://www.strobe-statement.org>
- TRIPOD-Transparent Reporting of a multivariable prediction model for individual Prognosis or Diagnosis <http://www.equator-network.org/reporting-guidelines/tripod-statement>
- SQUIRE-Standards for QUality Improvement Reporting Excellence <http://www.squire-statement.org>

13. b) The true-negative rate

The specificity (true-negative rate) of a test is defined as the proportion of negatives that are correctly identified as negatives (e.g. the percentage of healthy individuals correctly identified as not having a disease in a screening programme).

The sensitivity (true-positive rate) of a test is defined as proportion of positives that are correctly identified as positives (e.g. the percentage of people with a disease correctly identified as having the disease in a screening programme).

False-positive and false-negatives are also known are type 1 and type 2 statistical errors respectively. A type 1 error (false-positive; error of the first kind; α-error) occurs when a true null hypothesis is incorrectly rejected (e.g. a fire alarm rings when there is no fire). A type 2 error (false-negative; error of the second kind; β-error) occurs when a false null hypothesis is incorrectly accepted (e.g. a fire alarm fails to ring when there is a fire).

A p-value (probability value) is the probability of incorrectly rejecting the null hypothesis, if in fact it is true; nominally set by convention to be 'statistically significant' if <0.05 (i.e. less than 1 in 20 chance of incorrectly rejecting the null hypothesis—chance of a type 1 error).

Sensitivity, specificity and predictive value. In: Harris M and Taylor G (eds). *Medical Statistics Made Easy*, 3rd edn. Banbury: Scion Publishing Ltd, 2014, pp. 62–7.

14. e) *Administration of oxygen and IV fluids*

This patient has an acute abdomen and may well ultimately require surgical intervention. However, to ensure that he receives the appropriate treatment at the optimal time, he should be resuscitated with oxygen and IV fluids in the first instance prior to transfer to theatre, radiology, or high dependency unit. There should be no excuse for the basics of immediate emergency management to be omitted prior to moving this patient out of the emergency department. His tachycardia, elevated white cell count, and potential source of abdominal sepsis suggest a systemic inflammatory response syndrome (SIRS) and consideration should be given to the urgent administration of broad-spectrum antibiotics after blood cultures have been drawn. Only after the basics of resuscitation have been performed (including oxygen therapy, IV fluids, cardio-respiratory monitoring, placement of urinary catheter, administration of pain relief, etc.), should clinicians consider transferring for further investigation (e.g. CT scan), surgical management (e.g. theatre), or admission to an appropriate level of care bed (e.g. HDU or ICU).

Loftus I. Assessment of the critically ill surgical patient. In: Loftus I (ed.). *Care of the Critically Ill Surgical Patient,* 3rd edn. Boca Raton, FLA: CRC Press, 2010, pp. 1–10.

15. b) Upper abdominal ultrasound [handwritten: USS is always used in emergency setting; MRCP is used for confirmation]

In the absence of alcohol use, the most likely diagnosis in this patient is gallstone pancreatitis. An abdominal ultrasound is the most appropriate initial imaging modality where the presence of gallstones can be confirmed and the CBD diameter can be estimated. Further imaging is largely dependent on local surgical expertise with some surgeons preferring MRCP to confirm a clear CBD prior to laparoscopic cholecystectomy and others preferring laparoscopic cholecystectomy with intra-operative cholangiography +/– CBD exploration, which can be performed either directly or by a trans-cystic approach. Ideally, laparoscopic cholecystectomy should be performed within two weeks of presentation with gallstone pancreatitis. In patients with severe pancreatitis, cholecystectomy may be delayed until the patient has made a full recovery as recurrent acute pancreatitis in this setting is rare.

Working party on acute pancreatitis. UK guidelines for the management of acute pancreatitis. *Gut* 2005; 54 suppl 3:iii1–9.

16. e) CT abdomen/pelvis with IV contrast

The differential diagnosis in this patient includes an intra-abdominal collection/sepsis, early adhesional small bowel obstruction or unrecognized visceral injury at the time of the initial surgery. In this situation an ultrasound scan is unlikely to yield useful clinical information and proceeding directly to surgical intervention, either open or laparoscopically, without having established the cause of the patient's clinical condition may prove to be suboptimal. A good-quality contrast-enhanced CT in this setting will help establish the diagnosis and enable appropriate intervention. For example, a 6cm intra-abdominal collection in the right iliac fossa may settle with antibiotics or be amenable to percutaneous drainage, thus avoiding the potential morbidity associated with re-operation. The risks of ionizing radiation in young patients of child-bearing age should be borne in mind. However, the risk:benefit ratio associated with the clinical scenario is such that contrast-enhanced CT should be performed after appropriate consent from the patient is granted.

TA Salem et al. Prospective study on the role of the CT scan in patients with an acute abdomen. *Colorectal Disease* 2005; 7(5):460–6.

[handwritten: If localised clinically = CT scan. Soft but tender (rebound). Peritonitis - rigid board like as a push up conf. straight to theatre.]

17. a) Right hemicolectomy

[handwritten: Intussusception in adult 10 virtually always harbours malignancy]

This adult patient has an ileocolic intussusception. Up to 65% of adult cases are associated with a malignancy and therefore the lead point of an adult colonic intussusception has to be considered malignant until proven otherwise (i.e. by a pathologist!). Therefore, the optimal strategy is to perform a right hemicolectomy respecting the principles of an oncological resection. It is advisable that the intussuscepted bowel is not reduced perioperatively to avoid potential inadvertent intra-abdominal spread of malignant cells. The likely aetiology in this situation is a caecal cancer or polyp, inflammatory bowel disease, Meckel's diverticulum, or appendiceal lesion (e.g. low-grade appendiceal mucinous neoplasms (LAMN)). *[handwritten: = pathological lead point]*

Marinis A et al. Intussusception of the bowel in adults: a review. *World Journal of Gastroenterology* 2009; 15(4):407–11.

18. b) *Actinomyces israelii*

The description of a filamentous Gram-positive organism with presence of yellow sulphur granules here is pathognomonic for *Actinomyces spp*. Actinomycosis is a rare, granulomatous infection which usually presents in a chronic or sub-acute fashion. It is a normal commensal of the human GI and genital tracts and requires a breach or necrosis of normal tissue to become pathogenic. The most common presentation is cervicofacial actinomycosis occurring after oral surgery or because of poor dentition. It can also cause opportunistic infections such as pelvic actinomycosis in women with an intrauterine contraceptive device or pulmonary actinomycosis in smokers with dental caries. In this scenario, the patient has developed wound actinomycosis after his appendicectomy. This is best treated with wound debridement and a long course of antibiotics (usually penicillin-based) as directed by a microbiologist. Most commonly the diagnosis is only made post-operatively with the results of microbiological specimens. *[handwritten:) 6/52 abx .]*

Valour F et al. Actinomycosis: etiology, clinical features, diagnosis, treatment, and management. *Infection and Drug Resistance* 2014; 7:183–97.

19. e) Ruptured ovarian endometrial cyst

The intra-operative findings described in a female patient who is mid-cycle suggest a ruptured ovarian endometrial cyst ('chocolate' cyst). Endometrial cysts are caused by endometriosis and occur when the ectopic endometrial tissue bleeds within the ovaries. Over time this blood accumulates and turns a characteristic brown colour. When the cyst ruptures, it releases irritant fluid and content into the peritoneal cavity, causing acute severe lower abdominal pain but without a significant inflammatory response. Immediate surgical treatment at laparoscopy should be limited to peritoneal lavage and excision of redundant cyst wall while preserving the ovary. A ruptured corpus luteum cyst more typically occurs at the time of menstruation rather than mid-cycle.

Vercellini P et al. Endometriosis: pathogenesis and treatment. *Nature Reviews Endocrinology* 2014; 10:261–75.

20. c) Total colectomy and end ileostomy

The main points to consider with this scenario are that this elderly diabetic with cardio-respiratory comorbidity presented as an emergency with a malignant large bowel obstruction and compromise of the caecum. Only the brave (or foolish) would consider a restorative procedure in this setting. The distended right colon with CT proven intra-mural gas is a contraindication to performing only a Hartmann's procedure in this patient. Stenting could be considered if she was unfit for a general anaesthetic but one would have to consider strongly what options would be available if the stent failed, migrated, obstructed, or perforated the colon. The optimal surgical option here would be to perform a total colectomy and end ileostomy.

Schein M et al. *Schein's Common Sense Emergency Abdominal Surgery.* Shrewsbury: TFM Publishing Ltd, 2015.

21. b) IV antibiotics

The key with this question is in the wording of the question itself. The optimal initial treatment here would be to allow the small paracolic abscess a chance to settle with a conservative approach using antibiotics, IV fluids, close clinical observation, and patience. If the clinical condition improves then no further intervention will be required and the patient can be followed up in the outpatient clinic. If he fails to settle or his condition deteriorates then percutaneous drainage or surgical intervention is indicated. If surgery is being considered, recent evidence from the Ladies trial suggests that laparoscopic lavage is not superior to sigmoidectomy for Hinchey 3 diverticulitis.

Vennix S et al. Laparoscopic peritoneal lavage or sigmoidectomy for perforated diverticulitis with purulent peritonitis: a multicentre, parallel-group, randomised, open-label trial. *Lancet* 2016; 386:1269–77.

22. a) Gram positive anaerobic spore-forming bacillus

Clostridium difficile is a Gram-positive, anaerobic, spore-forming bacillus and shows optimum growth on blood agar. Its ability to form spores means that it can survive in extreme conditions that the active bacteria cannot tolerate. The bacterium is not eradicated by alcohol-based hand cleansers due to its spore-forming capability. *C. difficile* may be present in the human colon in 2–5% of the adult population and is transmitted via the faecal–oral route.

Pathogenic *C. difficile* strains produce multiple toxins but the most commonly recognized are enterotoxin (toxin A) and cytotoxin (toxin B). These toxins are responsible for inflammation and diarrhoea in infected patients.

23. c) MRI of natal cleft

It would be advantageous to obtain a more detailed assessment of the sinus anatomy in this situation especially in view of the pit near the anal margin and evidence of previous surgery. Further surgical intervention can then be tailored to the MRI results and patient characteristics. In this case it is important to distinguish between pilonidal disease, a complex fistula-in-ano or even hidradenitis suppurativa. MRI will be helpful in this setting to exclude any deep communication with the anorectum.

Taylor S et al. Pilonidal sinus disease: MR imaging distinction from fistula in ano. *Radiology* 2003; 226:662–7.

24. a) Reduction, Ladd's procedure, and appendicectomy

The description of the duodenojejunal flexure to the right of the midline on contrast imaging is diagnostic of a malrotation in the postnatal and early childhood period. Malrotation is a congenital abnormality that can lead to midgut volvulus around a short mesenteric root. This occurs due to a failure of the normal anticlockwise rotation of the bowel during foetal development. A volvulus in this setting can lead to vascular comprise of the SMA (superior mesenteric artery) and SMV (superior mesenteric vein) vessels in addition to small bowel obstruction and is therefore a surgical emergency. Surgery involves reduction (+/− resection), Ladd's procedure (division of Ladd's bands, widening of the midgut mesentery), and appendicectomy.

Davies D and Langer J. Paediatric surgical emergencies. In: Paterson-Brown S (ed.). *Core Topics in General and Emergency Surgery: A Companion to Specialist Surgical Practice*, 5th edn. Philadelphia, PA: Saunders Ltd, pp. 215–28.

25. e) P-POSSUM

In this situation, the P-POSSUM (Portsmouth—Physiology and Operative Severity Score for the enUmeration of Mortality and Morbidity) score would provide a preoperative estimate of risk. It uses 12 physiological and 6 operative parameters to provide a percentage estimate of perioperative morbidity and mortality. Originally described in 1991 as a score for surgical procedures in general, the POSSUM score has been revised, adapted and applied to many surgical specialties (e.g. V-POSSUM (vascular), CR-POSSUM (colorectal), or O-POSSUM (oesophagogastric)). The primary use in the preoperative setting is to enable informed discussion with patients and relatives and to allow surgeons to predict which patients may benefit from planned HDU/ICU post-operative care. It can also be used for benchmarking of performance for critical care units and as part of clinical governance procedures.

<http://www.riskprediction.org.uk>

26. c) MRCP

The aetiology of acute pancreatitis (AP) should be determined. In the majority of patients, the aetiology is clear from the history and initial investigations (lab tests and imaging). Gallstones or a strong alcohol history will be present in most patients. All patients should have an abdominal ultrasound as part of the initial assessment of AP. MRCP or EUS (endoscopic ultrasound) should be considered if the initial US does not demonstrate gallstones. In patients with unexplained pancreatitis and at risk of malignancy (age greater than 45, new onset diabetes, or weight loss) a CT pancreas should be performed. EUS is a useful adjunct in screening for malignancy, assessing ampullary lesions, determining presence of pancreatic duct dilatation and microlithiasis. EUS is often available only in centres specializing in pancreatic disease.

In patients with obstructive liver function, it is established practice to assess the bile duct prior to consideration of surgery. MRCP has the advantage over ERCP (endoscopic retrograde cholangiopancreatography) of being non-invasive, but with comparable sensitivity and specificity for detecting bile duct stones. If a duct stone is visualized on MRCP, an ERCP and stone extraction can be performed. A laparoscopic cholecystectomy can be performed on an elective basis although ideally this should be done on index admission. Although steroids can cause pancreatitis, it would be important in this case to rule out gallstone disease. Care should be taken before attributing pancreatitis to drug, infectious, or metabolic causes as these are much rarer and are frequently incorrectly implicated. Idiopathic pancreatitis should be investigated in centres specializing in pancreatic disease with a multidisciplinary approach.

Tenner S et al. American College of Gastroenterology guideline: management of acute pancreatitis. *American Journal of Gastroenterology* 2013; 108(9):1400–15.

27. c) US abdomen/pelvis

Acute appendicitis is the most common general surgical problem encountered in pregnancy. The clinical presentation is similar to non-pregnant women but the following should be borne in mind:

> Right lower quadrant pain is the most common symptom, but in late pregnancy the pain may be in the right mid- or upper abdomen. A mild leucocytosis can be a normal finding in pregnancy, so the raised WCC may or may not be a sign of appendicitis

If the diagnosis is not certain, imaging is required to establish an early diagnosis and avoid the implications of a negative appendicectomy. Ultrasonography may identify an inflamed appendix or reveal other pathology. However, it is less sensitive than in non-pregnant women due to the gravid uterus, maternal BMI, and operator skill. If inconclusive, magnetic resonance imaging (MRI) of the abdomen should be considered.

When the diagnosis of appendicitis is established, appendicectomy should be performed. No RCTs have been performed to suggest a benefit with either an open or laparoscopic approach. A meta-analysis in 2014 suggested a higher rate of foetal loss with laparoscopic appendicectomy but the results were not strong enough to abandon this approach.

Walker HG et al. Laparoscopic appendicectomy in pregnancy: a systematic review of the published evidence. *International Journal of Surgery* 2014; 12(11):1235–41.

28. c) Erect CXR

Rectal foreign bodies can present a diagnostic and management challenge. They can be caused by a variety of objects, leading to degrees of local trauma and associated with perforation or delayed injury. Patients are often unwilling to seek medical attention leading to a delay in presentation. Patients tend to be males between 30 and 40 years old.

The American Association for the Surgery of Trauma has proposed a Rectal Organ Injury Scale as follows:

- Grade I Contusion or hematoma without devascularization, or partial-thickness laceration (most common)
- Grade II Laceration ≤50% circumference
- Grade III Laceration >50% circumference
- Grade IV Full-thickness laceration with extension into the perineum
- Grade V Devascularized segment[1]

Patients should be assessed for signs of perforation or obstruction and if present they require surgical intervention. Plain films may be helpful to identify pneumoperitoneum or the presence of the object. If the foreign body is *in situ*, it should be removed in theatre with sedation. Most foreign objects can be removed transanally, depending on size and location. If the transanal approach is unsuccessful, laparoscopy or laparotomy may be required. This can allow the object to be 'milked' transanally or removed via a colotomy. It is recommended all patients undergo sigmoidoscopy after extraction to ensure no damage to the rectal mucosa.

Steele SR and Goldberg JE. Rectal foreign bodies: UpToDate. May 2015. <https://www.uptodate.com/contents/rectal-foreign-bodies>.

Koornstra JJ and Weersma RK. Management of rectal foreign bodies: description of a new technique and practice guidelines. *World Journal of Gastroenterology* 2008; 14(27):4403–6.

29. d) Anterior sternoclavicular dislocation

Patients with chest-wall trauma often have associated intrathoracic, intra-abdominal, or other life-threatening injuries. An initial assessment will identify abnormal vital signs, penetrating injury or the presence of chest-wall signs. It is helpful to establish the mechanism of injury as this can highlight any underlying serious injury.

[1] Reproduced from *Current Opinion in Critical Care*, 2, 6, Moore E, Cogbill T, Malangoni M et al., Scaling system for organ specific injuries. Copyright (1996) with permission from Wolters Kluwer Health, Inc.

Chest-wall injuries associated with significant intrathoracic or abdominal injury include multiple rib fractures, scapula fracture, sternal fracture, flail segment, and posterior sternoclavicular dislocation. A posterior sternoclavicular (SC) dislocation tends to be associated with mediastinal/tracheal injury and is less common than an anterior SC dislocation.

Patients may present with hypoxia or signs of respiratory difficulty, paradoxical respiratory movement (suggesting flail chest), seat-belt sign, tenderness across the chest wall, or abdominal tenderness.

The chest. In: Boffard KD (ed.). *Manual of Definitive Surgical Trauma Care*, 4th edn. Boca Raton, FLA: CRC Press, 2016, pp. 75–97.

30. c) 1500ml of immediate chest tube drainage

Most life-threatening thoracic injuries can be managed safely and effectively with decompression and/or insertion of an intercostal drain. Emergency department thoracotomy is rarely indicated in patients in extremis with penetrating trauma. This is performed to allow control of haemorrhage, pericardotomy, control of aortic outflow (cross-clamp aorta), or to perform internal cardiac massage. An anterior lateral thoracotomy in the fifth intercostal space is preferred, mostly in the left chest, particularly if this is for a resuscitative thoracotomy. However, this will depend on the pattern of injury.

The indications for thoracotomy in a patient with a massive haemothorax post-chest tube placement would be drainage of 1500mls immediately following insertion of a chest drain or an ongoing bleeding rate >200mL/hour. However, patient physiology should be the most important factor rather than simply absolute numbers.

The chest. In: Boffard KD (ed.). *Manual of Definitive Surgical Trauma Care*, 4th edn. Boca Raton, FLA: CRC Press, 2016, pp. 75–97.

31. d) Inject adrenaline and apply hemoclips

Non-variceal upper gastrointestinal bleeding remains a significant problem in the United Kingdom, with peptic ulcer disease being the most common cause. Upper GI bleeds in elderly or hospitalized patients continue to carry high mortality rates. Patients with upper GI bleeding should undergo prompt endoscopy, ideally by a specialist in endotherapy for GI bleeding. Unstable patients should have immediate endoscopy after resuscitation, while all others should have an endoscopy within 24 hours of admission.

Endoscopic therapy for bleeding peptic ulcers should consist of dual therapy rather than adrenaline injection alone—either mechanical (clips), thermal coagulation, or injection with fibrin or thrombin. High-dose intravenous PPI therapy (80mg omeprazole followed by 8mg/h for 72 hours) is recommended in patients with active bleeding or visible vessel at endoscopy.

Repeat endoscopy should be considered for patients at high risk of re-bleeding or who re-bleed within the first 24 hours. This may allow further endoscopic treatment or lead to referral to interventional radiology or surgery.

Recently, haemostatic powders have been introduced to facilitate control of active bleeding by delivering a powdered product over the bleeding site. This forms a solid matrix with a tamponade function. Evidence is limited and based on a number of small case series. However, these powders appear to be effective in controlling GI bleeding from a variety of sources. In particular, these appear to be effective in treating cancer-related haemorrhage and bleeding from areas that are difficult to access.

Bustamante-Balén M and Plumé G. Role of hemostatic powders in the endoscopic management of gastrointestinal bleeding. *World Journal of Gastrointestinal Pathophysiology* 2014; 5(3):284–92.

Dworzynski K et al. Management of acute upper gastrointestinal bleeding: summary of NICE guidance. *British Medical Journal* 2012; 344:e3412.

32. c) **Spurting vessel**

Stigmata of recent haemorrhage are endoscopically identified features with predictive value for further bleeding. However, they should be evaluated in context with the physiological condition of the patient and any comorbidities. The endoscopic findings are usually classified in order of decreasing risk of further haemorrhage:

I.   Active bleeding (spurting or oozing)

II. Non-bleeding visible vessel

III. Adherent clot

IV. Flat pigmented spot

V.   Clean ulcer base

There is wide variation in the literature regarding the predictive value of these signs, as variations may result from inter-observer variability and the vigour of washing the ulcer base or removing clot. However, these signs are useful and should encourage the endoscopist to proceed with endoscopic treatment.

Freeman ML. Value of stigmata in decision-making in gastrointestinal haemorrhage. *Baillieres' Best Practice & Research Clinical Gastroenterology* 2000; 14:411–25.

33. a) **Urgent CT angiogram**

Aortoenteric fistula is an uncommon but life-threatening condition. It can be classified as primary (arising *de novo* between the abdominal aorta and the GI tract) or secondary, following any aortic reconstruction, but most commonly after surgically placed grafts, including stent grafts. The most frequent site of fistulation is the duodenum.

Bleeding is the most common presentation. Patients often present with a herald bleed followed by a massive life-threatening bleed. This was first described by Sir Astley Cooper in 1829. The diagnosis is often delayed as the condition is not suspected and a high index of clinical suspicion is required. The management should be as follows:

- Haemodynamically unstable patients with massive bleeding and a known AAA should be transferred directly to theatre for control of bleeding and repair by the vascular team
- Haemodynamically stable patients with acute gastrointestinal bleeding should have an upper GI endoscopy—however, the fistula is only visible in 50% cases
- Haemodynamically stable patients with suspected bleeding and the possibility of a fistula should have an urgent CT angiogram

If there is any uncertainty, there should be a low threshold for involving the vascular team at an early stage in the management of these patients.

Busuttil SJ and Goldstone J. Diagnosis and management of aortoenteric fistulas. *Seminars in Vascular Surgery* 2001; 14(4):302–11.

34 c) **CT guided percutaneous drainage of collection**

A pelvic collection following colorectal resection is a sign of an anastomotic complication. Management depends on the clinical condition of the patient, the radiographic findings, and the feasibility of percutaneous drainage.

Generalized peritonitis → for of → theatre.

For patients with generalized peritonitis, resuscitative measures should be instituted and the patient transferred to theatre. The outcome will depend on operative findings but if there is evidence of full anastomotic breakdown, an end stoma should be performed.

For patients with no evidence of generalized peritonitis a CT scan will identify the collection. A water-soluble contrast enema is also helpful as this will show the presence of an ongoing leak. If the patient is well, and the collection is localized and amenable to an image-guided percutaneous drainage, this should be first-line therapy. For very low pelvic abscesses in continuity with the anastomotic leak, an examination under anaesthesia and trans-rectal drainage can be performed. Patients should continue on intravenous broad-spectrum antibiotic therapy. While some surgeons may treat the pelvic collection with antibiotics, the authors believe the majority would opt for percutaneous drainage, which is why this is deemed the most correct answer.

McDermott FD et al. Systematic review of preoperative, intraoperative and postoperative risk factors for colorectal anastomotic leaks. *British Journal of Surgery* 2015; 102(5):462–79.

35. b) Incision and drainage of the clot under local anaesthesia

A thrombosed external haemorrhoid presents as an acutely painful purplish/blue mass in the perineal area. These tend to resolve spontaneously after four or five days. The main argument in favour of a conservative approach with good analgesia, laxatives, and topical agents is that the surgical treatment for haemorrhoids is likely to be painful for the same time as natural healing. However, for those patients who present within 72 hours from the onset of pain, incision and evacuation of clot in the thrombosed haemorrhoid provides immediate relief. This is simple, safe, and can be performed in a ward setting. However, there is a higher rate of recurrence.

Cataldo P et al. Practice parameters for the management of haemorrhoids (revised). *Diseases of the Colon & Rectum* 2005; 48:189–94.

Greenspon J et al. Thrombosed external haemorrhoids: outcome after conservative or surgical management. *Diseases of the Colon & Rectum* 2004; 47(9):1493–8.

36. c) Contrast CT abdomen and pelvis

Anastomotic leak is a recognized complication following colorectal surgery. While an extensive leak may result in a rapid deterioration in the patient's condition with pyrexia, acute abdominal pain, and tenderness, a smaller leak or contained collection presents with more subtle signs. These may manifest as a post-operative ileus, cardiac arrhythmia (most commonly atrial fibrillation), or failure to progress. In these cases, a high index of suspicion is needed and appropriate investigation with a contrast-enhanced CT or water-soluble contrast enema performed. While it is important to rate control patients in fast AF, it is a sign of an underlying surgical problem in the majority of cases and often improves with management of the leak or collection. The treatment options will depend on the patient's condition and extent of the anastomotic leak.

Current evidence would support the use of contrast for CT in such a scenario as the benefit from early imaging outweighs the risk of contrast-induced nephropathy. However, patients should be treated with volume expansion and the lowest possible volume of contrast used.

Hyman N et al. Anastomotic leaks after intestinal anastomosis: It's later than you think. *Annals of Surgery* 2007; 242(2):254–8.

Post op complications off the sieve

37. b) Ileum

Radiation to the abdomen and pelvis can damage intestinal structures, particularly the ileum (radiation enteritis) and the rectum (radiation proctitis). The duodenum, jejunum, and colon are less commonly affected. Patients can present in the acute setting with an acute abdomen during radiotherapy, or with acute-on-chronic attacks years later.

The indications for surgical treatment of radiation enteritis are:

- Obstruction-Surgery is indicated for intractable symptoms. However, a non-operative policy is best in these patients if possible as laparotomy is fraught with difficulty due to dense adhesions, risk of small bowel injury, and poor healing.
- Fistula-Surgery is required if the fistula does not close with conservative measures.
- Perforation-The ileum is the most common site of perforation. This requires immediate surgical attention.
- Bleeding-The most common site for bleeding is the rectum although patients can present with refractory bleeding from the small bowel.
- Malnutrition-This can occur as a result of prolonged ileus or short bowel syndrome. Many of these patients require total parenteral nutrition and specialist care.

Sher MR and Bauer J. Radiation-induced enteropathy. *American Journal of Gastroenterology* 1990; 85(2):121.

Pironi L et al. ESPEN guidelines on chronic intestinal failure in adults. Home Artificial Nutrition & Chronic Intestinal Failure Special Interest Group of ESPEN. *Clinical Nutrition* 2016; 35(2):247–307.

38. c) Mesh implantation as sublay repair

The diagnosis of incisional hernia is usually obvious except in the very obese where CT can be helpful in identifying the size of the defect and the morphology of the abdominal musculature. A large number of surgical procedures are described in the literature, highlighting that no single technique is best for every case. The three most common types of mesh repair are inlay, onlay, or sublay. The sublay technique is perhaps more effective as the mesh is not only sutured in position but also held in place by intra-abdominal pressure. The anterior and posterior sheaths are both closed, with the mesh lying between these two layers and deep to the muscle. This view is supported by the results of meta-analyses which also suggest a lower rate of surgical site infection with the sublay technique.

The component separation technique, which is a type of rectus abdominis muscle advancement flap, is an alternative repair technique for large and complex abdominal wall defects. Primary closure may be achieved without a mesh, but a bridging mesh may be required if there is concern about tension or if the defect is too large.

A laparoscopic approach can be considered, but often for smaller hernias with a defect less than 10cm (see Figure 3.2).

Holihan JL et al. Mesh location in open ventral hernia repair: A systematic review and network meta-analysis. *World Journal of Surgery* 2016; 40(1):89–99.

De Vries Reilingh TS et al. *Hernia* 2004; 8:56–9.

De Vries Reilingh TS et al. 'Components separation technique' for the repair of large abdominal wall hernias. *Journal of the American College of Surgeons* 2003; 196:32.

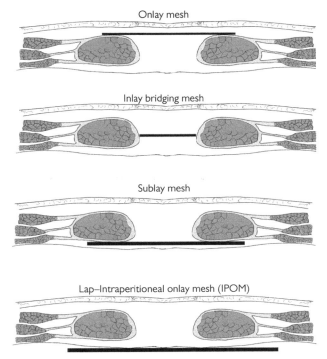

Fig. 3.2 Types of mesh repair of incisional hernias

39. d) Myocardial contusion

The causes of distended neck veins in trauma patients are tension pneumothorax, open pneumothorax, pericardial tamponade, and air embolism. It is important to remember that neck veins may not be distended in hypovolaemic patients with cardiac tamponade or tension pneumothorax.

Extended Matching Items

Evidence-based medicine

1. G. Paired t-test

As the research nurse wishes to compare pain scores (quantitative data) before and after an intervention (paired or matched data), each patient acts as their own control. These type of data are known as paired data. Assuming the data are normally distributed, then the use of the paired t-test allows for a reduction in inter-patient variability, therefore increasing statistical power compared to the unpaired t-test. If the data do not follow a normal distribution, they can either be transformed or a non-parametric test can be used (e.g. Wilcoxon signed rank).

t-tests and other parametric tests. In: Harris M and Taylor G (eds). *Medical Statistics Made Easy*, 3rd edn. Banbury: Scion Publishing Ltd, 2014, pp. 28–30.

2. A. Chi-squared test

The researcher wishes to compare the likelihood of developing a post-operative pelvic collection (binary data outcome) between open versus laparoscopic surgical groups (categorical data groups). Here there are 2 independent groups of patients who have either had or not had a specific outcome and so can be compared by using a simple 2 × 2 table. Therefore, the test of choice is the Chi-squared test.

Chi-squared test. In: Harris M and Taylor G (eds). *Medical Statistics Made Easy*, 3rd edn. Banbury: Scion Publishing Ltd, 2014, pp. 34–6.

3. I. Wilcoxon rank sum test *= Same as Mann-Whitney U trt.*

This surgical trainee wishes to compare post-operative CRP levels (continuous data) between two small groups of surgical patients (categorical data). Therefore, we have samples from two small independent groups containing some skewed data (not normally distributed). As the sample size is small and the data appear skewed, the test of choice is the Wilcoxon rank sum test.

Mann-Whitney and other non-parametric tests. In: Harris M and Taylor G. *Medical Statistics Made Easy*, 3rd edn. Banbury: Scion Publishing Ltd, 2014, pp. 31–3.

The acute abdomen

4. B. 2

The Glasgow–Imrie criteria scoring system uses 8 clinical and laboratory variables measured at 48 hours after the onset of symptoms to aid in the stratification and prognostication of acute pancreatitis. Described in the 1980s, it remains useful in identifying patients at high risk of developing acute severe pancreatitis who may benefit from admission to a level 2 or 3 clinical area for more intensive observation and management. It is calculated by measuring the following (note the handy PANCREAS acronym):

- PaO2 <8kPa/60mmHg
- Age >55years
- Neutrophils (WBC) >15 × 10^9/L
- Calcium <2mmol/L
- Renal function (urea) >16mmol/l
- Enzymes (AST/ALT >200iu/l or LDH >600iu/L)
- Albumin <32g/L
- Sugar (glucose) >10mmol/l

Each criterion scores 1 point. A score of 3 or more indicates acute severe pancreatitis. Other scoring systems commonly used are the Ranson criteria (for alcohol-related pancreatitis) or the APACHE score. Other variables such as raised CRP and high BMI have also been identified as independent predictors of outcome following admission with acute pancreatitis.

The Atlanta classification divides the severity of the inflammation into:

- Mild pancreatitis (oedematous or interstitial) is usually associated with parenchymal inflammation only and with no local complications or systemic involvement. It is usually self-limiting with an uneventful recovery. *Res. ds*

(handwritten: local complications + SIRS / MODS)

- Severe pancreatitis (necrotizing). This is associated with pancreatic parenchymal inflammation with local or systemic complications that has a protracted clinical course and a higher mortality rate. Typically defined by a Ranson criteria >3 or an APACHE II score >8. It is mostly associated with necrosis.

Blamey SL et al. Prognostic factors in acute pancreatitis. *Gut* 1984; 25(12):1340–6.

BMJ online. Best Practice guidelines for acute pancreatitis summarizes the diagnostic criteria. Available at: <http://bestpractice.bmj.com/best-practice/monograph/66/diagnosis/criteria.html>.

5. J. 10

The Alvarado scoring system can be used to aid in the diagnosis of acute appendicitis. It uses clinical (from history and examination) and laboratory variables to generate a score out of 10. The score can be calculated as follows:

- Signs:
  - Right lower quadrant tenderness (2 points)
  - Elevated temperature >37.3°C (1 point)
  - Rebound tenderness (1 point)
- Symptoms:
  - Migratory pain to right lower quadrant (1 point)
  - Anorexia (1 point)
  - Nausea +/− vomiting (1 point)
- Laboratory:
  - Leucocytosis >10,000 (2 points)
  - Leukocyte left shift (1 point)[2]

A score of <5 carries a 'low probability' of appendicitis; a score of 5 or 6 is 'compatible' with acute appendicitis; 7 to 8 suggests 'probable' appendicitis; and 9 to 10 suggests 'very probable' appendicitis. A modified version of the Alvarado score (leukocyte left shift removed and scored out of 9) can also be used when a differential full blood count cannot be obtained.

Alvarado A. A practical score for the early diagnosis of acute appendicitis. *Annals Emergency Medicine* 1986; 15(5):557–64.

Bowel obstruction

6. F. Gallstone ileus

As this is an elderly patient with an abdominal scar and no obvious herniae the most likely cause is an adhesional small bowel obstruction. However, the key detail in this scenario is an unusual gas pattern in the right upper quadrant (pneumobilia). On occasion the gallstone may also be visible. X-ray evidence of a visible gallstone in the RIF, small bowel obstruction, and pneumobilia are the classic features of Rigler's triad in a gallstone ileus.

Gallstone ileus develops when a large gallstone erodes through the body of the gall bladder causing a fistula with the proximal small bowel. The stone then passes into the small bowel where

---

[2] Adapted from *Annals Emergency Medicine,* 15, 5, Alvarado A. A practical score for the early diagnosis of acute appendicitis, pp. 557–64. Copyright © 1986 Published by Mosby, Inc.

it can become impacted, commonly toward the distal ileum, causing a mechanical obstruction. This requires surgical intervention to remove the stone (enterolithotomy) and can be performed as an open operation or laparoscopically. No attempt should be made to correct the underlying cholecystoduodenal fistula in the acute setting. It is also important to make sure that there are no other stones in the dilated proximal bowel as these can potentially become impacted after removal of the first stone.

Ravikumar R and Williams JG. The operative management of gallstone ileus. *Annals of the Royal College of Surgeons of England* 2010; 92(4):279–81.

7. C. Colon cancer

The most likely cause of large bowel obstruction in an older male patient with a microcytic anaemia is colon cancer until proven otherwise. Ideally, this patient should have an urgent CT scan of chest, abdomen, and pelvis both to confirm the clinical suspicion of colon cancer and stage the disease prior to further management. The use of self-expandable metal stents for obstructing colonic cancers as a bridge to surgery has fallen out of favour due to high complication rates and poorer longer-term survival. UK guidelines currently do not advocate a 'stent first' policy in non-palliative colonic cancer unless as part of a trial. *[handwritten: Genr or 'ostomy — do ostomy.]*

Scottish Intercollegiate Guidelines Network (SIGN). Diagnosis and management of colorectal cancer. Edinburgh: SIGN, December 2011 (SIGN publication No. 126). <http://www.sign.ac.uk/assets/sign126.pdf>

8. E. Femoral hernia

An elderly patient presenting with an acute bowel obstruction and tender lump in the groin has an obstructed or incarcerated groin hernia until proven otherwise. The most likely cause in this scenario is a femoral hernia. Female pelvic anatomy and the recent weight loss make this patient at higher risk of developing an acute hernia due to the relative widening of the femoral canal and subsequent herniation of a knuckle of small bowel. Immediate resuscitative measures should be employed prior to surgical intervention including reducing the hernia and inspecting the bowel to assess for viability. Bowel is resected if required and the femoral defect is repaired. Femoral hernia repair is traditionally performed via an open high approach (McEvedy) in the emergency setting and a low approach (Lockwood) electively but is increasingly performed laparoscopically.

Whalen HR et al. Femoral hernias. *British Medical Journal* 2011; 343:d7668.

Post-operative complications

9. F. Anastomotic leak   *[handwritten: Post op. ARDS = anastomotic leak]*

This patient has presented with signs of respiratory failure and sepsis after an elective colonic resection. The most likely diagnosis is a leak or dehiscence of the colonic anastomosis. Initial treatment should include resuscitation with oxygen, IV fluids, antibiotics, organ support, and further investigations to confirm the diagnosis. If the patient is haemodynamically stable, he may be transferred for a CT scan of the abdomen and pelvis in order to confirm the diagnosis. Local radiology departments vary in their enthusiasm for the use of rectal contrast in this setting. The main risk factors for anastomotic leak in this scenario are the history of heavy alcohol use and recent course of steroids.

McDermott FD et al. Systematic review of preoperative, intraoperative and postoperative risk factors for colorectal anastomotic leaks. *British Journal of Surgery* 2015; 102(5):462–79.

10. A. Abdominal compartment syndrome

This elderly, obese patient has developed abdominal compartment syndrome after an emergency laparotomy. The difficult abdominal wall closure using mesh has led to an increase in intra-abdominal pressure leading to abdominal hypertension. This in turn has caused a reduction in abdominal perfusion pressure leading to end-organ dysfunction manifest as acute renal failure and hypotension (reduced venous return). Additional respiratory embarrassment can also occur due to 'splinting' of the diaphragm, hypoventilation, and type I respiratory failure.

A better understanding has led to earlier recognition of abdominal compartment syndrome within emergency departments and intensive care units. It is now increasingly recognized as a major cause of morbidity such as metabolic acidosis, decreased urine output, and decreased cardiac output. The consequences of abdominal compartment syndrome may be easily mistaken for conditions such as hypovolaemia, and inappropriate correction may exacerbate rather than help the situation.

If left untreated, abdominal compartment syndrome has a very poor prognosis with a very high mortality rate. Even with treatment, the condition carries a mortality rate of up to 70%. However, the high mortality is not entirely related to the condition itself, as it tends to develop in patients with multiple organ failure where the primary pathology, such as severe polytrauma and peritonitis, also carries a high morbidity and mortality. A requirement for multiple transfusions is also a strong predictor of mortality as is a history of diabetes.

Treatment should be aimed at maximizing abdominal wall compliance (paralysis), ensuring intra-vascular volume is maintained (IV fluids), and early consideration of decompressive laparostomy.

Hunt L et al. Management of intra-abdominal hypertension and abdominal compartment syndrome: a review. *Journal of Trauma Management & Outcomes* 2014; 8:2.

11. G. Cystic duct stump leak

The most likely complication in this scenario is a leak from the cystic duct stump. This will cause bile to collect in the gall bladder fossa and right upper quadrant. This may give rise to local symptoms of pain, nausea and vomiting, and localized sepsis. More rarely it can cause a generalized biliary peritonitis. See Figure 3.3.

Treatment should include analgesia, antibiotics if signs of sepsis are present, and drainage of the collection (either laparoscopically or percutaneously). MRCP can be used to assess the biliary anatomy but some would prefer to perform ERCP and biliary stenting without further imaging. Cystic duct leaks are included in the Strasberg Classification of Biliary Injuries, as follows:

[handwritten annotation: MRCP = non-contrast = bile activity on contrast.]

Type A Cystic duct leaks or leaks from small ducts in the liver bed

Type B Occlusion of part of the biliary tree, typically clipped and divided right hepatic ducts

Type C Transection (but not ligation) of the aberrant right hepatic duct

Type D Lateral injuries to major bile ducts

Type E1 Common hepatic duct division, >2cm from bifurcation

Type E2 Common hepatic duct division, <2cm from bifurcation

Type E3 Common bile duct division at bifurcation

Type E4 Hilar stricture, involvement of confluence, and loss of communication between right and left hepatic duct

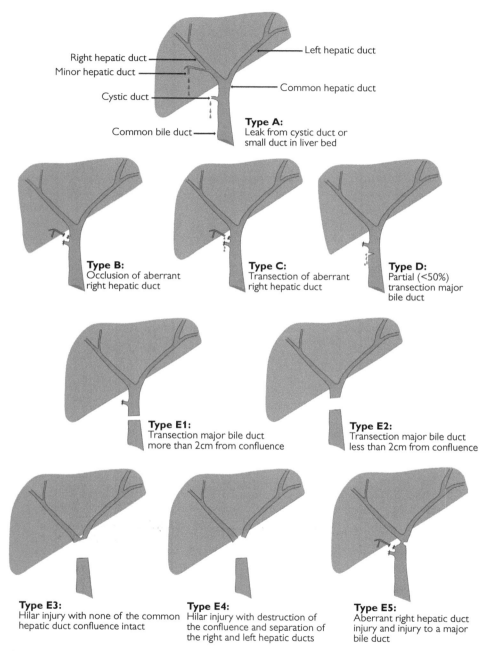

Fig 3.3 Strasbourg classification of bile duct injuries

Source data from *Journal of the American College of Surgeons*, 180, Strasberg SM, Hertl M, Soper NJ. An analysis of the problem of biliary injury during laparoscopic cholecystectomy, pp. 101–25, 1995.

Type E5 Involvement of aberrant right hepatic duct alone or with concomitant stricture of the common hepatic duct[3]

Strasberg SM et al. An analysis of the problem of biliary injury during laparoscopic cholecystectomy. *Journal of the American College of Surgeons* 1995; 180:101–25.

Rustagi T and Aslanian HR. Endoscopic management of biliary leaks after laparoscopic cholecystectomy. *Journal of Clinical Gastroenterology* 2014; 48(8):674–8.

Trauma scoring systems

12. F. 6

The American Society of Anesthesiologists (ASA) first introduced the ASA physical status classification system in 1963. It classifies patients preoperatively into six categories depending on the level of pre-existing co-morbidity. Originally described as five categories, this was modified to six to include patients declared brainstem dead who are undergoing organ donation. When surgery is performed as an emergency, grades I to V are suffixed with 'E'. The ASA score can be used to predict perioperative risk. Clinically this can be useful to predict which patients may benefit from level 2 or 3 care post-operatively. The ASA scoring system is as follows:

Class 1: A normal healthy patient

Class 2: A patient with mild systematic disease

Class 3: A patient with severe systemic disease that is not incapacitating

Class 4: A patient with an incapacitating systemic disease that is a constant threat to life

Class 5: A moribund patient who is not expected to survive for 23 hours with or without operation[4]

Owens WD et al. ASA physical status classification: a study of consistency of ratings. *Anesthesiology* 1978; 49:239–43.

13. M. 13

The Glasgow Coma Score is a clinical score to assess impairment of consciousness in response to defined stimuli. It includes assessment of eye opening, verbal and motor responses. A score based on the best possible response to each component of assessment is then generated. This can then be recorded to assess progress (or deterioration) over time (see Table 1.3).

This patient's best response was: eyes open to voice/sound = 3; verbal response was appropriate/orientated to person = 5; best motor response was to localize to painful stimulus = 5. This gave him a calculated GCS of 13/15.

Teasdale G and Jennett B. Assessment of coma and impaired consciousness. A practical scale. *Lancet* 1974; 304(7872):81–4.

[3] This article was published in *Journal of the American College of Surgeons*, 180, Strasberg SM, Hertl M, Soper NJ, An analysis of the problem of biliary injury during laparoscopic cholecystectomy, pp. 101–25. Copyright Elsevier (1995).

[4] Reproduced from *Anesthesiology*, 49, Owens WD, Felts JA, Spitznagel EL Jr., ASA physical status classification: a study of consistency of ratings, pp. 239–43. Copyright (1978) with permission from Wolters Kluwer Health, Inc.

14. B. 2

The American Association for the Surgery of Trauma (AAST) liver injury scale is most commonly scoring system to describe the appearance of liver parenchymal injury. It is most commonly used to describe the appearances of the liver on cross-sectional imaging. It can be graded as follows:

- Grade I:
  - Haematoma: subcapsular, nonexpanding, <10% surface area
  - Laceration: capsular tear, nonbleeding, <1cm parenchymal depth
- Grade II:
  - Haematoma: subcapsular, nonexpanding, 10–50% surface area
  - Haematoma: intraparenchymal nonexpanding, <10cm diameter
  - Laceration: capsular tear, active bleeding, 1–3cm parenchymal depth, <10cm length
- Grade III:
  - Haematoma: subcapsular, >50% surface area or expanding, ruptured subcapsular with active bleeding
  - Haematoma: intraparenchymal >10cm or expanding
  - Laceration: capsular tear >3cm parenchymal depth
- Grade IV:
  - Haematoma: ruptured intraparenchymal haematoma with active bleeding
  - Laceration: parenchymal disruption involving 25–75%hepatic lobe or involves 1–3 Couinaud's segments (within one lobe)
- Grade V:
  - Laceration: parenchymal disruption involving >75% of hepatic lobe or involves >3 Couinaud's segments (within one lobe)
  - Vascular: juxtahepatic venous injuries (e.g. retrohepatic vena cava)
- Grade VI:
  - Vascular: hepatic avulsion
  - If more than one injury is present, advance one grade for injuries up to Grade III[5]

Ahmed N and Vernick JJ. Management of liver trauma in adults. *Journal of Emergencies, Trauma and Shock* 2011; 4(1):114–19.

Wound management

15. J. Vascular reconstruction

Arterial ulceration and tissue loss is a definitive indication for revascularization by either endovascular techniques or surgical bypass. Key to the success of any attempt at revascularization is accurate preoperative imaging and aggressive post-operative management of risk factors.

---

[5] Reproduced from *Journal of Trauma—Injury Infection & Critical Care*, 38, 3, Moore EE, Cogbill T, Jurkovich G et al., Organ Injury Scaling: Spleen and Liver (1994 Revision), pp. 323–4. Copyright (1995) with permission from Wolters Kluwer Health, Inc.

16. A. Debridement

The physiological compromise and clinical picture in this scenario indicates necrotizing fasciitis. This is a surgical emergency which requires urgent aggressive debridement of compromised tissue. Achieving this can take more than one visit to the operating theatre. Close liaison with Microbiology is required as antimicrobial therapy should be tailored to the specific organisms identified by cultures as quickly as possible.

17. E. Negative pressure wound therapy

Negative pressure wound therapy (NPWT) is used to expedite healing in wounds left open intentionally or in chronic wounds that have failed to heal. Although the mechanism of action of NPWT is not entirely clear, it is thought that at the very least, the sealed dressing maintains optimal conditions for re-epithelialization.

Controversy has surrounded the use of NPWT in open abdominal wounds, given concern regarding the risk of inducing enteric fistulation. It is generally felt that NPWT should not be applied to an open abdomen with exposed bowel which has not yet fistulated. In these circumstances, NPWT should only be initiated and managed by medical teams with the requisite training, and the outcome of therapy should be rigorously audited.

18. I. Rotational flap

The most important aspect of pressure sore management should be regarded as prevention with identification of modifiable risk factors and protection of at-risk patients. Most ulcers are managed non-operatively using a multidisciplinary approach involving both primary and secondary care. Surgery is reserved for non-resolving cases in patients able to withstand general anaesthesia.

Either loco-regional musculocutaneous or fasciocutaneous flaps can be utilized. The type of flap that is required is decided on a case-by-case basis and is dependent on the site of the ulcer. Care must be taken to ensure that any suture lines are placed away from pressure points.

NICE Guidelines: Pressure sores: prevention and management. Clinical guideline. 2014. Available online at <https://www.nice.org.uk/guidance/cg179?unlid=206883283201610921513>.

Hunter IA and Davies A. Managing pressure sores. *Surgery* 2014; 32(9):472–9.

Microbiology

19. E. *Chlamydia trachomatis*

Pelvic inflammatory disease (PID) is infection of the upper genital tract resulting in endometritis, salpingitis, or oophoritis. It is a common condition in sexually active women, being responsible for 1 in 60 visits to primary care in women under 40. *Chlamydia trachomatis* is responsible for 50–65% of cases, with *Neisseria gonorrhoea* in 15%. It is likely to be under-diagnosed as symptoms may be minimal or absent. Treatment is based on local microbial policy.

Jivraj S and Farkas A. Gynaecological causes of abdominal pain. *Surgery* 2015; 33, 226–31.

20. F. *Campylobacter*

Campylobacter is the most common cause of food poisoning in the United Kingdom and accounts for nearly 300,000 cases per year. Of these cases around one-third are confirmed on microbiological culture. The most common cause is undercooked poultry in 80%. *Campylobacter* may be present in around 65% of chickens in the United Kingdom.

There are 17 different species of *Campylobacter* but *C. jejuni* and *C. coli* are the most common pathogens in human disease. The incubation period is between two and five days and symptoms usually last less than seven days. Symptoms include diarrhoea, which may be bloody, abdominal pain, fever, nausea/vomiting, and malaise. The condition is usually self-limiting and so does not normally require treatment other than fluid and electrolyte replacement. While *Salmonella* and *E. coli* can also be related to undercooked meat, they are statistically less likely.

21. C. *Yersinia enterocolitica*

Yersinia enterocolitica is a member of the Enterobacter family and is transmitted via contaminated food or water. In some areas it is responsible for more cases of bacterial enteritis than *Shigella* and *Salmonella*. The symptoms are mainly diarrhoeal but the predilection for terminal ileitis leads to the pseudoappendicitis syndrome of pyrexia, right lower quadrant pain, tenderness, and leucocytosis.

22. I. *Candida albicans*

Prolonged indiscriminate use of broad-spectrum antibiotics in the management of severe acute pancreatitis has led to the recognition of super-infection with *Candida* particularly *Candida albicans*. Most endpoints related to acute pancreatitis are negatively impacted upon by superimposed fungal infections, and most significantly mortality.

Major trauma

23. A. Mattox manoeuvre

The Mattox manoeuvre facilitates left retroperitoneal exposure. It is also described as a left-sided medial visceral rotation. It allows access and exposure over the entire abdominal aorta, left renal vessels, coeliac axis, and superior mesenteric artery as well as the left iliac arteries.

An extended incision is made in the peritoneum lateral to the left colon. Rather than continuing in the plane between the kidney and the left colon as one might perform for a left hemicolectomy, the incision and dissection continues posterior to the kidney which is reflected medially and anteriorly along with the spleen and tail of pancreas. The incision should start low down in the left lower quadrant, the colon is rotated medially, and incision extended upward. Dissection should sweep from below, upward, and medially.

Although superb access can be obtained along the major vessels, the manoeuvre may cause injury to the spleen or disruption of the left lumbar veins.

24. D. Pringle manoeuvre

In the context of trauma, physiological compromise of the patient is due to haemorrhage until proven otherwise. Patients are resuscitated in line with ATLS principles whilst attempting to identify the bleeding compartment. This may be obvious in single penetrating wounds but less so in blunt trauma, particularly if there are no external signs of injury.

If hepatic bleeding is not controlled by direct pressure, the in-flow can be controlled using the Pringle manoeuvre. This involves clamping or even manual pinching of the portal structures where they run in the gastro–duodenal ligament. Should bleeding continue, it is likely that the inferior vena cava or the hepatic vein have also traumatized. Temporary control of bleeding is suspicious of hepatic arterial or portal venous injury.

25. G. Damage control laparotomy

The intercostal drain has excluded a significant haemothorax therefore leaving the abdomen as the likely source of bleeding. The decision to proceed with a damage control procedure is based on a number of factors and does not need to be the intention of the procedure at the outset. Inability to achieve haemostasis or the development of the lethal triad (hypothermia, acidosis, and coagulopathy) should prompt attempts to terminate the procedure in a safe manner, whereby bleeding has been tamponaded by multi-quadrant packing and contamination is controlled. Certain intra-operative manoeuvres can aid with providing access or limiting inflow to allow identification of the bleeding source. Left (Mattox) and right (Cattall–Brasch) medial visceral rotation allow excellent exposure of the great vessels to allow repair as necessary. These are performed by sharply dividing the peritoneum laterally and bluntly mobilizing the spleen and colon on the left, or the colon and duodenum on the right to expose the cava or abdominal aorta and facilitate repair.

Bleeding related to pelvic trauma can be catastrophic and again patient physiology determines the method employed to gain control, if application of a pelvic binder has not done so. A stable patient or one who has responded to initial resuscitative measures affords the opportunity to employ angio-embolization which is superior to external fixation at controlling haemorrhage. Should these measures prove unsuccessful, attempts to control haemorrhage by extra-peritoneal pelvic packing should be employed.

26. H. Angio-embolization

Patients with high-energy pelvic fractures frequently have concomitant abdominal, head, and thoracic injuries which should also be considered as a source of ongoing bleeding. Between 60–80% of patients have musculoskeletal injuries, 12% have urogenital injuries, and 8% have lumbosacral injuries.

Aggressive fluid resuscitation is critical in the patient who is haemodynamically unstable. Displaced pelvic fractures can be stabilized temporarily by immobilization and partial reduction of displacement. A sheet can be tied around the pelvis, or the legs can be tied together in an internally rotated position.

Military anti-shock trousers (MAST) have been shown to be effective in the prehospital treatment of patients who are hypotensive and have pelvic fractures. However, they limit exposure to the lower abdomen and legs, decrease expansion of the lungs, and there is some evidence that they may increase the risk of developing compartment syndrome in under-perfused patients.

Bleeding from a significant pelvic bony injury is usually secondary to bleeding from cancellous bone at the fracture site or from a retroperitoneal lumbar plexus injury. Only a minority (20%) of deaths from pelvic haemorrhage can be attributed to major arterial injury.

Although haemorrhage from pelvic fractures can be catastrophic, care has to be taken not to miss bleeding from other sites as these patients usually have multiple injuries. Intra-abdominal and bladder injuries are not infrequent.

Continued unexplained blood loss despite fracture stabilization and aggressive resuscitation mandates angiographic exploration to look for continued arterial bleeding. Bleeding can be controlled using a number of angiographic techniques including embolization.

The timing of arteriography and embolization is controversial. Most authors recommend arteriography after the initial stabilization, laparotomy, or both. A skilled radiologist is critically important. Aggressive fluid resuscitation must be continued during angiography. Hypothermia may develop during a prolonged radiographic procedure if the patient is not adequately warmed and resuscitated.

Extraperitoneal pelvic packing (EPP) appears to be a safe and quick means of enhancing hemodynamic stabilization and reducing acute haemorrhage-related mortality in hemodynamically unstable pelvic fracture patients, in combination with optimal transfusion. It may be useful as a bridge to angio-embolization or other time-consuming procedures.

Boffard K. Part 4: Specific organ injury. In: Boffard K (ed.). *Manual of Definitive Surgical Trauma Care*, 2nd edn. London: Hodder Arnold, 2007, pp. 65–156

Hernias

27. B. Amyand's hernia

amyand = appendix.

Amyand's hernia is the eponymous condition where the appendix is included in the hernia sac which becomes incarcerated. It is a rare condition and accounts for less than 1% of inguinal hernias. The condition is named after the English surgeon, Claudius Amyand (1680–1740), who performed the first successful appendicectomy in 1735.

Amyand's hernia is commonly misdiagnosed as an ordinary incarcerated hernia. Symptoms mimicking appendicitis may occur. An inflamed appendix in the hernia sac may also be mistaken for strangulation. Treatment consists of a combination of appendicectomy and hernia repair.

Kingsnorth AN et al. Hernias, umbilicus and abdominal wall. In: Williams NS et al (eds). *Bailey & Love's Short Practice of Surgery*, 25th edn. London: Arnold, 2008, pp. 968–90

28. F. Petit's hernia

lumbar

Lumbar hernias are rare and can usually be classified into primary or secondary types. Primary hernias occur spontaneously whereas secondary hernias develop after trauma, infection or previous surgical procedures and constitute about 25% of all lumbar hernias.

Lumbar hernias tend to come through two weak areas within the posterolateral abdominal wall: the superior lumbar triangle of Grynfeltt is the more common site; less commonly a lumbar hernia may arise through the inferior lumbar triangle of Petit. Occasionally patients may present with a 'diffuse' hernia that is not confined to these triangles and is especially difficult to repair.

Petit's hernia is bounded anteriorly by the free margin of the external oblique muscle, medially and posteriorly by the latissimus dorsi, and inferiorly by the iliac crest. The neck is usually large which means that the hernia is thought to have a lower risk of strangulation compared to some other hernias. Colonic incarceration through the inferior lumbar triangle may occur and may give rise to intermittent obstructive symptoms. Petit's hernia is more common in males and more commonly occurs on the left side.

Meckel's = Littre's.

29. D. Littre's hernia

Littre's hernia is the protrusion of a Meckel's diverticulum through a potential opening in the abdominal wall. Although inguinal herniae are the most common site, the next most frequent site is para-umbilical.

Alexis de Littre (1700) initially described an 'ileal diverticula' which was thought to be due to traction. August Gottlieb Richter (1785) realized that these were congenital and Johann Friedrich Meckel (1809) postulated their embryologic origin. Sir Frederic Treves (1897) distinguished between Littre's and Richter's hernia.

The inguinal region is the most common site of a Littre's hernia (50%), followed by incarceration in an umbilical (20%) and femoral (20%) hernia. The hernia may contain both a Meckel's diverticulum and small bowel and both may undergo strangulation, necrosis, and perforation. In children, umbilical hernias not infrequently contain a Littre's hernia as the diverticulum is more prone to adhere to the sac.

Thoracic trauma

30. B. Left anterolateral thoracotomy

The left anterolateral thoracotomy is the incision of choice in the unstable patient. It allows the heart to be exposed, tamponade to be relieved, control of bleeding from the heart or pulmonary hilum, cardiac massage, and cross-clamping of the descending aorta. This is the approach of choice for injury to the left thorax or any injury above the nipple in the right thorax.

The chest. In: Boffard KD (ed.). *Manual of Definitive Surgical Trauma Care*, 4th edn. Boca Raton, FLA: CRC Press, 2016, pp. 73–96.

31. C. Clamshell thoracotomy

The clamshell thoracotomy allows the chest to be opened widely giving rapid access for trans-mediastinal or lung injury. It also gives excellent exposure to posterior injuries. See Figure 3.4.

32. C. Clamshell thoracotomy

The incision is extended across the sternum to make a clamshell thoracotomy for the reasons previously stated.

33. A. Median sternotomy

The median sternotomy is ideal for penetrating injury at the base of the neck (zone 1) and the thoracic outlet. It allows exposure of the heart and origins of the great vessels. It has the advantage of extending the incision up into the neck (Henry's incision), downward into a midline laparotomy or lateral extension for a supraclavicular approach.

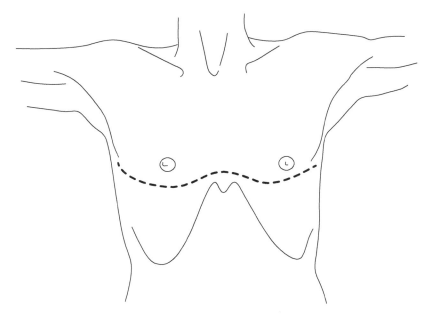

Fig. 3.4 Clamshell thoracotomy

Biologic agents

34. A. Bevacizumab

This recombinant humanized monoclonal antibody blocks angiogenesis by inhibiting the action of vascular endothelial growth factor A (VEGF-A). The drug is sold under the trade name of Avastin. It is primarily used to prevent new vessel formation in a variety of cancers. It is usually reserved for advanced disease when combined with standard chemotherapy in the management of metastatic colon, lung, renal, and ovarian cancers. It has also been used in wet age-related macular degeneration.

35. E. Basiliximab

Basiliximab is a chimeric (human-murine) monoclonal antibody that is used as an immunosuppressive agent to prevent immediate transplant rejection in patients undergoing kidney transplants. It is sold under the trade name of Simulect. It is usually used in combination with other immunosuppressive drugs. It is frequently used as alternative therapy to ciclosporin. It is active against the alpha chain (CD25) of the IL-2 receptor of T-cells. This prevents T-cells from replicating and it also impairs their ability to activate B cells. It therefore also indirectly inhibits antibody formation.

36. F. Trastuzumab

Trastuzumab is a monoclonal antibody that interferes with the HER2/neu receptor. It inhibits over expression of HER2. The HER (human epidermal growth factor receptor) cell membrane receptors are activated by epidermal growth factors and signal protein synthesis. The HER2 receptor may be over-expressed in certain cancers and it mediates cell reproduction. Trastuzumab (brand name Herceptin) may be used particularly in patients with breast cancer who have been shown to over-express the HER2 receptor. The drug is of no benefit, and may cause harm, if administered to patients with breast cancer who do not over-express HER2.

37. D. Vedolizumab

Vedolizumab is a gut-selective monoclonal antibody that is used in the treatment of both ulcerative colitis and Crohn's disease. It binds integrin $\alpha 4\beta 7$ (LPAM-1, lymphocyte Peyer's patch adhesion molecule 1). The $\alpha 4\beta 7$ integrin-expressing T-cell is an important leucocyte in the pathogenesis of both Crohn's disease and ulcerative colitis. When activated, these T-cells preferentially adhere to endothelial surfaces within the GI tract and associated lymphoid tissue. Vedolizumab (trade name Entyvio) works by preventing activation of these T-cells, which significantly attenuates leukocyte extravasation into the GI tract. This results in gut-selective anti-inflammatory therapy.

The drug has been used as second- or third-line monoclonal therapy in patients with Crohn's disease and ulcerative colitis when they are no longer responsive to anti-TNF (tumour necrosis factor) therapy or where anti-TNF therapy is contraindicated (e.g. active tuberculous infection).

38. H. Cetuximab

Cetuximab (trade name Erbitux) is a chimeric (mouse–human) monoclonal antibody active against epidermal growth factor receptor (EGFR). It is used in the treatment of metastatic colorectal cancer, metastatic non-small-cell lung cancer, and head and neck cancer. It is indicated for the treatment of colon cancer with wild-type KRAS, either in isolation or in combination with conventional chemotherapy. The EGFR is responsible for signalling that induces cells to divide. The downstream pathway following EGFR activation includes the protein KRAS. KRAS mutations may occur in some cancers, which can lead to uncontrolled cell division irrespective of whether the EGFR has been blocked by cetuximab. If KRAS is normal (wild-type) cetuximab may work. However, if mutated it is unlikely that cetuximab will work because the mutated KRAS gene is continuously active, irrespective of whether the EGFR has been blocked or not.

COLORECTAL SURGERY

QUESTIONS

Single Best Answers

1. **A 73 year old male presents with left iliac fossa pain and diarrhoea. On examination he has LIF peritonism and inflammatory markers are raised with a WCC 18 × 10⁹/L and CRP 240mg/L. A CT scan confirms diverticulitis with a pelvic abscess. This is classified as:**

   a) Hinchey I
   b) Hinchey II
   c) Hinchey III
   d) Hinchey IV
   e) Cannot be classified with this information

2. **A 57 year old male has been diagnosed with a rectal cancer 10cm from the anal verge after a positive bowel screening test. A staging CT demonstrates localized disease and MRI stages the tumour as cT3a with a circumferential resection margin (CRM) of 3mm. The most likely management recommendation following MDT discussion is:**

   a) Short course radiotherapy followed by early surgery
   b) Long course chemotherapy and radiotherapy followed by surgery
   c) Early surgery
   d) Long course radiotherapy followed by surgery then adjuvant chemotherapy
   e) Further tests are required to make the decision on treatment

3. **A 59 year old male is referred by gastroenterology with a biopsy proven anterior rectal cancer, 8cm from the anal verge. CT and MRI show tumour lying 1mm from the mesorectal fascia anteriorly. There is a mesorectal node 2mm from the mesorectal fascia and a 15mm external iliac node. The next step in management should be**

   a) Anterior resection
   b) Anterior resection and defunctioning loop ileostomy
   c) Neoadjuvant chemoradiotherapy
   d) CT PET
   e) AP resection

4. **A 29 year old female presents with a 24hr history of right iliac fossa pain, localized peritonism, and raised inflammatory markers. Diagnostic laparoscopy confirms appendicitis and an appendicectomy is performed. Subsequent pathology reveals a 2.2cm carcinoid tumour at the tip of the appendix, 1.2mm from the proximal resection margin. What is the next most appropriate step in this patient's management?**
    a) Regular six-monthly clinic follow-up
    b) Yearly CT scans for the first three years
    c) Colonoscopy
    d) Right hemicolectomy
    e) Octreotide scan

5. **A 22 year old female with familial adenomatous polyposis coli undergoes a restorative proctocolectomy with defunctioning loop ileostomy. Her post-operative course is complicated due to a leak from the ileal pouch-anal anastomosis. At EUA, a 1cm posterior defect in the pouch-anal anastomosis is noted. A pelvic MRI displays a 3cm presacral cavity. What is the most appropriate next step in her management?**
    a) Immediate revision of the ileal pouch-anal anastomosis
    b) Permanent non-reversal of ileostomy
    c) Reversal of ileostomy at three months
    d) Vacuum-assisted closure device therapy
    e) EUA and curettage of cavity

6. **A 21 year old male with a family history of colon cancer is informed he is a mismatch repair gene carrier and is 'at risk of HNPCC'. Which of the following screening recommendations should be applied?**
    a) Colonoscopy and upper GI endoscopy every five years starting now
    b) Two-yearly colonoscopy from age 25 and 2-yearly upper GI endoscopy from age 50
    c) Annual colonoscopy and two-yearly upper GI endoscopy starting now
    d) Colonoscopy every 3 years from age 30 and upper GI endoscopy every 3 years from age 40
    e) Colonoscopy every 5 years and upper GI endoscopy every 10 years starting now

7. **A 42 year old lady presents with recurrent retroperitoneal sarcoma. In her thirties she was treated for breast cancer and colon cancer. Genetic testing confirms a germline mutation in which of the following genes?**
    a) *RET*
    b) *TP53*
    c) *APC*
    d) *KRAS*
    e) *MLH1*

8. **Ten years after a diagnosis of Crohn's colitis, a 52 year old male undergoes a check colonoscopy. High-grade dysplasia is noted in four of ten biopsies. The biopsies were taken from an elevated area in the left colon that was not endoscopically resectable. What is the most appropriate next step in this patient's management?**
   a) Repeat colonoscopy in six months
   b) Review his medication and consider adding Infliximab
   c) Proctocolectomy and ileal pouch
   d) Consider colectomy and ileorectal anastomosis
   e) Total proctocolectomy and end ileostomy

9. **A routine CT of chest, abdomen and pelvis performed in a patient who is two years after abdomino-perineal resection for an early distal rectal cancer, shows an unsuspected parastomal hernia containing a loop of small intestine. How is this best managed?**
   a) Consider early repeat CT scan to see if it is progressing
   b) Transposition of the stoma to the other side of the abdomen
   c) Local repair of the hernia plus or minus using mesh
   d) Laparoscopic repair using a Sugarbaker technique
   e) Reassurance and standard follow-up

10. **A 30 year old male presents with a 6-month history of bloody diarrhoea. At colonoscopy a florid colitis is identified. There is rectal sparing. A diagnosis of Crohn's disease is made. Which of the following statements is consistent with the diagnosis?**
    a) There will be no long-term increased risk of colorectal cancer because the diagnosis is Crohn's disease rather than ulcerative colitis
    b) The prevalence of Crohn's disease is 150 per 100,000 in the United Kingdom
    c) The prevalence of Crohn's disease has been stable over the last 30 years
    d) Colitis with rectal sparing is pathognomonic of Crohn's disease.
    e) There is a much-reduced risk of developing toxic megacolon because the diagnosis is Crohn's disease rather than ulcerative colitis.

11. **A 67 year old gentleman presents with a 2-day history of colicky abdominal pain and diarrhoea. Clinical examination is unremarkable. Routine bloods show a CRP of 175mg/L and a WCC of 15×10^9/L. What is the single next-best diagnostic test to evaluate this gentleman?**
    a) Faecal calprotectin
    b) Stool for culture and sensitivity and *C. difficile* toxin
    c) Abdominal ultrasound
    d) Colonoscopy with full preparation
    e) CT scan

12. **Which of the following statements is incorrect in relation to gastrointestinal stromal tumours (GIST)?**
    a) Arise from the interstitial cells of Cajal
    b) Can be differentiated from leiomyosarcomas of bowel by staining positively for CD117 antigen (C-KIT)
    c) Surgical resection with clear margins is associated with 5-year survival of >90%
    d) Prognosis is related to the size of the tumour and the number of mitoses per high power field on histology
    e) Rarely metastasize to lymph nodes

13. **You are asked to review a 35 year old man with a 5-year history of colitis. He has been on the gastroenterology ward for five days and his acute colitis has failed to respond to IV steroids over this time. He has previously been stable on azathioprine and he is keen to avoid a stoma. Currently, his stool frequency is 9/day, the CRP is 150mg/L, and his albumin is 25g/L. What is the most appropriate management?**
    a) Anti-TNF therapy
    b) Add in IV antibiotics and continue IV steroids for a further 48 hours
    c) Emergency panproctocolectomy with ileal pouch and loop ileostomy
    d) Emergency subtotal colectomy and end ileostomy
    e) Emergency subtotal colectomy and ileorectal anastomosis

14. **A 56 year old patient presents 4 weeks after undergoing a small bowel resection and stricturoplasty for recurrent Crohn's disease. There is an open wound which is producing at least 700mls of intestinal fluid/ day. A CT scan shows a fistula track arising from a 6cm abscess cavity in the region of the recent ileocolic anastomosis. What is the most appropriate management plan?**
    a) Laparotomy
    b) Percutaneous drainage of the abscess followed by a laparotomy
    c) TPN, IV antibiotics, and octreotide
    d) Supportive therapy including antibiotics, drainage of the abscess, and discuss biologic therapy with the Gastroenterology team to treat a presumed Crohn's-related fistula
    e) Percutaneous drainage, TPN, IV antibiotics, and a contrast small bowel study to define the site of the fistula

15. **Which of the following statements is correct in relation to anal or anogenital warts?**
    a) HPV types 16 and 18 are most frequently the cause of anal warts
    b) HPV types that cause anal warts are considered high risk for progression to cancer
    c) Only a minority of unaffected partners of patients with warts develop them within one year
    d) HPV infections tend to be lifelong and the virus is rarely cleared from the body
    e) The Gardasil HPV vaccine protects against HPV types that are associated with both a high risk of cancer and against anal warts

16. A 22 year old female presents 4 months following incision and drainage of a perianal abscess. On examination, she has a 5mm area of granulation tissue at the site of the previous surgery in the 11 o'clock position. A subcutaneous ridge is palpable extending from the incision site towards the anal margin. Pressure leads to expression of a bead of pus from the opening. What is the next step in her management?
    a) EUA and drain persistent perianal abscess
    b) MRI of the perineum
    c) Prescribe a two-week course of antibiotics to treat a persistent perianal abscess
    d) EUA and lay open anal fistula
    e) Advise that perianal abscesses can take some time to settle and review in three months

17. Which of the following statements is correct in relation to rectal prolapse?
    a) Over the age of 50 years, the incidence of rectal prolapse is similar in males and females
    b) A minority of adults who present with rectal prolapse also report faecal incontinence
    c) Constipation is rarely an issue in patients with true rectal prolapse
    d) Rectal prolapse in children may be associated with cystic fibrosis
    e) Conservative management is rarely successful in children aged less than four years

18. A 27 year old male presents with a 6-month history of rectal dissatisfaction, a feeling of incomplete evacuation, and passing blood and mucus per rectum. At flexible sigmoidoscopy he is noted to have multiple areas of ulceration affecting the anterior rectal wall at 7–10cm from the anal verge. Biopsies show thickening and disruption of the muscularis mucosa and the lamina propria is replaced with smooth muscle. Displaced mucus glands are also reported deep within the submucosa. What is the most likely diagnosis?
    a) Crohn's disease
    b) Solitary rectal ulcer syndrome (SRUS)
    c) Ulcerative proctitis
    d) Lymphogranuloma venereum (LGV) rectal infection
    e) Rectal lymphoma

19. Calprotectin is a calcium-binding protein that exhibits antibacterial and antifungal activity. Which of the following statements is not correct in relation to calprotectin?
    a) Constitutes 60% of neutrophil cytosolic protein
    b) Is an abundant protein found in all body fluids in relation to the degree of inflammation
    c) Is degraded by bacteria in the gut
    d) Elevated faecal concentrations are found in patients with colorectal carcinoma and to a lesser extent those with adenomatous polyps
    e) Elevated faecal calprotectin is not specific for inflammatory bowel disease

20. **A 30 year old female with a history of liver transplant for sclerosing cholangitis and panproctocolectomy and ileal pouch for ulcerative colitis presents with a 4-day history of abdominal pain, cramps, nausea, vomiting, blood-stained diarrhoea, and pyrexia. What is the most appropriate next step in her management?**
    a) Commence metronidazole
    b) Check CMV serology
    c) Urgent CT scan of abdomen and pelvis
    d) Contact the liver transplant team to discuss concern that she is showing signs of rejection of her liver transplant
    e) Pouchoscopy/biopsy and stool for culture and sensitivity

21. **A 45 year old female with a 10-year history of Crohn's disease presents with small bowel obstruction that has not resolved after 3 days of intravenous steroids. Prior to admission she had been treated with an 8-week course of oral steroids because of obstructive symptoms. Her CRP is 40mg/L, WCC 12 × 10⁹/L, and albumin 27g/L. She is taken to theatre and at operation an inflammatory phlegmon involving 15cm of terminal ileum and caecum is identified. There is a 3cm abscess alongside this. What is the most appropriate management?**
    a) Drain abscess and ileocolic anastomosis to bypass the inflammatory phlegmon
    b) Drain abscess, washout, and defunctioning proximal ileostomy
    c) Ileocolic resection with primary anastomosis
    d) Ileocolic resection with primary anastomosis and proximal defunctioning stoma
    e) Ileocolic resection with end ileostomy

22. **The following is correct regarding the risk of colorectal cancer in patients with inflammatory bowel disease**
    a) The risk of colorectal cancer is higher in Crohn's disease compared to ulcerative colitis, given a similar extent and duration of disease
    b) All patients with inflammatory bowel disease should have a screening colonoscopy ten years after the onset of colonic symptoms
    c) Screening colonoscopy should never be performed when the disease is active
    d) The identification of high-grade dysplasia within an adenomatous polyp is an indication for colectomy
    e) The severity of inflammation is not an independent risk factor

23. **Which of the following factors increases the risk of developing colorectal cancer in patients with inflammatory bowel disease?**
    a) Primary sclerosing cholangitis
    b) Crohn's disease affecting 50% of the colon
    c) Biologic therapy, for example Infliximab
    d) Late disease onset
    e) Long-term azathioprine

24. **Which of the following is correct with regard to large bowel surveillance in Lynch syndrome?**
    a) Total colonic surveillance should commence at age 25 and occur every 5 years until age 75
    b) Total colonic surveillance should commence at age 25 and occur every 2 years until age 75
    c) Total colonic surveillance should commence at age 25 and occur yearly until age 75
    d) Total colonic surveillance should commence at age 45 and occur every 5 years until age 75
    e) Total colonic surveillance should commence at age 45 and occur every 2 years until age 75

25. **Which of the following is incorrect regarding Peutz–Jeghers syndrome?**
    a) Upper GI endoscopy is recommended every two years
    b) The risk of colorectal cancer is 75% at age 70
    c) Females are at greater risk of developing cancer
    d) The risk of gastric malignancy is 25%
    e) Inactivating mutations in *STK11* gene are identifiable in >90% cases

26. **The immunohistochemical profile of anal adenocarcinoma is as follows**
    a) CK7+ve, CK20–ve
    b) CK7–ve, CK20+ve
    c) CK7–ve, CK20–ve
    d) CK7+ve, CK20+ve

27. **Which of the following factors does not influence prognosis in anal cancer?**
    a) Gender
    b) Tumour stage
    c) Histological subtype
    d) Nodal involvement
    e) Response to chemoradiotherapy

28. **Which of the following has been shown to be an independent risk factor for anastomotic leak in rectal cancer surgery?**
    a) Low weight/cachexia
    b) Use of a pelvic drain
    c) Long operating time
    d) Presence of a defunctioning stoma
    e) Preoperative use of NSAIDs

29. **In Lynch syndrome (HNPCC or hereditary non-polyposis colorectal cancer) which of the following statements is true?**
    a) Accounts for 10% of colonic carcinomas
    b) Often affects the proximal colon
    c) Genetics referral is not indicated
    d) Three-yearly colonoscopy is recommended
    e) Affects chromosome 5q21

30. **A 45 year old male is diagnosed with a squamous cell carcinoma following examination under anaesthesia and biopsy of an anal lesion. The next most appropriate management step is**
    a) Fluorouracil (5-FU) and mitomycin C (MMC)
    b) 5-FU, MMC, and radiotherapy
    c) Radiotherapy
    d) Abdominoperineal resection
    e) Wide local excision of the lesion

31. **In relation to primary colonic lymphoma (PCL) which of the following is true?**
    a) Is more common in females
    b) Classically occurs in patients in their third to fourth decade of life
    c) T-cell lymphomas are the most common histological type
    d) Most commonly involves the caecum
    e) Surgical resection is contraindicated

32. **Which of the following is the most important risk factor in relation to 30-day post-operative mortality after colorectal cancer surgery?**
    a) Emergency operations
    b) Stage of disease
    c) Elderly patients
    d) Socioeconomic deprivation
    e) Comorbidity (Charlson comorbidity score of ≥3)
    f) Surgeon experience

33. **A 60 year old male presents with a rectal cancer at 8cm. CT and MRI show no distant disease and a T3 primary tumour, 1mm from the anterior margin, with a large node within the mesorectum abutting the mesorectal fascia. The next most likely step in his management is**
    a) PET scan to assess for metastatic disease
    b) Proceed to anterior resection
    c) Neoadjuvant 5-FU and radiotherapy (45Gys, 25 fractions)
    d) Radiotherapy (45Gys, 25 fractions)
    e) Short course neoadjuvant radiotherapy (25Gys, 5 fractions)

34. **In metastatic colorectal cancer, cetuximab is most appropriate in which of the following circumstances?**
    a) KRAS wild-type patients
    b) Patients with liver metastases
    c) Patients with peritoneal disease
    d) KRAS-mutated patients
    e) All patients with lung metastases

35. **Which of the following is true of small bowel adenocarcinoma?**
    a) It is commoner in Eastern societies
    b) Crohn's disease is the most important risk factor
    c) Not related to the adenoma–carcinoma sequence
    d) Occurs more commonly in females
    e) Most commonly affects the ileum

36. **Which of the following drugs is used in the treatment of gastrointestinal stromal tumours (GIST)?**
    a) Cetuximab
    b) Imatinib
    c) Interferon
    d) Adalimumab
    e) Paclitaxel

37. **A 45 year old male attends for a colonoscopy for investigation of diarrhoea. A 22mm sessile lesion is identified in the upper rectum. A successful endoscopic mucosal resection (EMR) is performed and histology shows a completely excised neuroendocrine tumour with a high Ki-67 index. The most important step in his further management will be**
    a) Check flexible sigmoidoscopy in three months
    b) CT scan
    c) Anterior resection
    d) Transanal excision of the EMR site
    e) Endoscopic ultrasound

38. **In the management of appendiceal carcinoids, appendicetomy is adequate in which of the following scenarios:**
    a) 22mm tumour confined to the tip of the appendix
    b) 12mm tumour with deep invasion into the mesoappendix
    c) 10mm tumour present at the appendix base resection margin
    d) 14mm tumour located near the base of the appendix
    e) 12mm tumour in the tip of the appendix with lymphovascular invasion

39. **What is the most common side effect of cetuximab?**
    a) Immediate infusion reaction
    b) Skin reaction
    c) Eye irritation
    d) Peripheral neuropathy
    e) Insomnia

40. **A 60 year old man has a 2cm pedunculated polyp excised from his sigmoid colon. The pathology confirms a focus of adenocarcinoma extending to junction of the polyp and stalk. This is classified as**
    a) Haggitt level 1
    b) Haggitt level 2
    c) Haggitt level 3
    d) Haggitt level 4
    e) None of the above

41. **A 70 year old female presents with diarrhoea. A colonoscopy reveals a flat sessile polyp at 25cm. She undergoes endoscopic mucosal resection of the lesion and pathology reveals evidence of adenocarcinoma extending to, but not involving, the muscularis propria. This is pathologically staged as:**
    a) Kikuchi Sm1a
    b) Kikuchi Sm1b
    c) Kikuchi Sm1c
    d) Kikuchi Sm2
    e) Kikuchi Sm3

42. **A 50 year old female presents with RIF pain and raised inflammatory markers. A diagnosis of appendicitis is made. At laparoscopy she is found to have an enlarged appendix with mucinous material present and perforation at the tip of the appendix. Mucin is present in the pelvis. The correct next step is**
    a) Appendicetomy and washout
    b) Conversion to laparotomy and right hemicolectomy
    c) Laparoscopic right hemicolectomy
    d) Removal of mucin for histopathology
    e) Conversion to laparotomy and removal of all disease

43. **A 55 year old male presents with a 3-day history of increasing pain in the right iliac fossa. This occurs against a background of a month history of abdominal pain with alteration in bowel function. His WCC is 14×10^9/L and CRP is 70mg/L. At laparoscopy the appendix is acutely inflamed but the inflammation appears to extend into the base of the caecum, with neovascularization and induration.**
    a) Appendicectomy
    b) On-table colonoscopy and proceed based on the results
    c) Right hemicolectomy and washout, taking fluid for C&S
    d) Send the appendix for a frozen section and proceed based on the results
    e) Close the wound with a view to further investigations once recovered

44. **Which of the following statements is not part of the Amsterdam II clinical criteria for families with Lynch syndrome?**
    a) Three or more relatives with an associated cancer (colorectal cancer, endometrial cancer, small intestinal cancer, cancer of the ureter/renal pelvis)
    b) Two or more successive generations affected
    c) Two or more relatives diagnosed before the age of 50 years
    d) Familial adenomatous polyposis (FAP) should be excluded in cases of colorectal cancer
    e) Tumours should be verified by pathological examination

45. **A 45 year old woman presents with 2 mucinous cancers in the right colon. A staging CT scan also suggests a concomitant uterine cancer. Her mother died from ovarian cancer. Which of the following genes is likely to be responsible?**
    a) *p53*
    b) *MSH2*
    c) *APC*
    d) *C-Myc*
    e) *KIT*

46. **When performing a proctectomy and ileoanal pouch in patients with ulcerative colitis, why would one consider performing a concomitant mucosectomy?**
    a) Technically easier to perform the anastomosis
    b) Improves pouch function and continence
    c) Reduces the risk of inflammation in the anal transition zone
    d) Reduces the risk of dysplasia in the anal transition zone
    e) Abolishes the risk of malignancy in the anal transition zone

Extended Matching Items

Management of anorectal conditions

    A. GTN ointment
    B. Flexible sigmoidoscopy
    C. Colonoscopy
    D. Injection of Botox®
    E. Endoanal US and anorectal manometry
    F. Examination under anaesthetic
    G. MRI perineum
    H. Lateral internal sphincterotomy
    I. Topical diltiazem ointment

For each of the following scenarios, please select the most appropriate next step in management. Each option may be used once, more than once, or not at all.

1. A 25 year old male presents with bright red rectal bleeding. There is associated perianal discomfort. He is passing mucus per rectum and has an intermittent increase in stool frequency up to eight times per day. He has been feeling generally lethargic with one-half stone in weight loss over the preceding three months.

2. A 30 year old female returns to the outpatient clinic following a second trial of Botox® injection for an anal fissure. She reports a small improvement in symptoms for a month following Botox®. However, she now feels are as bad as ever with excruciating pain on defaecation. Examination confirms a posterior fissure.

3. A 65 year old male is referred with a suspected anal fissure. He has a history of increasing anal pain and rectal bleeding over the preceding six weeks. It is not possible to do a rectal examination in the clinic due to spasm/pain.

Suspected acute appendicitis

A. Open resection of terminal ileum, caecum, and appendix
B. Laparoscopic resection of terminal ileum, caecum, and appendix
C. Washout, taking fluid for C&S
D. Open biopsy of terminal ileum
E. Laparoscopic appendicectomy and washout
F. Right hemicolectomy and washout
G. Frozen section of appendix and proceed based on the results
H. Open biopsy of caecum
I. Biopsy mesenteric nodes

For each of the following scenarios, please select the most appropriate next step in management. Each option may be used once, more than once, or not at all.

4. A 25 year old female with a 6-month history of weight loss presents with a 1-day history of central abdominal pain localizing in the right iliac fossa. A preoperative scan showed no pelvic pathology but free fluid in the pelvis. At laparoscopy, the terminal ileum is thickened, congested, and shows fat encroachment. The appendix also looked somewhat congested.

5. A 30 year old male is taken to theatre for a laparoscopy, having presented with a 48-hour history of right iliac fossa pain. At operation the appendix is inflamed with some free pus. At the tip, just beyond a point of perforation, there is a 0.5cm yellow tumour.

6. A 19 year old female presents with a 48-hour history of abdominal pain, WCC of 17 × 10^9/L, and CRP of 50mg/L. At laparoscopy, there is marked erythema and congestion with adherent fibrin on the fallopian tubes, ovaries, and uterus. There is free fluid in the pelvis.

Extra-intestinal manifestations (EIM) of inflammatory bowel disease (IBD)

A. Arthritis
B. Erythema nodosum
C. Spondylitis
D. Peripheral arthropathy
E. Sweet's syndrome
F. Pyoderma gangrenosum
G. Primary sclerosing cholangitis
H. Uveitis
I. Apthous stomatitis
J. Rheumatoid arthritis
K. Episcleritis
L. Cardiomyopathy

For each of the following question, please select the most appropriate answer from the preceding list. Each option may be used once, more than once, or not at all.

7. Which condition is associated with an increased risk of pouchitis?

8. What is the most common extra-intestinal manifestation in children with inflammatory bowel disease?

9. More than 50% of patients with this extra-intestinal manifestation are HLA-B27-positive.

Anal pain

A. Chronic pelvic pain
B. Proctalgia fugax
C. Chronic proctalgia/levator ani syndrome
D. Anal fissure
E. Intersphincteric abscess
F. Pudendal neuralgia
G. Haemorrhoids
H. Perianal abscess
I. Coccygodynia
J. Perianal Crohn's disease
K. Anal cancer
L. Behçet's disease

For each of the following scenarios, please select the most likely diagnosis. Each option may be used once, more than once, or not at all.

10. A 40 year old female presents with a 12-month history of deep anal pain, described as if she was sitting on a ball and worse on sitting down. Episodes of pain last at least 30 minutes and are unrelated to defaecation. Pain is mostly felt on the left side of the perineum.

11. A 25 year old male presents with a 6-month history of severe anal pain. This is transient and lasts 10–20 minutes. It can wake the patient from sleep and is associated with an intense desire to defaecate, which usually relieves the pain. Rectal examination is unremarkable.

12. A 29 year old male presents with a 2-day history of increasing anal pain, a fever, and general malaise. Examination of the perianal tissues reveals no tenderness, induration or abscess. Rectal examination is not possible due to tenderness and spasm. What is the most likely diagnosis?

Constipation

A. Slow-transit constipation
B. Pseudo-obstruction
C. Rectal cancer
D. Diverticular stricture
E. Ischaemic stricture
F. Constipation-predominant IBS
G. Hypothyroidism
H. Hirschsprung's disease
I. Inflammatory bowel disease-related stricture
J. Drug-related constipation
K. Hypercalcaemia
L. Lack of dietary fibre

For each of the following scenarios, please select the most likely diagnosis from the preceding list. Each option may be used once, more than once, or not at all.

13. You are asked to review a 55 year old female who is in the high-dependency unit of the cardiothoracic ward. She is day 5 post-CABG (coronary artery bypass graft). She has not been eating for several days. She has a past history of hypothyroidism but is on T4 replacement therapy. Her abdominal X-ray shows massive colonic distention down to the rectum.

14. A 25 year old is seen at clinic complaining of bloating, abdominal pain, and 'terrible constipation'. She states that she is only moving her bowel every two to three weeks. Her diet is poor. A colonic transit study is performed which shows 50% of the markers remain in the colon on day 3 and 10% of the markers remain on day 5.

15. A 75 year old man with a past history of ischaemic heart disease presents with a 3-month history of increasing constipation. Nine months prior to assessment he had an acute admission with rectal bleeding. At colonoscopy, sigmoid diverticular disease is noted. More proximally in the splenic flexure, a smooth stricture is encountered.

Faecal incontinence

A. Radiation enteritis
B. Malabsorption
C. Laxative abuse
D. Occult sphincter injury at childbirth
E. Pudendal nerve neuropathy
F. Overflow incontinence
G. Diabetic neuropathy
H. Full-thickness rectal prolapse
I. Previous anorectal surgery
J. Previous rectal surgery
K. Idiopathic
L. Age-related degeneration of the anal sphincter
M. Rectal mucosal prolapse

For each of the following descriptions, choose the single most likely cause of the faecal incontinence from the list above. Each option may be used once, more than once, or not at all.

16. A 75 year old, para 3+0, female presents with passive faecal incontinence for the last 6 months. She is a type 2 diabetic of 20 years duration. Clinical examination shows a patulous anus and solid stool on her underclothes. On straining, a 5cm prolapse with concentric mucosal folds is seen.

17. A 29 year old, para 1+0, female with type 2 diabetes of 3 years' duration presents with a 1-year history of both urge and passive faecal incontinence.

18. A 25 year old, para 1+0, female with a BMI of 21 presents with episodic faecal incontinence. A faecal calprotectin is 45 and random colonic biopsies are reported as showing melanosis coli.

Emergency presentations

A. Appendicitis
B. Meckel's diverticulum
C. CMV colitis
D. Crohn's colitis
E. Ulcerative colitis
F. Colonic lymphoma
G. Indeterminate colitis
H. Mesenteric ischaemia
I. *Clostridium difficile* colitis
J. Collagenous colitis
K. Typhlitis/ileocaecal syndrome
L. Mesenteric adenitis

For each of the following descriptions, choose the single most likely diagnosis from the preceding list. Each answer can be used once, more than once, or not at all.

19. A 15 year old female undergoing chemotherapy for acute myeloid leukaemia presents with a short history of diarrhoea, with severe crampy abdominal pain. She is febrile and tachycardic. Examination reveals tenderness and signs of local peritoneal inflammation in the right iliac fossa.

20. A 58 year old female with a history of rheumatoid arthritis presents with a 6-month history of watery diarrhoea. She is systemically well. A colonoscopy is mostly unremarkable through to the caecum but the terminal ileum could not be intubated.

21. A 47 year old male who is 4 years post-liver transplant for cryptogenic cirrhosis presents with an 8-week history of bloody diarrhoea, crampy abdominal pain, and general malaise. At colonoscopy there is a generalized increase in vascularity with focal ulceration in the caecum and ileocaecal valve.

Polyposis syndromes

A. Desmoid tumour
B. Peutz–Jeghers syndrome
C. Li–Fraumeni syndrome
D. HNPCC
E. Familial adenomatous polyposis
F. Juvenile polyposis
G. Lynch syndrome
H. Hyperplastic polyposis syndrome
I. Turcot's syndrome
J. Muir–Torre syndrome
K. Gardner syndrome

For each of the following scenarios, choose the single most likely diagnosis from the preceding list. Each option may be used once, more than once, or not at all.

22. A 25 year old male is found to have multiple colonic and duodenal polyps. His only significant past history is of dental interventions for multiple impacted and supernumerary teeth.

23. A 25 year old female, who has had a previous right hemicolectomy for cancer, now presents with a glioblastoma.

24. A 14 year old male presents with anaemia. Investigations reveal several intestinal polyps and no evidence of mucocutaneous pigmentation.

Anal intraepithelial neoplasia (AIN)

A. Reassure and discharge from clinic
B. Review every six months
C. Review at six months and discharge
D. Review every 12 months
E. Wide local excision
F. Wide local excision and reconstruction with a flap
G. Local excision and mapping
H. Imiquimod 5% cream
I. Cryotherapy ablation
J. CO_2 laser ablation
K. Perform regular anal cytology screening

For each of the following scenarios, please select the most appropriate management plan from the preceding list. Each option may be used once, more than once, or not at all.

25. A 30 year old HIV-positive man requests screening for AIN as he has a friend who has been diagnosed with anal cancer and another friend undergoes screening in the United States. He is asymptomatic and clinical examination reveals no overt abnormality.

26. A 40 year old female presents with an isolated area of the perianal skin which is slightly raised. Excision biopsy shows AIN 1 (LSIL) with clear margins.

27. A 32 year old HIV-positive man presents with extensive multifocal change in the perianal skin encompassing more than 90% of the circumference on the anus. Biopsies confirm AIN 3 (HSIL).

Side-effects of chemotherapy for colorectal cancer

A. Folinic acid
B. Gabapentin
C. Cetuximab
D. Radiotherapy
E. Oxaliplatin
F. Mitomycin C
G. Radiotherapy
H. 5-fluorouracil
I. Capecitabine

Select the drug that is most likely to account for the problem described in each of the following scenarios. Each option may be used once, more than once, or not at all.

28. A 50 year old man is receiving post-operative adjuvant treatment for Duke's C cancer of the right colon. He presents to his GP seven days after his last treatment with redness and swelling of the palms and soles of his feet.

29. A 60 year old lady with colon cancer is undergoing chemotherapy at her local oncology centre. She presents to her GP with an acne-like rash affecting her face, neck and trunk. She started a new drug two weeks previously.

30. A 50 year old male with metastatic rectal cancer is undergoing palliative chemotherapy. When reviewed in the surgical clinic, he complains of numbness, tingling, and cramping of the hands and feet. This is particularly triggered by exposure to the cold.

Bowel cancer screening programme

A. 0.01–0.02%
B. 0.1–0.2%
C. 0.5%
D. 1–3%
E. 5%
F. 10–25%
G. 30–40%
H. 50%
I. 60–80%

For each of the following scenarios, choose the most accurate answer from the preceding list. Each option may be used once, more than once, or not at all.

31. What percentage of cancers detected through screening will be a polyp cancer?

32. What proportion of males who are invited to participate in the screening programme will return a completed test?

33. For the first round of screening, what is the likelihood that an individual will be asked to attend for colonoscopy due to a positive test?

Rectal cancer

A. Low Hartmann's procedure
B. Anterior resection +/− defunctioning loop ileostomy
C. Abdomino–perineal resection
D. Extra-levator abdomino–perineal resection
E. Pelvic exenteration
F. Defunctioning stoma
G. Palliative radiotherapy
H. No treatment
I. Neoadjuvant chemotherapy and then restage
J. Colonic/rectal stent

For each of the following scenarios, please select the most appropriate next step in management. Each option may be used once, more than once, or not at all.

34. A 75 year old man presents with rectal bleeding and tenesmus. Digital rectal examination revealed poor anal tone and a cancer with the distal margin at 7cm. CT colonography showed no other gross abnormalities but colonic distension was poor due to inability to retain gas. The tumour threatened the circumferential margin on MRI so he was treated with down-staging preoperative chemoradiation. His post-treatment scans show a good response and the margin is no longer threatened.

35. An 80 year old man, on home nebulisers for COPD, presents with rectal bleeding and symptomatic anaemia. Colonoscopy reveals a tumour at 6cm. Imaging and biopsies are consistent with a locally advanced rectal cancer encroaching on the levators.

36. A 50 year old male presents with a T4 low rectal cancer invading the prostate and bladder neck, which has increased in size on neoadjuvant treatment. CT confirms a PET-positive primary lesion but no other thoracic or abdomino–pelvic disease.

Polyp cancers

A. Repeat colonoscopy in three months
B. Colonoscopy and tattoo
C. Transanal excision
D. Endoscopic mucosal resection
E. Right hemicolectomy
F. Anterior resection
G. Subtotal colectomy and ileorectal anastomosis

For each of the following scenarios, please select the most appropriate next step in management. Each option may be used once, more than once, or not at all.

37. A 45 year old male presents with rectal bleeding. A colonoscopy reveals a sessile 23mm polyp at 12cm. Endoscopic mucosal resection is performed and the area is marked with a tattoo. Pathology reveals a polyp adenocarcinoma extending through to the middle third of the submucosa with poor differentiation and lymphovascular invasion.

38. A 70 year old female has been referred to the clinic by a nurse endoscopist who identified a large 3cm flat lesion in the transverse colon. It was noted to be a '3cm sessile lesion in the transverse colon, attempts to raise unsuccessful, biopsies taken'. Histology shows high-grade dysplasia. Should surgery be required the patient wishes to have a laparoscopic resection.

Pelvic tumours

A. Epidermoid cyst
B. Dermoid cyst
C. Teratoma
D. Rectal duplication cyst
E. Chordoma
F. Desmoid tumour
G. Meningocoele
H. Retroperitoneal sarcoma

For each of the following scenarios, please select the most likely diagnosis. Each option may be used once, more than once, or not at all.

39. A 40 year old male complains of weight loss and a 3-year history of slowly increasing back and pelvic pain. The pain is positional and he also complains of impotence. A CT of chest, abdomen, and pelvis reveals a malignant looking 15cm lesion at the saccrococcygeal junction which is invading bone. There are lung metastases.

40. A 4 year old child presents with a history of constipation and difficulty in micturition. A plain abdominal X-ray is reported as showing the 'scimitar sign' with anterior displacement of the rectum.

41. A 45 year old female presents with a feeling of tenesmus. A pelvic MRI demonstrates a retrorectal 10cm multiloculated cyst with several other small cysts present nearby.

Single Best Answers

1. b) Hinchey II

Diverticulosis is common in the Western world with a prevalence of 10% at 40yrs rising to 60–80% at 80yrs. Around one in ten patients develops symptoms or complications. CT is the current gold-standard investigation for suspected complicated diverticulitis. In this way the condition can be divided into four groups – the Hinchey classification is summarized as follows.

- I—Pericolic or mesenteric abscess/phlegmon
- II—Pelvic/remote intra-abdominal/retroperitoneal abscess
- III—Purulent peritonitis
- IV—Faeculent peritonitis

Non-operative management with intravenous antibiotics is currently recommended for patients in Hinchey I. The majority of patients with a localized abscess can also be managed with antibiotics. Radiologically guided percutaneous drainage can also be considered for these patients. The use of laparoscopic peritoneal lavage remains controversial but is carried out in some centers for patients in Hinchey stage II or III. Operative management for patients with generalized peritonitis includes faecal diversion or colonic resection with or without primary anastomosis. See Figure 4.1.

Hinchey EJ et al. Treatment of perforated diverticular disease of the colon. *Advances in Surgery* 1978; 12:85–109.

Vennix S et al. Laparoscopic peritoneal lavage or sigmoidectomy for perforated diverticulitis with purulent peritonitis: A multi centre, parallel group, randomised, open label trial. *Lancet* 2015; 386:1269–77.

Schulz J et al. Laparoscopic lavage vs primary resection for acute perforated diverticulitis: The SCANDIV randomised control trial. *Journal of the American Medical Association* 2015; 314(13):1364–75.

2. c) Early surgery

All patients diagnosed with rectal cancer should have thorough preoperative staging unless contraindicated. Colonoscopy and biopsy is the initial investigation of choice. CT colonography may be used to exclude synchronous lesions if colonoscopy is incomplete due to stricturing of the lumen. For rectal cancer, an MRI of pelvis should also be carried out to determine the local extent of the tumour, in addition to a CT of chest, abdomen, and pelvis.

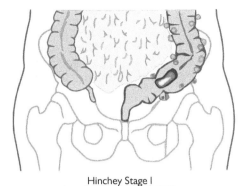

Hinchey Stage I
Localised pericolic abscess

Hinchey Stage II
Mesenteric or distant abscess

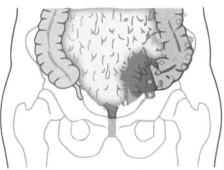

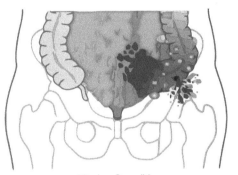

Hinchey Stage III
Perforation (gas and purulent peritionitis)

Hinchey Stage IV
Free perforation with faeculent peritionitis

Fig. 4.1 Hinchey staging of diverticulitis

Source data from *Advances in Surgery*, 12, Hinchey EJ, Schaal PG, Richards GK, Treatment of perforated diverticular disease of the colon, pp. 85–109, 1978.

N.B. T3 = in low rectal ↑ stage.

There is a high risk of local recurrence in patients where the resection margin/mesorectal fascia is threatened (<1mm), or in patients with low tumours encroaching on the inter-sphincteric plane or levators. These patients should be considered for chemoradiotherapy prior to surgical resection. Patients with moderate risk of local recurrence without margin threat (T3b, suspicion of involved mesorectal nodes or extramural vascular invasion on MRI) could be considered for preoperative radiotherapy. Patients in the low-risk category can proceed directly to surgery.

In the situation described in Figure 4.2, the patient has a mid-upper rectal tumour which has extended <1mm beyond the bowel wall and is not encroaching on the surgical margin (3mm). The risk of local recurrence is low and the patient should be considered for early surgery.

Taylor FG et al. One millimetre is the safe cutoff for magnetic resonance imaging prediction of surgical margin status in rectal cancer. *British Journal of Surgery* 2011; 98(6):872–9.

Colorectal cancer: The diagnosis and management of colorectal cancer. NICE guideline CG131. December 2014. <http://www.guidance.nice.org.uk/cg131>.

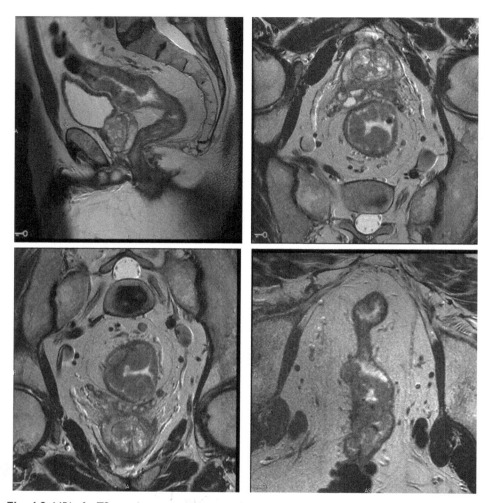

Fig. 4.2 MRI of a T3 rectal cancer which is not threatening the circumferential margin.

Reproduced from Colorectal assessment. In MacKay GJ, Dorrance HR, Molloy RG, and O'Dwyer PJ, *Colorectal Surgery*, 2010, figure 2.3, with permission from Oxford University Press.

CT–PET for all occult metastatic disease

3. d) CT PET

A CT–PET scan should be considered for patients with suspicion of occult metastatic disease as this may render them inappropriate for surgical resection or alter patient management. In the patient discussed, the enlarged external iliac node is outside the plane of a standard total mesorectal excision and so a CT–PET may alter management. CT–PET should also be considered in patients with isolated lung or liver metastases prior to resection, ablation, or cytoreductive chemotherapy.

Scottish Intercollegiate Guidelines Network. Diagnosis and management of colorectal cancer. SIGN Guideline No. 126. December 2011. <http://www.sign.ac.uk/assets/sign126.pdf>.

→ Non-regional nodes = CT PET. for all GI cancers.

4. d) Right hemicolectomy

Carcinoid tumours are the most common tumours of the appendix. They are diagnosed in 3–9 of every 1000 appendicectomy specimens, often as an incidental finding. Size and location of the tumour are the best predictors of prognosis. Appendicectomy is usually sufficient for tumours <1cm with no other adverse features. Current guidelines recommend more extensive resection for tumours >2cm, tumours at the base of the appendix, positive resection margins, deep invasion of the mesoappendix (>3mm), lymphovascular invasion, or a high mitotic index. Right hemicolectomy should be considered for these patients. Management of tumours sized 1–2cm remains controversial.

Pape U-F et al. ENETS consensus guidelines for the management of patients with neuroendocrine neoplasms from the jejuno–ileum and the appendix including goblet cell carcinomas. *Neuroendocrinology* 2012; 95:135–56.

5. d) Vacuum-assisted closure device therapy

This is a difficult situation for both the surgeon and patient and preservation of a pouch with good functional result may be challenging. Over the last decade, there have been many reports of successful treatment of colorectal, coloanal, or pouch-anal anastomotic leakage with the use of endoluminal vacuum-assisted closure devices. The aim of such treatment is to promote healing enough that luminal integrity can be restored and to prevent the development of chronic presacral collections or sinuses. These devices work by providing continuous transanal drainage via a sponge plug placed within the cavity and attached to a suction unit. This acts to promote granulation and to reduce the size of the defect. Treatment is usually required for 4–6 weeks with a successful closure rate of between 50–60%. In the scenario presented this is likely to give the optimal chance of saving the anastomosis with the lowest chance of morbidity for the patient.

Keskin M et al. Effectiveness of endoluminal vacuum-assisted closure therapy (Endosponge) for the treatment of pelvic anastomotic leakage after colorectal surgery. *Surgical Laparoscopy, Endoscopy & Percutaneous Techniques Journal* 2015; 25(6):505–8.

6. b) Two-yearly colonoscopy from age 25 and 2-yearly upper GI endoscopy from age 50

Hereditary non-polyposis colon cancer (Lynch syndrome) is an autosomal dominant condition associated with an elevated risk of cancer. The most common genetic mutation affects DNA mismatch repair genes conferring a lifetime risk of colorectal cancer of 60–80%. Tumours are frequently multiple, often present earlier, with a large proportion found in the proximal colon.

Regular colonoscopy has been shown to reduce the risk of colorectal cancer in patients with HNPCC by 80%. Colonoscopy is recommended from age 25, or 5 years before the youngest affected relative, depending on which comes first. This should be performed at 18–24 monthly intervals until age 75. Extra-colonic tumours associated with HNPCC include endometrial, gastric, ovarian, and renal. Screening for extra-colonic tumours includes: upper GI endoscopy biannually from age 50; annual trans-vaginal ultrasound, endometrial sampling and CA125; and annual renal tract ultrasound.

Cairns S et al. Guidelines for colorectal cancer screening and surveillance in moderate and high risk groups. *Gut* 2010; 59:666–90.

7. b) TP53

Li–Fraumeni syndrome is a rare autosomal dominant syndrome due to germline mutations in the *TP53* tumour suppressor gene. The syndrome is characterized by the early onset of multiple tumour types at different sites. 50% of carriers will develop malignancy by the age of 30 years. The commonest associated malignancies are breast, sarcoma, brain, and adrenal tumours. Many other tumour types are reported in Li–Fraumeni families including gastrointestinal cancers.

Germline mutations in the *RET* proto-oncogene are associated with hereditary cancer syndrome, Multiple endocrine neoplasia (MEN) 2A and 2B. MEN2 is an autosomal dominant cancer syndrome characterized by medullary thyroid carcinoma, phaeochromocytoma, and primary hyperparathyroidism. An inherited inactivating mutation of the APC tumour suppressor gene is associated with familial adenomatous polyposis (FAP). FAP is an autosomal dominant condition affecting 1 in 10,000 and accounting for <1% of all colorectal cancers. Somatic mutations of the KRAS proto-oncogene occur in many solid malignancies including lung, breast, pancreatic, and colorectal carcinomas. Germline mutations in KRAS are associated with Noonan syndrome (cardiac abnormalities, short stature, characteristic facies), which is not in itself a hereditary cancer syndrome. *MLH1* is a mismatch repair gene with mutations occurring in 30% of HNPCC families, predisposing to colorectal and endometrial cancer.

Malkin D. Li–Fraumeni syndrome. *Genes Cancer* 2011; 2(4):475–84.

8. e) Total proctocolectomy and end ileostomy

Patients with ulcerative colitis and Crohn's colitis face an increased lifetime risk of developing colorectal cancer. Factors associated with increased risk include long duration of colitis, extensive colonic involvement, primary sclerosing cholangitis, and a family history of colorectal cancer. Some studies also suggest that early age at disease onset and uncontrolled or severe disease with active inflammation may be independent risk factors for the development of colorectal cancer.

Patients with low- or high-grade dysplasia found in a discrete adenoma-like polyp, but nowhere else, can be safely managed with polypectomy and accelerated surveillance. However, dysplasia of any grade found in an endoscopically non-resectable polyp and high-grade dysplasia found in flat mucosa are both strong indications for proctocolectomy.

Because of the multifocal nature of dysplasia in Crohn's colitis, total proctocolectomy and end ileostomy are recommended in good-risk patients. In specific circumstances, such as poor-risk patients, especially in the setting of low-grade dysplasia, close endoscopic surveillance or alternatively segmental or subtotal colectomy and close post-operative endoscopic surveillance may be considered.

Kiran RP et al. Dysplasia associated with Crohn's colitis: segmental colectomy or more extended resection. *Annals of Surgery* 2012; 256(2):221–6.

9. e) Reassurance and standard follow-up

Unfortunately, parastomal hernias are seen following all forms of stoma, but patients with a colostomy are most at risk. Predisposing factors include a large aperture, age >70 years, a BMI of >25 kg/m^2, diabetes, and chronic elevation of intra-abdominal pressure.

Many patients with a parastomal hernia are asymptomatic and given the less than perfect results of surgery, are best observed. Patients may develop symptoms ranging from discomfort to significant abdominal pain. The appearance of the untidy bulge can also be distressing to patients. More serious complications include the development of obstruction and strangulation of bowel within the parastomal hernia, difficulty in applying a stoma appliance, and skin damage through leakage of faeces. Surgical repair is difficult and a number of techniques have now been shown to be associated with a very high recurrence rate. In particular, local suture repair is associated with a recurrence rate of up to 70%. Transposition or relocation of the stoma is associated with a recurrence rate of at least 30%. In addition, there is also risk of an incisional hernia at the old stoma site. A mesh repair is considered to be the gold standard and should be considered in symptomatic patients. A biologic mesh is usually only indicated if there is contamination of the wound, given its high cost.

Systematic reviews have shown no significant difference in outcome between any of the various techniques described for a mesh repair of a parastomal hernia. However, there are advantages to a laparoscopic repair. There is low-grade evidence to suggest that a laparoscopic Sugarbaker technique may be the procedure of choice. Prevention by inserting a mesh at the time of fashioning of the primary stoma perhaps offers the best long-term solution to this problem.

Hansson BME. Parastomal hernia: treatment and prevention; where do we go from here? *Colorectal Disease* 2013; 15:1467–70.

10. b) The prevalence of Crohn's disease is 150 per 100,000 in the United Kingdom

Crohn's disease (CD) and ulcerative colitis (UC), collectively referred to as inflammatory bowel disease (IBD), are characterized by chronic inflammation of the gastrointestinal tract. There is a multifactorial aetiology. However, genetics/family history and environmental factors appear to play a role in their development.

Together these long-term conditions are estimated to affect about 240,000 people in the United Kingdom, approximately 400 patients per 100,000 population. The point prevalence of Crohn's disease is around 150 per 100,000 population with an annual incidence around 8–10 per 100,000.

There has been a fourfold increase in the incidence of Crohn's disease in the Western world over the last 30 years, whereas the incidence of ulcerative colitis appears to be stable.

The precise incidence of toxic megacolon is unknown. The incidence in ulcerative colitis and Crohn's disease was approximately 1–5% three decades ago but has gradually decreased because of earlier recognition and intensive management of severe colitis. There does not appear to be a significant difference in the risk of developing toxic megacolon in Crohn's versus ulcerative colitis.

Steed H et al. Crohn's disease incidence in NHS Tayside. *Scottish Medical Journal* 2010; 55(3):22–5.

Grieco MB et al. Toxic megacolon complicating Crohn's colitis. *Annals of Surgery* 1980; 191:75.

Rubin GP et al. Inflammatory bowel disease: epidemiology and management in an English general practice population. *Alimentary Pharmacology & Therapeutics* 2000; 14(12):1553–9.

Inflammatory bowel disease. In: MacKay GJ et al. (eds). *Colorectal Surgery*. Oxford: Oxford University Press, 2010, pp. 109–94.

11. b) Stool for culture and sensitivity and *C. difficile* toxin

The short history is suggestive of infection. Possible causes include *C. difficile* colitis, *Campylobacter*, and *Salmonella* infection. Although flexible sigmoidoscopy with enema prep may need to be considered in this patient, the first and easiest assessment is to obtain a stool sample for culture and sensitivity and *C. difficile* toxin.

Clostridium difficile infection can be associated with a severe illness. Moderately severe *C. difficile* infection is associated with non-bloody diarrhoea, abdominal discomfort/tenderness, nausea with occasional vomiting, dehydration, WCC > 15,000 × 10^9/L, and evidence of acute kidney injury.

Severe *C. difficile* infection should be recorded in the presence of severe or bloody diarrhoea, a pseudomembranous colitis, severe abdominal pain, vomiting, ileitis, temperature >38.9°C, WCC >20,000 × 10^9/L, hypoalbuminaemia, and acute kidney injury.

Leffler DA and Lamont T. *Clostridium difficile* infection. *New England Journal of Medicine* 2015; 372:1539–48.

12. c) Surgical resection with clear margins is associated with a 5-year survival of >90%

Gastrointestinal stromal tumours (GIST) are the most common mesenchymal tumour of the intestinal tract. The tumours are located typically in the submucosa of the stomach and the small and large intestines although they can arise in the oesophagus, greater omentum, and mesenteric adipose tissue. It was initially thought that many of these tumours were leiomyomas and leiomyosarcomas but electron microscope studies show no smooth muscle differentiation.

The tumours arise from the interstitial cells of Cajal and the genetic basis of GIST growth is a mutation of the KIT and PDGFRA gene, which leads to constitutional activation of receptor tyrosine kinase. The KIT and PDGFRA oncoprotein therefore serves as a crucial diagnostic and therapeutic target. *highly recurrent*

Surgery offers the only curative option and forms the mainstay of initial management in suitable patients. At best the 5-year survival with clear surgical resection margins is 40–50% and <10% when the margins are involved. GISTs do not metastasize to lymph nodes and the goal of treatment is to achieve macroscopic clearance of tumour without perforation. Risk factors for recurrence include surgical factors such as incomplete resection, intraperitoneal rupture or bleeding, and tumour-associated factors such as tumour size, mitotic index, or location.

Adjuvant therapy with tyrosine kinase inhibitors (imatinib, sold under the trade name of Glivec®) is recommended for high-risk patients after complete resection, or for those with unresectable and advanced GISTs.

Beham AW et al. Gastrointestinal stromal tumours. *International Journal of Colorectal Disease* 2012; 27(6):689–700.

13. d) Emergency subtotal colectomy and end ileostomy

There are a number of factors to be considered when assessing this gentleman. He has already been on an immunomodulator for a number of years and has now failed to respond to five days of intravenous steroids. The stool frequency is high, CRP is elevated, and his albumin is low. A number of indexes have been developed to try and predict the risk of steroid failure in acute colitis. Truelove and Witt's criteria for acute exacerbations in ulcerative colitis measure frequency of stools, blood in the stool, temperature, heart rate, haemoglobin, and ESR (erythrocyte sedimentation rate). The Travis risk index estimates the risk of steroid failure and the requirement for colectomy. It is performed between day 3 and day 5. A stool frequency of >8 provides an 85% positive predictive value for requiring colectomy. The World Health Organization index for predicting risk of steroid failure is also performed between days 3 and 5. Mean stool frequency, the presence or absence of colonic dilatation, or the presence of hypoalbuminaemia are measured.

This gentleman has a high predicted risk of steroid failure and requirement for colectomy. This occurs against a background of immunosuppression with azathioprine and a well-established diagnosis of colitis over the preceding three-year history. Prior exposure to thiopurines appears to limit the efficacy of IV cyclosporine, although this does not seem to affect the outcome of patients treated with infliximab. However, factors which may adversely affect outcome with infliximab include a baseline CRP >20 mg/L, concomitant steroid use, and disease duration >3 years.

Most patients are keen to avoid a stoma but it must be explained to the patient that a stoma can be life-saving in this circumstance. The correct option here is emergency subtotal colectomy and end ileostomy. Consideration can be given to a completion proctectomy and ileal pouch once the patient has recovered from his surgery. Usually this will be more than six months after the index colectomy. Even if the patient did not want to consider an ileal pouch, a subtotal colectomy and end ileostomy (leaving the rectum in place) is the correct option in the emergency setting.

Kedia S et al. Management of acute severe ulcerative colitis. *World Journal of Gastrointestinal Pathophysiology* 2014; 5(4):579–88.

14. e) Percutaneous drainage, TPN, IV antibiotics, and a contrast small bowel study to define the site of the fistula

Type 2 intestinal failure describes the condition of intestinal failure that occurs in association with septic, metabolic, and complex nutritional complications. Typically, this may occur following a laparotomy. It is usually associated with intra-abdominal sepsis. Given the relatively late presentation in this case, the patient has localized the source of sepsis (by forming an abscess) which then discharged through the abdominal wall, causing a high-volume fistula.

A multidisciplinary approach is important. The management plan should use an algorithm including management of sepsis in the first instance, followed by correction of nutritional deficiencies which frequently requires parenteral nutrition. More specialized imaging is then performed in order to define the anatomy of the fistula before consideration can be given to developing a surgical plan for repair (SNAP: i.e. attention to Sepsis, Nutrition, Anatomy, and then a Plan for surgery).

The development of an intra-abdominal abscess and fistula within a few weeks of a surgical resection in a patient with Crohn's disease should be treated as a surgical complication. Biologic therapy is unlikely to help and may predispose to further sepsis.

Calvert CR and Lal S. Approaches to intestinal failure in Crohn's disease. *The Proceedings of the Nutrition Society* 2011; 70(3):336–41.

15. e) The Gardasil HPV vaccine protects against HPV types that are associated with both a high risk of cancer and against anal warts

Human papilloma virus (HPV) types 6 and 11 cause genital warts, while types 16 and 18 cause cervical cancer. In 99% of cases, cervical cancer occurs as a result of a history of infection with high-risk types of HPV (16 and 18). Around 75% of unaffected partners of patients with warts develop them within 8 months. The body clears approximately 90% of HPV infections within 2 years of infection.

The Gardasil vaccine (produced by Merck & Co.) protects against HPV types 6, 11, 16, and 18. The vaccine is preventive and must be given before exposure to the virus in order to be effective. Ideally, it should be administered before individuals become sexual active. The vaccine is approved in the United States for use in both males and females as early as nine years of age.

In the United Kingdom, Gardasil replaced Cervarix in September 2012. Cervarix had been used routinely in young females from its introduction in 2008 but was only effective against the high-risk HPV types 16 and 18, neither of which typically causes warts. Gardasil vaccine will also therefore protect against ano–genital warts.

Department of Health. 'Your guide to the HPV vaccination from September 2012'. January 2013. <https://www.gov.uk/government/publications/your-guide-to-the-hpv-vaccination-from-september-2012>.

16. b) MRI of the perineum

10–40% of patients who present with a perianal abscess will have persistent discharge from the wound and ultimately go on to develop a fistula-in-ano. Given the preceding history and clinical findings it is likely that this young lady has developed a fistula. The sphincter mechanism in females is less well developed and the anal canal is shorter compared to males. As a consequence, females have less sphincter reserve when considering laying open of a fistula-in-ano. In addition, the anal sphincter complex is somewhat thinner anteriorly compared to posteriorly.

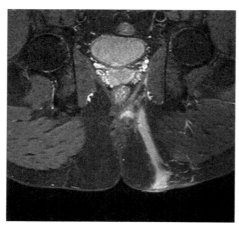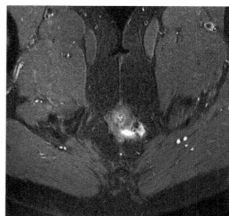

Fig. 4.3 MR of fistula-in-ano

MRI can be helpful in delineating the site and number of tracks, especially with a complex fistula. Although some surgeons might not routinely perform an MRI in all patients presenting with a new simple fistula-in-ano, one should also take into account that females of child-bearing age are at risk of sustaining an additional sphincter injury during parturition. It is therefore better to err on the side of caution in terms of management of this fistula. In such circumstances, an MRI should be performed before proceeding to EUA (examination under anaesthetic; see Figure 4.3). The MRI will assess the track and also enable a reasoned judgment on the depth of involvement of the sphincter. Consideration can then be given at EUA to laying open a subcutaneous or low intersphincteric fistula. However, given her age and the site of the fistula, it is most likely that a newly identified fistula will be treated with a loose Seton drain in the first instance with a view to performing definitive surgery at a later stage.

Fistulograms and sinograms are no longer used as a routine in patients with a suspected fistula-in-ano. Anorectal manometry and endorectal ultrasound are also not used routinely in first-line management although these investigations may have a role in patients with complex fistulas or in those who have had a previous sphincterotomy or other invasive anorectal procedures.

Whiteford MH. Perianal abscess/fistula disease. *Clinics in Colon and Rectal Surgery* 2007; 20(2):102–9.

17. d) Rectal prolapse in children may be associated with cystic fibrosis

Rectal prolapse, internal intussusception, and solitary rectal ulcer syndrome comprise a spectrum of anatomical abnormalities involving descent of full- or partial-thickness rectal wall associated with pelvic floor dysfunction. Overall, rectal prolapse affects relatively few people (2.5 cases/100,000 people). This condition affects mostly adults, and women over 50 years of age are 6 times as likely as men to develop rectal prolapse. Most women with rectal prolapse are in their sixth decade, while the few men who develop prolapse are much younger, averaging 40 years of age or less. At least half of all adults who present with rectal prolapse also report faecal incontinence. 25–50% of patients will report constipation.

Risk factors in children include cystic fibrosis (can affect up to 20% of children with cystic fibrosis). Other risk factors in children include chronic constipation, diarrhoea, coughing, malnutrition, and

Hirschsprung's disease. Conservative treatment is usually successful in children aged less than four years.

Varma M et al, Practice parameters for the management of rectal prolapse. *Diseases of the Colon & Rectum* 2011; 54:1339–46.

18. b) Solitary rectal ulcer syndrome (SRUS)   *Fibromuscular obliteration of lamina propria*

Solitary rectal ulcer syndrome (SRUS) is also referred to as mucosal prolapse solitary rectal ulcer syndrome (MPSRUS). The term is misleading as lesions may not be solitary or ulcerated or even confined to the rectum. The main presentation is rectal bleeding in association with mucus discharge, tenesmus, straining, and rectal pain. There is often a history of self-digitation.

Endoscopy may show single or multiple ulcers or simply an area of erythematous mucosa. Macroscopically, the most florid changes are usually seen anteriorly in the distal rectum from 5–10cm from the anal verge. The mucosa may be heaped up and the appearances at endoscopy can be suggestive of a tumour. It can also be misdiagnosed as proctitis or secondary to rectal infection

Histologically, the condition may mimic proctitis and the reactive atypia and smooth muscle fibre extensions into the crypts may be mistaken for true dysplasia. Fibromuscular obliteration of the lamina propria is a pathognomonic finding. In addition, the hypertrophic muscularis mucosa demonstrates extension of muscle fibres upwards between the crypts.

Patient education and behaviour modification are important in managing early-stage SRUS. Behaviour modification techniques are important to reinforce the need to avoid repeated attempts to defaecate and self-digitation. Biofeedback can also be helpful. Local excision or banding of the inflamed areas are unlikely to help and have a very high recurrence rate. Topical treatments with anti-inflammatory drugs have been tried but have not been found to be consistently helpful. If there is evidence of full thickness rectal prolapse or circumferential internal intussusception consideration can be given to a rectopexy. Rarely an anterior resection or a defunctioning stoma is considered in severe cases.   *Lamina propria contains vessels + lymph nodes*

Zhu Q et al. Solitary rectal ulcer syndrome: Clinical features, pathophysiology, diagnosis and treatment strategies. *World Journal of Gastroenterology* 2014; 20(3):738–44.   *very significant for breech love — Tr disease*

19. c) Is degraded by bacteria in the gut

Calprotectin is relatively stable in faeces for up to one week at room temperature as the protein is resistant to bacterial degradation within the gut. This makes it eminently suitable as a marker for gastrointestinal inflammation. Higher levels tend to be found in inflammation in the colon compared to the small intestine.

Faecal calprotectin is evenly distributed throughout the faeces. Many studies have shown significant differences in faecal calprotectin concentrations between healthy volunteers and patients with inflammatory bowel disease. The cut-off concentration of faecal calprotectin considered significant is 50µg/g. Faecal calprotectin is also used as a screening tool to predict abnormal small bowel radiology in patients with abdominal pain or diarrhoea who present to a gastroenterology clinic.

An elevated faecal calprotectin, however, is not specific for inflammatory bowel disease and elevated concentrations are found in patients with colorectal cancer and, to a lesser extent, those with adenomatous polyps. Other factors associated with an elevated faecal calprotectin are increasing age, obesity, the use of non-steroidal anti-inflammatory drugs, and physical inactivity.

Sutherland AD et al. Review of fecal biomarkers in inflammatory bowel disease. *Diseases of the Colon & Rectum* 2008; 51:1283–91.

20. e) Pouchoscopy/biopsy and stool for culture and sensitivity

Although the history is very suggestive of pouchitis it is important to remember that up to 30% of cases of pouchitis are secondary to other factors including the use of non-steroidal anti-inflammatory drugs, C. difficile infection, Candida albicans, CMV infection, ischaemia, radiation injury, chemotherapy, and collagen deposition. *Always exclude c-diff + cmv*

In this scenario the patient has a liver transplant and will therefore be immunosuppressed. Infection with either C. difficile or CMV is a distinct possibility and needs to be excluded.

Although metronidazole has been the most commonly used antibiotics to treat acute pouchitis, up to 10% of patients may have pouchitis refractory to metronidazole. Ciprofloxacin alone or in combination with metronidazole is often successful in this setting. Ciprofloxacin also appears to be better than metronidazole at reducing the overall pouch disease activity index and is generally associated with fewer side effects. In experimental models, ciprofloxacin appears to have an anti-inflammatory effect rather than just an antibacterial effect, which may favour its use in inflammatory bowel disease patients.

In the longer term, probiotics may prevent the development of pouchitis and reduce relapse rates. VSL#3 has been proven to maintain remission following antibacterial treatment of acute pouchitis. It may also reduce the risk of developing pouchitis, if given for the first year following fashioning of an ileal pouch. More recently, therapies such as anti-TNF based treatments have also been shown to be effective, albeit in small patient populations.

Coffey JC et al. Pouchitis: an evolving clinical enigma—a review. *Diseases of the Colon & Rectum* 2009; 52:140–53.

21. e) Ileocolic resection with end ileostomy

Intra-abdominal septic complications, such as an anastomotic leak, fistula, or intra-abdominal abscess formation, develop in 10–20% of patients undergoing surgery for Crohn's disease. Risk factors include a low albumin level, preoperative use of steroids, and the presence of an abscess or fistula at the time of laparotomy. Yamamoto showed that there was a 50% risk of septic complications if all 4 risk factors were present, with a 29% risk of septic complications when 3 risk factors were present, and around a 15% risk of complications if 1 or 2 risk factors were present. There was a 5% risk of septic complications in patients who had none of these risk factors. Factors that did not affect the incidence of septic complications included age, duration of symptoms, number of previous bowel resections, site of disease, type of operation (resection, strictureplasty, or bypass), covering stoma and number, site or method of anastomosis.

A more recent meta-analysis of observational studies by Huang and colleagues reported that risks factors for post-operative intra-peritoneal septic complications in Crohn's disease included the preoperative use of steroids, a preoperative abscess, previous surgical history, and low albumin levels. In this meta-analysis, previous surgical history was also found to be a risk factor for intra-abdominal septic complications. There was no association between the anastomotic method or the use of immunomodulators and the risk of septic complications.

It is unclear if biologic therapy is associated with an increased risk of septic complications. Huang's paper suggested that biologic therapy was not clearly associated with an increase in septic complications whereas a review by Ahmed and colleagues in 2014 reported a significant association between use of anti-TNF drugs and the risk of post-operative wound infection and septic shock. This paper also failed to show an association between the use of thiopurines or combined immunomodulatory drugs and post-operative complications.

agree with tripple abx

In the current scenario, the patient's risk factors for post-operative intraperitoneal septic complications included the preoperative use of steroids, a low albumin, and the presence of an abscess. She has at least a 30% chance of an anastomotic leak/septic complication. Performing an anastomosis in this circumstance should be viewed as being higher risk and would not be the procedure of choice. Resection of the diseased segment and fashioning an end ileostomy, with a view to performing an ileocolic anastomosis at some point in the future, would be the procedure of choice.

Huang W et al. Risk factors for postoperative intra-abdominal septic complications after surgery in Crohn's disease: A meta-analysis of observational studies. *Journal of Crohn's and Colitis* 2015; 9(3):293–301.

Yamamoto T et al. Risk factors for intra-abdominal sepsis after surgery in Crohn's disease. *Diseases of the Colon & Rectum* 2000; 43(8):1141–5.

Ahmed Ali U et al. Impact of preoperative immunosuppressive agents on postoperative outcomes in Crohn's disease. *Diseases of the Colon & Rectum* 2014; 57(5):663–74.

22. b) All patients with inflammatory bowel disease should have a screening colonoscopy ten years after the onset of colonic symptoms

Patients with long-standing inflammatory bowel disease are at increased risk of colorectal cancer. Data from the St Mark's surveillance program suggests the risk is 7.7% at 20 years and 15.8% at 30 years, with an increasing cancer risk associated with the length of disease. The ACPGBI guidelines suggests classification of patients into low-, moderate-, and high-risk groups. Here is a summary of the guidelines:

Low risk: Five-yearly colonoscopy is recommended for

- Extensive colitis with no endoscopic/histological active inflammation on the previous colonoscopy
- Left-sided colitis (any grade of inflammation) or Crohn's colitis affecting <50% of the surface area of the colon

Intermediate risk: Three-yearly colonoscopy is recommended for:

- Extensive colitis with mild endoscopic/histological active inflammation on the previous surveillance colonoscopy
- Post-inflammatory polyps ✳
- Family history of colorectal cancer in a first-degree relative aged 50 years or over

Higher risk: Yearly colonoscopy is recommended for:

- Extensive colitis with moderate or severe endoscopic/histological active inflammation on the previous surveillance colonoscopy
- Stricture within past five years
- Confirmed dysplasia within past five years in a patient who declines surgery
- Primary sclerosing cholangitis/post-orthotopic liver transplant for primary sclerosing cholangitis
- Family history of colorectal cancer in a first-degree relative aged <50 years

Extensive colitis is defined as ulcerative colitis extending proximal to the splenic flexure or Crohn's colitis affecting at least 50% of the surface area of the colon. The protocol for colonoscopy is either chromoendoscopy with biopsy of targeted areas, or 2–4 biopsies taken every 10cm throughout the colon. Minimum = 36 biopsies

Guidelines for colorectal cancer screening and surveillance in moderate and high risk groups (update from 2002), *Gut* 2010; 59:666–90. doi:10.1136/gut.2009.179804.

Rutter MD et al. Thirty-year analysis of a colonoscopic surveillance program for neoplasia in ulcerative colitis. *Gastroenterology* 2006; 130(4):1030–8.

Eaden JA et al. The risk of colorectal cancer in ulcerative colitis: A meta-analysis. *Gut* 2001; 48:526–35.

23. a) Primary sclerosing cholangitis

Several risk factors for the development of colorectal cancer in inflammatory bowel disease have been identified. These include:

- Duration and extent of disease
- Primary sclerosing cholangitis — *high risk surveillance*.
- Family history of sporadic colorectal cancer — *medium → high risk surveillance*.
- Young age at diagnosis of colitis

Patients with a first-degree relative with colorectal cancer have a twofold increase in their risk. Those with a first-degree relative diagnosed with colorectal cancer before 50 years of age have a ninefold increased risk.   *>50 = x2 risk <50 = x9 risk*

Those with a prolonged period of inflammation are also at increased risk of development of colorectal cancer. Therefore, if active inflammation is seen at colonoscopy medical therapy should be increased and surveillance intervals should be tightened.

Ekbom A et al. Ulcerative colitis and colorectal cancer. A population-based study. *New England Journal of Medicine* 1990; 323:1228–33.

Askling J et al. Family history as a risk factor for colorectal cancer in inflammatory bowel disease. *Gastroenterology* 2001; 120:1356–62.

Rutter MD et al. Cancer surveillance in longstanding ulcerative colitis: endoscopic appearances help predict cancer risk. *Gut* 2004; 53:1813–16.

24. b) Total colonic surveillance should commence at age 25 and occur every 2 years until age 75

Total colonic surveillance (at least biennial) should commence at age 25 years and be carried out at 2-yearly intervals until age 75. It has been shown that even at this interval there is a risk of developing interval cancers. Surveillance has been shown to increase life expectancy in those with Lynch syndrome by seven years.   *↓ Cancer by 80%.*

Vasen HF et al. Interval cancers in hereditary non-polyposis colorectal cancer (Lynch syndrome). *Lancet* 1995; 345:1183.

Guidelines for colorectal cancer screening and surveillance in moderate and high-risk groups (update from 2002). *Gut* 2010; 59:666–90. doi:10.1136/gut.2009.179804.

25. e) Inactivating mutations in *STK11* gene are identifiable in >90% cases

Peutz–Jeghers syndrome is an autosomal dominant condition defined by hamartomatous polyps of the small intestine, colon, and rectum, in conjunction with mucocutaneous pigmentation. Those affected are at risk of developing gastro-oesophageal, small bowel, pancreatic, and colorectal cancers with an overall risk of 85–90% by the age of 70. In females there is a 50% lifetime risk of breast cancer, therefore all female patients should undergo active breast screening.

In 20–63% of cases, inactivating mutations can be identified in the gene <u>STK11</u>. There have also been genetic mutations identified on chromosome 19q1

Large bowel surveillance is recommended 2-yearly from age 25 years. Upper gastrointestinal surveillance is recommended 2-yearly from age 25 years. It is also recommended that patient undergo intermittent screening for small bowel carcinomas. This is usually performed by the use of small bowel MRI to avoid repeated high-dose radiation exposure in young patients.

Guidelines for colorectal cancer screening and surveillance in moderate and high-risk groups (update from 2002). *Gut* 2010; 59:666–90.

26. a) CK7+ve, CK20–ve

It is important to differentiate anal cancer from low rectal cancer as the management strategy differs significantly. The primary treatment for anal cancer is usually radiotherapy in combination with chemotherapy. Tumours involving the anorectal junction should be classified as rectal cancers if the centre is more than 2cm proximal to the dentate line and as anal cancers if the centre is 2cm or less from the dentate line.

Those tumours which arise in the perianal skin at the anal margin are biologically similar to other skin tumours and are staged according to the classification for cancers of the skin. Primary tumours of the anal margin constitute 15–20% of anal squamous cell carcinoma. They have high cure rates with wide local excision alone. This is often the primary treatment for tumours of the anal margin which are less than 3cm, well-differentiated, and superficial.

Immunohistochemistry can be useful in differentiating colorectal from anal adenocarcinoma in those tumours high in the anal canal. Anal lesions tend to be CK7+ve/CK20–ve on immunoprofile, whilst colorectal adenocarcinomas are usually CK7–ve/CK20+ve.

It also important to consider rectal invasion from tumours arising in the prostate. These tend to stain CK7–ve and CK20–ve.

Hobbs CM et al. Anal gland carcinoma. *Cancer* 2001; 15:2045–9.

ACPGBI Position Statement for Management of Anal Cancer. *Colorectal Disease* 2011; 13(Suppl 1):1–52.

27. c) Histological subtype

In anal squamous carcinoma the histological subtype is thought to have minimal relevance to the prognosis. However, tumours with prominent basaloid features and small tumour cell size have been linked to 'high-risk' human papilloma virus infection. The following independent factors have been identified as predictive of outcome in anal squamous carcinoma:

- Sex (females appear to have better prognosis)
- Tumour stage
- Nodal involvement
- Response to radio- or chemoradiotherapy

ACPGBI Position Statement for Management of Anal Cancer. *Colorectal Disease* 2011; 13(Suppl 1):1–52.

Das P et al. Prognostic factors for squamous cell cancer of the anal canal. *Gastrointestinal Cancer Research* 2008; 2(1):10–14.

28. c) Long operating time

A number of studies have looked at risk factors after both open and laparoscopic rectal cancer surgery. The following have been identified as risk factors for anastomotic leak:

- Obesity
- Male versus female patients — *difficult, male, pelvis.*
- Post-radiotherapy patients
- Long operating time
- Not using a pelvic drain — *↑ risk of leak!! - always leave a drain.*
- Not using a defunctioning stoma
- Multiple firings of a linear stapler across the rectal stump
- Lower one-third anastomosis versus mid and upper rectal anastomoses — *closer to anal verge the risk ↑.*

Other factors (e.g. smoking and heavy use of alcohol) have also been shown in isolated studies to have a negative impact on anastomotic healing. A number of studies have assessed the impact of NSAID drugs, although most studies have concentrated on post-operative administration (for pain relief) rather than preoperative use of this class of drugs. In some studies, the post-operative use of NSAIDs has been shown to increase the risk of anastomotic leak, although this seems to relate particularly to Diclofenac. The data come mainly from retrospective population-based studies. In one recent prospective audit of 1500 patients NSAIDs had no effect on anastomotic leak and were actually associated with reduced complications.

Sorenson LT et al. Smoking and alcohol abuse are major risk factors for anastomotic leakage in colorectal surgery. *British Journal of Surgery* 1999; 86:927–31.

Pommergaard HC et al. Preoperative risk factors for anastomotic leakage after resection for colorectal cancer: a systematic review and meta-analysis. *Colorectal Disease* 2014; 16(9):662–71.

Rullier E et al. Risk factors for anastomotic leakage after resection of rectal cancer. *British Journal of Surgery* 1998; 85:355–8.

Qu H et al. Clinical risk factors for anastomotic leakage after laparoscopic anterior resection for rectal cancer: a systematic review and meta-analysis. *Surgical Endoscopy* 2015; 29(12):3608–17.

STARSurg Collaborative. Impact of postoperative non-steroidal anti-inflammatory drugs on adverse events after gastrointestinal surgery. *British Journal of Surgery* 2014; 101(11):1413–23.

29. b) Often affects the proximal colon

Lynch syndrome (HNPCC or hereditary non-polyposis colorectal cancer) is an autosomal dominant genetic condition that has a high risk of colon cancer and other cancers including endometrial cancer ovary, gastric, small intestine, hepatobiliary tract, upper urinary tract, brain, and skin. The increased risk for these cancers is due to inherited mutations that impair DNA mismatch repair.

Individuals with HNPCC have about an 80% lifetime risk for colon cancer. Two-thirds of these cancers occur in the proximal colon. The mean age of colorectal cancer diagnosis is 44 (for members of families that meet the Amsterdam criteria). Also, women with HNPCC have an 80% lifetime risk of endometrial cancer. The average age of diagnosis of endometrial cancer is about 46 years.

The hallmark of HNPCC is defective DNA mismatch repair, leading to microsatellite instability. This is also known as MSI-H (the H denotes 'high'). HNPCC is associated with mutations in a number of genes involved in the DNA mismatch repair pathway. The most important of these is MSH2 (60%), MLH1 (30%), MSH6 (7–10%), with others occurring less frequently.

Patients who are mutation carriers should undergo 1–2-yearly colonoscopy from age 25 until 75 years of age.

Vasen HFA et al. Revised guidelines for the clinical management of Lynch syndrome (HNPCC): recommendations by a group of European experts. *Gut* 2013; 0:1–13.

30. b) 5-FU and mitomycin C and radiotherapy

Anal cancer is an uncommon malignancy which accounts for around 4% of malignancies of the lower GI tract. The incidence of anal cancer in increasing. This is thought to be due to lifestyle changes, which have resulted in an increased risk of human papilloma virus infection (HPV). Certain lifestyle choices such as receptive anal intercourse and a high number of lifetime sexual partners can increase the risk of HPV infection, which is strongly associated with the risk of anal cancer and may be a necessary step in its carcinogenesis.

Radiation therapy alone is associated with a 5-year survival rate in excess of 70%. However, such monotherapy requires high-dose (≥60Gy) radiotherapy which is frequently associated with necrosis and fibrosis. Combination therapy with 5-FU and cisplatin, concurrent with lower-dose radiation therapy, has a 5-year survival rate in excess of 70% with low levels of acute and chronic morbidity. The optimal dose of radiation with concurrent chemotherapy to optimize local control and minimize the toxic effects appears to be in the 45–60Gy range.

The Anal Cancer Trial (ACT-1) demonstrated the superiority of chemoradiation with 5-FU and mitomycin C (MMC) over radiation alone (reduced likelihood of local failures and cancer-related mortality). In long-term follow-up, for every 100 patients treated with chemoradiation compared to radiation alone, there were 25 fewer locoregional relapses and 12.5 fewer anal cancer deaths. However, there was a 9.1% increase in non-anal cancer deaths in the first 5 years following chemoradiation.

Epidermoid anal cancer: results from the UKCCCR randomised trial of radiotherapy alone versus radiotherapy, 5-fluorouracil, and mitomycin. UKCCCR Anal Cancer Trial Working Party. UK Coordinating Committee on Cancer Research. *Lancet* 1996; 348:1049–54.

National cancer institute information on anal cancer: Health professional version: <http://www.cancer.gov/types/anal/hp/anal-treatment-pdq#section/_36>.

31. d) Most commonly involves the caecum

Primary colonic lymphoma (PCL) is a rare condition accounting for less than 1% of all colonic cancers. Non-Hodgkin's lymphoma is the most common type and of these a diffuse large B-cell lymphoma is the most common histological type. The median age at diagnosis is 55 years. They occur more commonly in males. The caecum is the most common site. Diagnosis can be difficult and endoscopy and CT scan are not always helpful and certainly imaging can be confused with other diagnoses such as tuberculosis (TB) or Crohn's disease. Endoscopy and enteroscopy may simply reveal a non-specific colitis or ulceration. Mass lesions are uncommon. Morphologically, PCL may present with a stricturing lesion, circumferential infiltration, ulceration, mucosal fold thickening, or a cavitating mass. On occasion, surgery is required for open biopsy or biopsy of associated lymphadenopathy. However, if there is significant dubiety about the diagnosis, resection should be considered rather than simple open biopsy as the differential diagnosis includes Crohn's disease, small-bowel or colonic carcinoma, and TB.

The rate of intestinal perforation with chemotherapy is >30%, which has led to suggestions that surgery should be considered for primary colonic lymphoma disease that is confined to the bowel. Following successful resection, chemotherapy can be considered. There is no role for surgery in disseminated disease. For fit patients, chemotherapy consists of a combination of CHOP (cyclophosphamide, doxorubicin, vincristine, and prednisone) combined with rituximab. Such a regimen has also been used in patients with disseminated disease and has been shown to improve survival.

Chang SC. Clinical features and management of primary colonic lymphoma. *Formosan Journal of Surgery* 2012; 45:73–7.

32. e) Comorbidity (Charlson comorbidity score of ≥3)

A number of studies have looked in detail at specific risk factors for 30-day mortality including: surgeon experience and training; the number of cases going through an individual hospital; and a range of patient-centred data. The most recent UK-based review of post-operative mortality used data extracted from the National Cancer Data Repository. This large study analysed data from more than 160,000 individuals who underwent major resection in English hospitals between 1998 and 2006. The overall mortality was 6.7% but this decreased over time and was 5.8% in 2006. Specific risk factors that were identified included the following:

- Socioeconomic deprivation: most deprived quintile (7.8%)
- Stage of disease: Dukes D tumours (9.9%)
- Operative urgency: patients undergoing emergency resection (14.9%)
- Increasing age: for those >80 years (15%)
- Comorbidity: Charlson comorbidity score of ≥3 (24.2%)

Morris EJ et al. Thirty-day postoperative mortality after colorectal cancer surgery in England. *Gut* 2011; 60(6):806–13.

33. c) Neoadjuvant 5-FU and radiotherapy (45Gys, 25 fractions)

All patients with rectal cancer should undergo a complete assessment with a CT scan of chest, abdomen, and pelvis as well as an MRI scan of the pelvis. The pathology and imaging findings should be discussed at a multidisciplinary team meeting (MDT). Patients can be grouped into having a low, moderate, or high risk of recurrence based on the result of the MRI. This patient has an enlarged node which is threatening the surgical resection margin. The tumour is also 1mm from the resection margin. This patient is therefore staged as being at high risk of local recurrence and should be considered for preoperative chemoradiation. Long-course down-staging chemoradiation should be considered to allow tumour shrinkage before surgery in patients that are borderline between moderate and high risk. Short-course preoperative radiotherapy should be considered in moderate-risk patients who have operable rectal cancer.

cT1/T2 rectal cancers with no overt node involvement should be regarded as low-risk tumours and most patients will go straight to surgery. Preoperative long-course chemoradiotherapy should be considered where tumour breaches or threatens the margin (<1 mm margin) or for low tumours which encroach the intersphincteric plane or those who have levator involvement.

The management of patients with moderate-risk tumours often leads to more difficult management decisions. Patients with cT3b tumours (direct tumour invasion into the mesorectum), those with overt node involvement or those with extramural vascular invasion fall into this so-called moderate-risk group. Long-course chemoradiotherapy or short-course radiotherapy may be considered. However, many centres no longer tend to use the short-course regimen. When considering the management options for an individual patient, the height of the tumour from the anal margin is also relevant. It is also important to remember that nodal involvement, even if close to, or threatening a surgical margin is perhaps not as important a risk factor for recurrence compared to the extent of direct tumour invasion into the mesorectum and the presence of absence of overt vascular invasion.

Neoadjuvant treatment. In: MacKay GJ et al. (eds). *Colorectal Surgery.* Oxford: Oxford University Press, 2010:328–9.

NICE guidelines on the management of colorectal cancer. <https://www.nice.org.uk/guidance/cg131/chapter/1-Recommendations#management-of-local-disease>.

34. a) **KRAS wild-type patients**

Cetuximab is a chimeric monoclonal antibody that is active against epidermal growth factor receptor (EGFR). It is used in the treatment of metastatic rectal cancer, metastatic non-small cell lung cancer, and head and neck cancer. The EGFR signals through the mitogen-activated protein kinase (MAPK) pathway. The KRAS protein is part of this pathway. Cetuximab is designed to block the EGFR signal pathway. However, the KRAS protein, which is downstream of EGFR, may be either normal/'wild-type' or mutated. If mutated, KRAS signalling is increased and uncoupled from EGFR control. Blocking EGFR with cetuximab is not helpful in this circumstance and may even be harmful. Cetuximab is therefore only indicated for EGFR-expressing, KRAS wild-type metastatic rectal cancer, either in combination with chemotherapy or as a single agent in patients who have failed oxaliplatin- or irinotecan-based therapy. A diagnostic immunohistochemistry test is performed on tumour material to assess for EGFR expression. Approximately 75% of patients with metastatic colorectal cancer have an EGFR-expressing tumour and are therefore considered eligible for treatment with cetuximab.

In the United Kingdom, cetuximab is indicated for patients with metastatic colorectal cancer where liver metastases cannot be removed surgically before treatment; the patient would be fit enough for liver resection if it becomes possible following cetuximab; and the primary tumour is either removed or is deemed surgically resectable. Cetuximab is also now used first-line in combination with FOLFOX or FOLFIRI for patients with extensive metastatic disease.

The most correct answer to this question is that cetuximab is most appropriate for KRAS wild-type patients. While cetuximab is used in certain patients with liver metastases it is not suitable in all situations. This type of question is common in the examination where the candidate has to judge which is the most correct answer. See Figure 4.4.

Hoyle M et al. The clinical effectiveness and cost-effectiveness of cetuximab (mono- or combination chemotherapy), bevacizumab (combination with non-oxaliplatin chemotherapy) and panitumumab (monotherapy) for the treatment of metastatic colorectal cancer after first-line chemotherapy. *NIHR Health Technology Assessment* 2013; 17 (14):1–237.

National Institute for Health and Care Excellence. Cetuximab for the first-line treatment of metastatic colorectal cancer. NICE Guidance [TA176], August 2009. <https://www.nice.org.uk/Guidance/ta176>.

35. b) **Crohn's disease is the most important risk factor**

Small bowel adenocarcinoma (SBA) is a rare tumour which accounts for <5% of all gastrointestinal cancers. The incidence is around 10–20/million persons. There is some evidence that the incidence is increasing. SBA accounts for 40% of small bowel tumours. Neuroendocrine tumours, GISTs, and lymphomas account for the remainder. The duodenum is the most common location. A predisposing disease or genetic syndrome accounts for around 20% of cases in total: Crohn's disease (8.6%), FAP (3%), Lynch syndrome (3%), coeliac disease (1.5%), and Peutz–Jeghers syndrome (0.8%). Alcohol consumption and smoking have also been associated with an increased risk of SBA.

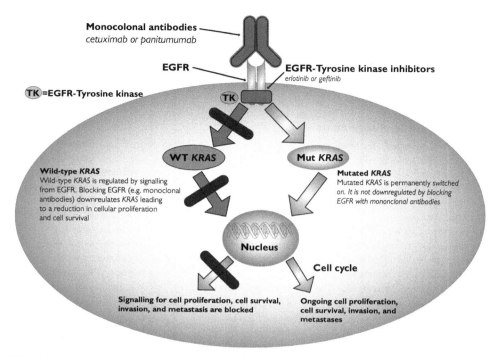

Fig. 4.4 Diagramatic representation of targets for anti-EGFR therapy and relevance to *KRAS* mutations

Population studies have estimated that a diagnosis of Crohn's disease is associated a 20–40fold increase in the relative risk of SBA compared to the general population. The cumulative risk is estimated to be 0.2% after 10 years of Crohn's disease and 2.2% after 25 years.

The diagnosis of SBA can be difficult. Many patients present with abdominal pain. Others may present with obstruction or GI bleeding. Obstruction is most common in jejunal or ileal tumours. The diagnosis may only be made after resection of a symptomatic stricture in a patient with an established diagnosis of Crohn's disease. The mainstay of management is surgical resection, possibly combined with post-operative adjuvant chemotherapy. Platinum-based chemotherapy seems to be the most effective.

Aparicioa T et al. Small bowel adenocarcinoma: Epidemiology, risk factors, diagnosis and treatment. *Digestive and Liver Disease* 2014; 46:97–104.

36. b) Imatinib

GI stromal tumour (GIST) is an uncommon cancer affecting 10–15/million per year. GISTs are impervious to standard chemotherapy. However, the discovery that at least 75% of these tumours have a KIT mutation led to the development of targeted chemotherapy. The KIT gene encodes the *tyrosine* kinase protein receptor, which is also known as proto-oncogene c-*Kit, tyrosine*-protein kinase *Kit*, CD117, or mast/stem cell growth factor receptor (SCFR).

Imatinib mesylate is a tyrosine kinase inhibitor with activity against KIT. Its structure mimics adenosine triphosphate (ATP) and it binds competitively to the ATP binding site of the target kinases. This prevents phosphorylation and signalling and thus inhibits proliferation and improves survival. Patients with an advanced GIST who are treated with imatinib show a 35–49% 9-year survival. The presence and type of KIT or PDGFRA mutation is predictive of response to imatinib.

Surgery is the primary treatment for all tumours which can be resected without significant morbidity. If this is not the case, then preoperative imatinib should be considered. Imatinib is effective in reducing the size of the tumour prior to resection, increasing the likelihood of negative margins and without significant morbidity.

Other tyrosine kinase inhibitors have been developed including sunitinib malate. This is an orally administered, multi-targeted receptor tyrosine kinase inhibitor which has shown significant and sustained clinical benefit in patients with imatinib-resistant or imatinib-intolerant GIST.

37. b) CT scan

Rectal carcinoid tumours are uncommon. Typically, they are discovered incidentally. At endoscopy they may present as a small sessile lesion or mass. On occasion the mass appears to be yellow or golden in colour. They are usually diagnosed at an earlier age compared to colonic carcinoid tumours (average age at diagnosis is 48–52 years). The 5-year survival rate ranges from 90–98%. Fewer than 20% of rectal carcinoids have evidence of metastatic disease at presentation. The size of the carcinoid tumour closely correlates with the likelihood of metastases. Tumours <1cm in size rarely show evidence of metastatic disease. Around 25% of tumours between 1–2cm in size and 70% of tumours >2cm show evidence of metastatic disease.

The Ki-67 proliferation index is used for both diagnosis and to assess the prognosis. Tumours with a high proliferation index are much more likely to have evidence of metastatic disease with some studies suggesting this to be the case in up to 100% of patients with a high proliferation index.

The main concern with the patient in this scenario is that they have a very high likelihood of metastatic disease given the tumour is >2cm in size and the Ki-67 proliferation index is high. At the very least, a CT scan should be performed and consideration should also be given to an octreoscan. If there is evidence for metastatic disease, aggressive surgery may not be indicated.

Miller HC et al. Role of Ki-67 proliferation index in the assessment of patients with neuroendocrine neoplasias regarding the stage of disease. *World Journal of Surgery* 2014; 38(6):1353–61.

Chung TP and Hunt HR. Carcinoid and neuroendocrine tumors of the colon and rectum. *Clinics in Colon and Rectal Surgery* 2006; 19(2):45–8.

38. d) 14mm tumour located near the base of the appendix

Most current guidelines suggest that a simple appendicectomy is adequate and curative treatment for appendiceal neuroendocrine tumours (NETs) of less than 1cm in size. Simple appendicectomy is also adequate treatment of tumours between 1–2cm in size, although such patients should be followed up for 5 years. A formal right hemicolectomy should be considered for higher-risk tumours. Features denoting higher risk include the following:

- tumour size >2cm
- tumour at the base of the appendix
- infiltration of the caecum
- positive surgical margins
- invasion of the appendiceal mesentery
- metastatic infiltration of appendiceal lymph node
- poor or undifferentiated tumour
- the presence of goblet cells

Most guidelines recommend that right hemicolectomy and lymph node dissection is considered for tumours <2cm when high-risk features are present; for example, vascular invasion, high proliferation index, deep mesoappendiceal invasion, positive, or unclear margins.

In the current scenario, the only tumour that is adequately treated is the 14mm tumour which is located near the base. This patient only requires surgical follow-up. All other patients should undergo right hemicolectomy because they fall into the higher risk category.

Griniatsos J and Michail O. Appendiceal neuroendocrine tumors: Recent insights and clinical implications. *World Journal of Gastrointestinal Oncology* 2010; 2(4):192–6.

39. b) Skin reactions

Side effects are not uncommon in patients taking cetuximab. Common side effects include some type of skin reaction, which affects up to 80% of patients. At least 15% of patients will have a severe skin rash. Patients may present with an acne-type rash which develops within the first two weeks of therapy. Skin reactions can last for up to 28 days after stopping therapy. Other skin reactions include skin peeling, redness, inflammation, and itchy or dry skin.

Other common side effects include weight loss, diarrhoea, nausea, abdominal pain, stomatitis, and peripheral neuropathy. Less frequent side effects include insomnia, fever, confusion, chills, hypocalcaemia, and bone and joint pain. Infusion reactions can also occur.

40. b) Haggitt level 2

A number of classification systems have been described which are based on endoscopic, morphologic, and histology findings in order to predict the risk of malignancy and metastatic disease in colorectal polyps. The depth of invasion into a polyp has been shown to correlate well with prognosis. Non-protruding lesions can be divided into those that are flush/slightly elevated lesions, laterally spreading lesions, and depressed lesions. Depressed lesions are considered more aggressive. For example, Kudo showed that depressed lesions of 6–10mm in diameter show submucosal invasion in approximately 24% of cases compared to 1.3% in protruding lesions and 0.5% in flush/slightly elevated lesions. The risk for submucosal invasion also increases with the size of the lesion. The Haggitt classification is based on the extent of invasion of the protruding malignant colorectal polyps (see Figure 4.5).

Haggitt RC et al. Prognostic factors in colorectal carcinomas arising in adenomas: implications for lesions removed by endoscopic polypectomy. *Gastroenterology* 1985; 89(2):328–36.

Kudo S et al. Endoscopic diagnosis and treatment of early colorectal cancer. *World Journal of Surgery* 1997; 21(7):694–701.

Management of polyps. In: MacKay GJ et al. (eds). *Colorectal Surgery.* Oxford: Oxford University Press, 2010, pp. 294–9.

41. e) Kikuchi Sm3

In early colorectal cancer, the depth of submucosal invasion is an important predictor for the risk of spread to regional lymph nodes. There is a strong relationship between the depth of submucosal invasion and the potential for spread to regional lymph nodes and distant organs. The submucosa may be divided into three layers from Sm1 to Sm3. Sm1 lesions are limited to the upper third of the submucosa, Sm2 lesions to the middle third, and Sm3 to the lower third of the submucosa. Sm1 lesions are further subdivided into three categories (a, b, and c). This sub-classification relates to the degree of horizontal involvement of the upper submucosal layer (ratio of the invading front to the width of the lesion). Overall, the risk of lymph node metastasis in Sm1 lesions is 2%, for Sm2

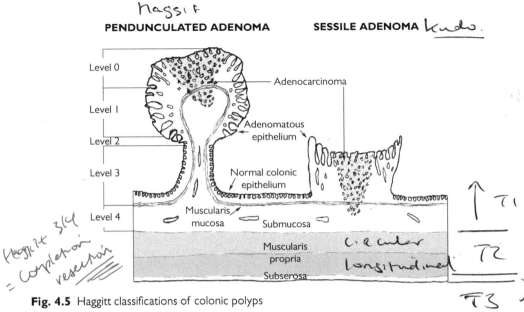

haggit

PENDUNCULATED ADENOMA   **SESSILE ADENOMA** Kudo.

Haggit 3/4
= Completion
resection

Fig. 4.5 Haggitt classifications of colonic polyps

Source data from *Gastroenterology*, 89, Haggitt RC, Glotzbach RE, Soffer EE, Wruble LD, Prognostic factors in colorectal carcinomas arising in adenomas: implications for lesions removed by endoscopic polypectomy. pp. 328-336, 1985.

tumours it is 8%, and it is 23% for Sm3 lesions. Extension into the muscularis propria makes the tumour a pT2 cancer (see Figure 4.6).

Kashida H and Kudo SE. Early colorectal cancer: concept, diagnosis, and management. *International Journal of Clinical Oncology* 2006; 11(1):1–8.

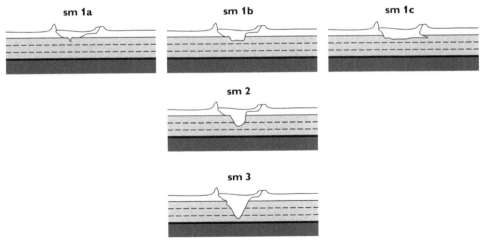

Fig. 4.6 Diagramatic representation of the Kikuchi staging of early colorectal cancer

Source data from *Diseases of the Colon & Rectum*, 38, 12, Kikuchi R, Takano M, Takagi K et al. Management of early invasive colorectal cancer. Risk of recurrence and clinical guidelines, pp. 1286–95, 1995.

Kikuchi R et al. Management of early invasive colorectal cancer. Risk of recurrence and clinical guidelines. *Diseases of the Colon & Rectum* 1995; 38(12):1286–95.

42. a) Appendicectomy and washout

This scenario raises concern that the diagnosis is that of a perforated mucinous cystadenoma or cyst adenocarcinoma of the appendix. Perforated appendiceal epithelial tumours are the likely primary pathology in the majority of patients who present with pseudomyxoma peritonei (PMP), an uncommon 'borderline malignancy'. Although there is considerable controversy regarding the pathophysiology of the primary tumour and how this relates to prognosis, it is clear that optimal treatment involves a combination of cytoreductive surgery with hyperthermic intra-peritoneal chemotherapy (HIPEC), performed by surgical oncologists who specialize in treating PMP.

In the current scenario a definite diagnosis of a perforated tumour within the appendix is not possible based on the simple finding of mucin near the appendix and some mucin in the pelvis. In addition, a right hemicolectomy is not going to alter the prognosis if there has already been intra-peritoneal dissemination of tumour cells. The best scenario therefore is to perform an appendicectomy, washout, and await definitive histology. If this confirms a perforated mucinous tumour of the appendix, a CT scan and assessment of the entire abdomen should be performed. Such patients should be followed up for at least four to five years with a regular CT scan. It is not certain whether all such patients will proceed to develop pseudomyxoma. If there is any evidence of a developing abnormality within the abdomen that might be consistent with early PMP referral to an appropriate specialist centre for consideration of cytoreductive surgery with HIPEC would be appropriate.

Bevan KE et al. Pseudomyxoma peritonei. *World Journal of Gastrointestinal Oncology* 2010; 2(1):44–50.

43. c) Right hemicolectomy and washout, taking fluid for C&S

The most likely diagnosis is that this patient has developed acute appendicitis secondary to a carcinoma in the caecum or base of the appendix. If this is suspected, consideration should be given to performing an open operation to assess the caecum directly. Appropriate experienced help should be sought. If there is any ongoing concern, a right hemicolectomy should be performed rather than attempting to perform an appendicectomy and possibly cut through the tumour at the base of the appendix.

44. c) Two or more relatives diagnosed before the age of 50 years

The Amsterdam criteria are used to help identify families who are likely to have Lynch syndrome which is also known as hereditary non-polyposis colorectal cancer (HNPCC). One of the few changes in the revised criteria is that only one or more relative needs to be diagnosed before the age of 50 years.

Umar A et al. Revised Bethesda Guidelines for hereditary nonpolyposis colorectal cancer (Lynch syndrome) and microsatellite instability. *Journal of the National Cancer Institute* 2004; 96 (4):261–8.

45. b) MSH2

This scenario describes a young patient who develops multiple right colon cancers and a uterine cancer. They also have a family history of colorectal cancer and it is likely that this patient has Lynch syndrome (HNPCC). This is an autosomal dominant condition where patients have a high risk of colon cancer as well as endometrial cancer, ovarian, stomach, small intestinal, upper urinary tract, brain, and skin. The increased risk of cancer is secondary to inherited mutations in DNA mismatch repair.

The colon cancers are typically poorly differentiated right-sided cancers which are frequently mucinous. Adenocarcinomas which show intraepithelial lymphocytes should also raise suspicion of a Lynch syndrome cancer. Patients have an 80% lifetime risk of colon cancer and the mean age at diagnosis of colon cancer is 44 years. Patients also have an 80% lifetime risk of endometrial cancer (mean age at diagnosis is 46 years).

Defects in DNA mismatch repair leads to microsatellite instability (MSI-H where H stands for high). The condition arises due to mutations in genes in the DNA mismatch repair pathway. MSH2 accounts for approximately 60% of cases, followed by MLH1 (30%), MSH6, and others.

Lynch HT et al. Review of the Lynch syndrome: history, molecular genetics, screening, differential diagnosis, and medicolegal ramifications. *Clinical Genetics* 2009; 76(1):1–18.

46. d) Reduces the risk of dysplasia in the anal transition zone

Although there has been considerable debate regarding the benefits of performing a mucosectomy when fashioning an ileal pouch for ulcerative colitis and FAP, it is now clear that functional outcome is substantially better in patients who have a double-stapled anastomosis rather than those who undergo a concomitant mucosectomy and hand-sewn anastomosis. Patients who undergo a concomitant mucosectomy appear to have lower resting and squeeze pressures and an increase in daytime and particularly night-time seepage of stool, compared to non-mucosectomy patients. Although mucosectomy theoretically reduces the risk of inflammation in the anal transition zone (termed 'cuffitis'), the evidence for this is not overwhelming and most surgeons would not consider this as a valid reason for performing a mucosectomy, given the poorer functional outcomes with this procedure.

Some centres have advocated mucosectomy for all patients and in experienced hands, good results can be obtained. However, rather poorer functional results are obtained when the procedure is performed by surgeons who routinely perform a double-stapled technique and only perform the occasional mucosectomy for specific indications.

The primary indication for performing a mucosectomy in colitis patients is to remove the anal transition zone, thereby theoretically reducing the risk of subsequent malignancy. Although a mucosectomy probably does reduce the risk of subsequent dysplasia, there is no hard evidence that it reduces the risk of malignancy and indeed many cases of malignancy developing within ileal pouches have occurred in patients where a mucosectomy was performed. It is thought that a mucosectomy rarely if ever completely removes the distal rectal and transition zone mucosa down to the dentate line. Islands of rectal mucosa inevitably remain which carry neoplastic potential.

The main indication for performing mucosectomy is in patients who are at increased risk of developing cancer if residual anal transition zone remains; that is, patients who already have developed a rectal cancer or who have been shown to have rectal dysplasia. Of course, these are also the patients who are going to be at increased risk of developing cancer within the any retained islands of rectal mucosa following a mucosectomy.

Mucosectomy may also be considered in patients who have FAP. This is especially so if the rectum contained numerous polyps. Patients who have relative rectal sparing may be considered for a double-stapled technique or even an ileorectal anastomosis. All FAP patients who have undergone an ileal pouch procedure will require regular follow-up to look for polyps either in the anal transition zone, in around the pouch-anal anastomosis, and also micropolyps within the pouch and terminal ileum (although the former do no tend to cause problems). FAP patients will also require upper GI endoscopy as part of their surveillance for duodenal adenomas which have a malignant potential.

Chambers WM and McC Mortensen NJ. Should ileal pouch-anal anastomosis include mucosectomy? *Colorectal Disease* 2007; 9(5):384–92.

Extended Matching Items

Management of anorectal conditions

1. C. Colonoscopy

A number of features of this scenario suggest this is more than just simple rectal bleeding. His history is suggestive of inflammatory bowel disease. He should undergo a workup in accordance with the BSG guidelines for assessment and management of inflammatory bowel disease and should be referred to a gastroenterologist for further care. He requires stool cultures ×3 to exclude an infective component, a faecal calprotectin, and blood tests to allow severity assessment as per the Truelove and Witt's criteria. A colonoscopy should be arranged with random colonic biopsies and biopsies of any inflamed segments. Terminal ileal intubation should also be performed.

2. E. Endoanal USS and manometry — *female's* *check sphincter injury/damage*

The patient has followed the standard sequence of treatment options for management of an anal fissure. Topical treatment (i.e. GTN/diltiazem) combined with a stool softener as first-line therapy. It should be stressed to the patient that they must be compliant with treatment and rigorously apply this twice a day for six to eight weeks. If this fails, injection of 25 units of Botox® into the intersphincteric space at the 3 and 9 o'clock position has been shown to improve healing rates for those fissures that have failed to heal on topical therapy. *unacceptable rate of complication .*
Lateral internal sphincterotomy (LIS) can be considered if Botox® does not improve symptoms. However, complications include a 10–15% risk of some impairment of bowel continence. In females, it is imperative to ensure that there has been no obstetric injury to the sphincter complex and that the fissure is indeed a high-pressure fissure. Therefore, endoanal US and anorectal manometry should be performed first prior to considering LIS. *Low pressure - anal advancement flap.*

Samin M et al. Topical diltiazem versus botulinum toxin a for the treatment of chronic anal fissure: a double blind randomised control trial. *Annals of Surgery* 2012; 255(1):18–22.

3. F. Examination under anaesthetic

This gentleman is rather old for a first-time presentation of an anal fissure. One has to be suspicious of other pathology. Although it might be reasonable to start topical therapy for a suspected anal fissure in younger patients, in this circumstance one has to exclude sinister pathology (e.g. anal or rectal cancer) in the first instance. Although an MRI might be helpful in excluding an occult abscess or tumour, it will not diagnose an anal fissure. Ultimately this gentleman will have to come to EUA.

This patient's medications should also be examined in order to exclude nicorandil-induced anal ulceration. Nicorandil can also be associated with the development of anal fistulas and can give rise to deep-seated anal pain, possibly in association with anal ulceration. These symptoms resolve on cessation of nicorandil whereas dose reduction does not seem to help.

Vella M and Molloy RG. Nicorandil-associated anal ulceration. *Lancet* 2002; 360:1979.

Suspected acute appendicitis — *Remember - must purify pus etc.*

4. C. Washout, taking fluid for C&S

The preceding history of weight loss combined with the findings at laparoscopy are suggestive of Crohn's disease. Although the appendix is somewhat congested, she clearly does not have a perforated or gangrenous appendicitis or obstruction. The finding of a terminal ileitis at operation for suspected appendicitis is non-specific and it is virtually impossible to differentiate between Crohn's disease and infectious enteritis (e.g. Yersinia). Rather than proceeding to resection of the

[handwritten margin note, left side, vertical:] High pressure fissure = sphincterotomy/flap. Low pressure = advancement flap

terminal ileum, and given that she has not had an opportunity to undergo medical therapy, ideally one would consider a washout with a view to investigating further when she has recovered from the laparoscopy.

Benoist S et al. Laparoscopic ileocecal resection in Crohn's disease: a case-matched comparison with open resection. *Surgical Endoscopy* 2003; 17:814–18.

Dignass A et al. The second European evidence-based Consensus on the diagnosis and management of Crohn's disease: Current management. *Journal of Crohn's and Colitis* 2009; 12:28–62 (ECCO statement 7E Terminal ileitis resembling Crohn's disease found at a laparotomy for suspected appendicitis should not routinely be resected).

[handwritten: Carcinoid – yellow]
[handwritten: 2 main tumours of app – Mucinos agr adenoma]

5. E. Laparoscopic appendicectomy and washout, taking fluid for C&S

This patient clearly has an acute perforated appendicitis. The 0.5cm yellow tumour is likely to be a carcinoid. Well-differentiated carcinoid tumours <1cm in size which are well clear of the resection margin (R0) should be treated with appendicectomy with no need for further follow-up. A right hemicolectomy is justified in tumours which are >2cm in size, those with a positive or unclear margin, or in tumours with deep mesoappendiceal invasion.

[handwritten: Goblet cell – Mucinos]
[handwritten: Approach – appendicectomy washout]

Plöckinger U et al. Consensus guidelines for the management of patients with digestive neuroendocrine tumours: Well-differentiated tumour/carcinoma of the appendix and goblet cell carcinoma. *Neuroendocrinology* 2008; 87:20–30.

6. C. Washout, taking fluid for C&S

The most likely diagnosis is pelvic inflammatory disease (PID). It is appropriate to take fluid for culture, washout, and not perform an appendicectomy. There is some debate as to the utility of performing an appendicectomy in this circumstance. However, if there is a definite diagnosis of PID, the addition of an incidental appendicectomy may slightly increase the risk of complications with little or no benefit and should probably not be performed. Appropriate antibiotic therapy should be discussed with the microbiology service but commonly prescribed antibiotics to treat PID include ofloxacin, metronidazole, ceftriaxone, and doxycycline.

Extra-intestinal manifestations (EIM) of inflammatory bowel disease (IBD)

7. G. Primary sclerosing cholangitis *[handwritten: – 5/7%]*

Primary sclerosing cholangitis (PSC) is a condition characterized by diffuse inflammation and fibrosis of the intra- and extra-hepatic bile ducts. It complicates 5–7% of patients with ulcerative colitis with a 2:1 male:female ratio. Patients typically present in their 40s with jaundice, pruritus, fatigue and weight loss. The condition slowly progresses to cirrhosis and liver transplant may need to be considered. Medical therapy does not appear to have an effect on survival. PSC is associated with an increased risk of cholangiocarcinoma and colorectal cancer. One meta-analysis reported a fourfold increased risk for the development of colorectal cancer. The cumulative risk of pouchitis is doubled in patients with PSC who have had an ileal pouch-anal anastomosis for ulcerative colitis.

Penna C et al. Pouchitis after ileal pouch-anal anastomosis for ulcerative colitis occurs with increased frequency in patients with associated primary sclerosing cholangitis. *Gut* 1996; 38(2):234–9.

Soetikno RM et al. Increased risk of colorectal neoplasia in patients with primary sclerosing cholangitis and ulcerative colitis: a meta-analysis. *Gastrointestinal Endoscopy* 2002; 56:48.

8. B. Erythema nodosum *[handwritten: – Skin changes 12%]*

Erythema nodosum occurs in up to 4% of patients with ulcerative colitis and up to 15% of patients with Crohn's disease. It is the most common EIM in children. Erythema nodosum may precede the

[handwritten: reflective of disease status whereas pyoderma is not]

diagnosis of IBD. It commonly occurs in women aged 20–30 years. Clinically it presents as sudden onset of warm, tender, red nodules on the shins with fever, malaise, and joint pains. It can last for up to six weeks. Treatment is with local symptomatic measures and treatment of the underlying inflammatory bowel disease. *Biopsy panniculitis* ·

Erythema nodosum may also occur in association with *streptococcal* infections, some drugs including the oral contraceptive pill, lymphoma, sarcoidosis, and autoimmune diseases.

Inflammatory bowel disease. In: MacKay GJ et al (eds). *Colorectal Surgery*. Oxford: Oxford University Press, 2010, pp. 109–4.

9. C. Spondylitis   *Crohn's (IBD ⇒ ant Gonads +++*

Axial arthropathy consists of two syndromes, spondylitis and isolated sacroiliitis. As an EIM of IBD, spondylitis is indistinguishable from ankylosing spondylitis, other than the fact that it is common in females (40%) and the male to female ratio for primary ankylosing spondylitis is 8:1. Spondylitis affects 2–6% of patients with IBD and is 20–30 times more prevalent than in the general population. More than 50% of patients with spondylitis are HLA-B27 positive. Patients typically present with low back pain which is prominent in the morning and usually relieved by exercise.

Symptomatic disease is usually treated with methotrexate and recent evidence suggests that anti-TNF drugs may also be of benefit. Asymptomatic sacroiliitis is commonly seen on X-rays and when present in isolation is not usually associated with HLA-B27 positivity.

Inflammatory bowel disease. In: MacKay GJ et al (eds). *Colorectal Surgery*. Oxford: Oxford University Press, pp. 182.

Anal pain

10. C. Chronic proctalgia/levator ani syndrome   *differential Coccygodynia (hard + free)*

Chronic proctalgia is a term that is used to describe chronic or recurrent pain in the anal canal/rectum. There are a number of synonymous terms including chronic idiopathic proctalgia, levator ani syndrome, puborectalis syndrome, chronic idiopathic perianal pain, and the piriformis syndrome. The key feature is that the pain is of at least 20-minutes duration as shorter episodes are suggestive of proctalgia fugax.

Proctalgia fugax is defined as a sudden severe deep-seated anal pain of less than 20-minutes duration that disappears completely (whereas chronic proctalgia persists throughout the day). Chronic proctalgia is divided into two subtypes according to the Rome III criteria: levator ani syndrome and unspecified functional anorectal pain. This separation is based on the presence or absence of tenderness in the levator muscle when palpated during digital rectal examination.

Although it was thought that this condition is due to a tendinitis, local steroid injection is not particularly effective in chronic proctalgia. Many patients report previous pelvic surgery, anal surgery, and childbirth as precipitating factors. High rates of anxiety, depression, and stress are reported in patients with chronic proctalgia.

Chiarioni G et al. Chronic proctalgia and chronic pelvic pain syndromes: New etiologic insights and treatment options. *World Journal of Gastroenterology* 2011; 17(40):4447–55.

11. B. Proctalgia fugax

Proctalgia fugax or functional recurrent anorectal pain is part of a spectrum of functional gastrointestinal disorders defined by the Rome III diagnostic criteria as episodes of sharp, fleeting pain that recur over weeks, are localized to the anus or lower rectum, and last from seconds to several minutes with complete resolution of pain between attacks. Although usually described as not having any diurnal variation, many patients describe getting sudden attacks at night when they can be woken from sleep. The presumption is that the attacks are precipitated by dreaming. Other precipitating factors include sexual activity, stress, constipation, defaecation, and menstruation. In addition, there may be no precipitating factor.

The condition should be differentiated from chronic proctalgia, which is a functional anorectal pain disorder with a vague, dull ache or pressure sensation high in the rectum. Chronic proctalgia is often worse when sitting than when standing or lying down and lasts at least 20 minutes.

Although the cause of proctalgia fugax is not certain, it does tend to occur in situations of increased stress and anxiety and it may be that spasm of the anal sphincter is a factor in the development of the pain. It is also associated with other functional disorders such as irritable bowel syndrome.

Many treatments are designed to relax anal spasm. This may be mechanical by self-digitation and massage of the puborectalis muscle, insertion of suppositories, or drug-induced using oral diltiazem or topical diltiazem/GTN. The effectiveness of such measures have never been properly assessed with a randomized controlled trial. A single study also reported that inhaled salbutamol may be of help.

Eckardt VF et al. Treatment of proctalgia fugax with salbutamol inhalation. *American Journal of Gastroenterology* 1996; 91:686–9.

12. E. Intersphincteric abscess

The short history in combination with fever and general malaise suggests the development of an acute problem such as an abscess. With no obvious findings in the perianal region and tenderness on rectal examination, or inability to perform a rectal examination because of spasm, the strong suspicion is of an intersphincteric abscess.

Such patients should be managed by performing an EUA. Not infrequently, intersphincteric abscesses spontaneously discharge through the internal opening of the anal gland at the level of the dentate line. However, if a bulge is identified within the anal canal this can be aspirated to dryness with a large-bore needle. Recurrent intersphincteric abscess may require formal drainage by performing a limited internal sphincterotomy over the abscess.

Constipation

13. B. Pseudo-obstruction

Ogilvie syndrome is the syndrome of acute dilatation of the colon in the absence of any mechanical obstruction. It is a serious condition with mortality rates as high as 30%. The high mortality rate reflects, at least in part, the fact that this condition occurs in critically ill patients, rather than the syndrome itself being lethal.

Colonic pseudo-obstruction is characterized by massive dilatation of the caecum and right colon. Caecal distention may exceed 10cm. It is a type of megacolon, sometimes referred to as 'acute megacolon' to distinguish it from toxic megacolon. The condition is named after the British surgeon Sir William Heneage Ogilvie (1887–1971) who first described it in 1948. Ogilvie's syndrome may occur after surgery, especially following CABG and total joint replacement. Drugs that disturb colonic motility (e.g. anticholinergics or opioid analgesics) contribute to the development of this condition.

It usually resolves with conservative therapy including correction of electrolyte abnormalities, avoiding oral intake, and insertion of a nasogastric tube. On occasion, colonoscopic decompression is necessary. This is successful in 70% of cases. Neostigmine may be considered prior to colonoscopic decompression. The use of neostigmine is not without risk since it can induce bradyarrhythmia and bronchospasm. Therefore, atropine should be within immediate reach when this therapy is used. Although described, neostigmine is rarely used in practice.

Maloney N and Vargas HD. Acute intestinal pseudo-obstruction (Ogilvie's syndrome). *Clinics in Colon and Rectal Surgery* 2005; 18(2):96–101.

14. F. Constipation-predominant IBS

Constipation is a frequent presenting symptom at clinic. It is important to identify what the patient means by the term 'constipation', as the word can mean different things to different people—even doctors. Doctors usually define constipation as passing hard pellet-like stools. Individuals usually think of constipation as infrequent stools, difficulty or straining at stools, a feeling of being unable to completely empty during a bowel movement, or the sensation of wanting to go but not being able to. There is also significant overlap with symptoms of irritable bowel syndrome.

By definition, true slow-transit constipation is present when a colonic transit study shows that more than 20% of the markers are retained at day 5 after ingestion. Most studies report that around one-third of IBS patients have diarrhoea-predominant IBS (IBS-D) and one-third have constipation-predominant IBS, the remainder having a mixed bowel pattern (IBS-M) with both loose and hard stools. Some individuals, now called 'alternators', switch subtype over time.

Jadallah JA et al. Constipation-predominant irritable bowel syndrome: A review of current and emerging drug therapies. *World Journal of Gastroenterology* 2014; 20(27):8898–909.

15. E. Ischaemic stricture

The most likely diagnosis here is an ischaemic stricture. Typically, these are smooth and most commonly occur in the region of the splenic flexure. There is often a preceding history of ischaemic colitis as suggested by this gentleman's history of having had an acute admission with rectal bleeding.

Ischaemic colitis is the most common form of gastrointestinal ischaemia and accounts for just over half of all cases. Ischaemic colitis occurs as a result of hypoperfusion of the colon, which in turn leads to mucosal injury or even full-thickness necrosis. Most patients recover without longer-term sequelae. The acute symptoms or pain, diarrhoea, and lower GI bleeding resolve in two to three days and the colon heals in one to three weeks. Rarely, after severe injury, healing may be delayed for up to six months. Less than 5% develop colonic gangrene, which present with signs of sepsis and peritonitis.

Colonic strictures may develop as a late complication in up to 10% of patients following an episode of ischaemic colitis. Some of these strictures may dilate over weeks or months, while others result in obstructive symptoms or an overt large bowel obstruction.

Washington C and Carmichael JC. Management of ischemic colitis. *Clinics in Colon and Rectal Surgery* 2012; 25(4):228–35.

Faecal incontinence

16. H. Full thickness rectal prolapse

50–70% of patients with rectal prolapse complain of faecal incontinence. The exact mechanism is not clear but it is likely to be related to a combination of stretching of the anal musculature and physiological changes, which include an impaired rectoanal inhibitory reflex with intermittent high-pressure rectal motor activity. Repair of the prolapse leads to an improvement in continence in 30– 70% of patients.

Farouk R et al. Restoration of continence following rectopexy for rectal prolapse and recovery of the internal anal sphincter electromyogram. *British Journal of Surgery* 1992; 79(5):439–40.

17. D. Occult sphincter injury at childbirth

10–25% of females report new faecal incontinence post-partum. Associated risk factors include:

- Forceps delivery
- Primiparous delivery

- Previous sphincter injury
- Episiotomy
- Augmented labour

The mechanism of injury is often multifactorial and includes direct sphincter injury from tears and episiotomy, occult sphincter injury, a pudendal nerve traction injury, and stretching of the perineum. Diabetic autonomic neuropathy is rarely a cause for faecal incontinence in isolation and usually only presents as a problem after five to ten years following the diagnosis of diabetes.

18. C. Laxative abuse

Patients who abuse laxatives may do so in order to lose weight although they may not be forthcoming in describing the use of laxatives in their history. This female had a low BMI, a normal faecal calprotectin, and random colonic biopsies showed melanosis coli, which is consistent with the use of laxatives of the anthranoid group including senna and rhubarb derivatives.

Emergency presentations

19. K. Typhlitis/ileocaecal syndrome

This condition is known by a number of names including typhlitis, neutropenic enterocolitis, and the ileocaecal syndrome. Typically, it affects patients undergoing chemotherapy for haematological malignancies but has also been described in patients undergoing high-dose chemotherapy for solid organ malignancies and also those with AIDS.

Patients present with fever, abdominal pain +/− peritonism in the right iliac fossa. It is usually associated with a neutropenia although not always. The terminal ileum and caecum are most commonly involved and local signs such as peritonism can be elicited. Treatment is with broad-spectrum antibiotics +/− granulocyte colony-stimulating factor (GCSF) to increase the white cell count. If there is evidence for perforation, laparotomy and a resection may be required. Mortality is usually greater than 50% in the presence of perforation and sepsis.

Benign colonic conditions. In: MacKay GJ et al. (eds). *Colorectal Surgery*. Oxford: Oxford University Press, pp. 195–248.

20. J. Collagenous colitis — *female (associated ē autoimmune disease*

Collagenous colitis is a subtype of microscopic colitis and typically presents with a history of *watery* watery diarrhoea with normal findings at colonoscopy. Symptoms are often of extended duration but the disease may have a relapsing course. The diagnosis is made at colonoscopy and biopsy. Histology typically shows a thickened band of sub-epithelial collagen in association with a chronic inflammatory cell infiltrate. The female:male ratio is 8:1 with a median onset in the sixth decade. Many cases are associated with coeliac disease, thyroid disease, diabetes, and rheumatoid arthritis. Budesonide induces a remission in around 85% of patients although the relapse rate is high.

21. C. CMV colitis

Cytomegalovirus (CMV) infection is very common and usually asymptomatic in the immune-competent patient. However, symptomatic infection or reactivation of asymptomatic infection can occur in transplant and HIV patients who are immunocompromised. CMV colitis leads to diarrhoea with GI bleeding. The infection is usually most prominent in and around the caecum, although the entire GI tract from mouth to anus can be affected. Severe cases can give rise to deep ulceration. Histology shows CMV inclusions. CMV PCR or immunohistochemistry may be necessary where there is a high clinical suspicion and classic viral inclusion bodies are not seen on H&E (haemotoxylin and eosin) staining. Ganciclovir is the first-line treatment.

[handwritten: Transplant + watery/bloody Caecal diarrhoea = CMV]

Polyposis syndromes

22. K. Gardner syndrome

[handwritten: – Desmoid + FAP = Gardner.]

Gardner syndrome is determined by the autosomal dominant familial polyposis coli gene (APC) which is present on chromosome 5. In addition to classic FAP features of multiple adenomatous polyps of the colon and duodenum, the syndrome is associated with dental abnormalities including multiple impacted and supernumerary teeth, multiple jaw osteomas, and congenital hypertrophy of the retinal pigment epithelium (CHRPE). Osteomas of the skull, thyroid cancer, epidermoid cyst, and fibromas have also been described. Up to 15% of patients will suffer from a desmoid tumour. The condition is also associated with aggressive fibromatosis (Desmoid tumours) of the retroperitoneum.

The aponeurosis of the rectus abdominis muscle is the most common site of desmoid tumours. These tumours occur more commonly in multiparous women. Extra-abdominal desmoid tumours are rare and most commonly occur in the breast or may occur as an extension of the lesion arising from the muscles of the chest wall. Mammary desmoid tumours account for less than 0.5% of primary breast neoplasms. In Gardner syndrome, the incidence of mammary desmoid tumours ranges from 4–17%.

Gardner syndrome at NIH's Office of Rare Diseases. <https://rarediseases.info.nih.gov/diseases/6482/disease>.

23. I. Turcot syndrome

Turcot syndrome is characterized by the presence of multiple colonic polyps in association with a primary brain tumour. It can also be associated with the presence of café-au-lait spots on the skin, multiple lipomas, and/or the development of basal cell carcinomas.

Turcot syndrome is rare and is considered to be a variant of two more common syndromes associated with polyp formation, Lynch syndrome and familial adenomatous polyposis (FAP). In families with glioblastomas and other features of Lynch syndrome, mutations have been found in the MLH1 and PMS2 genes. This is sometimes referred to as Turcot syndrome type 1 or 'true' Turcot syndrome. It is inherited as an autosomal recessive trait. In families with medulloblastoma and other features of FAP, mutations have been found in the APC gene (type 2 form of Turcot syndrome). This is inherited as an autosomal dominant condition.

Turcot syndrome; CNS tumors with Familial polyposis of the colon at NIH's Office of Rare Diseases. <https://rarediseases.info.nih.gov/diseases/420/disease>.

24. F. Juvenile polyposis

[handwritten: Differential FAP + Peutz Jegher.]

Juvenile polyposis syndrome is characterized by the presence of multiple polyps throughout the intestinal tract. Histologically the polyps are described as being juvenile. The term does not refer to the age of the affected patient. The polyps are non-neoplastic, hamartomatous, and benign but the condition is associated with a cumulative lifetime risk of colorectal cancer of 40%. Two genes (BMPR1A and SMAD4) are associated with juvenile polyposis syndrome.

The condition can occur sporadically or may be inherited in an autosomal dominant manner. Typically, patients present with bleeding, abdominal pain, and/or diarrhoea. The polyps usually begin appearing before the age of 20. The diagnosis is made if:

- Five or more juvenile polyps are identified within the colon or rectum
- Juvenile polyps are identified throughout the gastrointestinal tract
- Any juvenile polyps are found in a person with a family history of juvenile polyposis

Brosens LAA et al. Juvenile polyposis syndrome. *World Journal of Gastroenterology* 2011; 17(44):4839–44.

Anal intraepithelial neoplasia (AIN)   Line Das breast cancer Similar.

25. A. Reassure and discharge from clinic

Anal intraepithelial neoplasia (AIN) is a precursor for invasive squamous cancer. These precursor lesions are also referred to as squamous intraepithelial lesions (SILs) which may by low grade (LSIL) or high grade (HSIL). It is a multifocal disease and associated with the HPV virus. The exact prevalence in the general population is less than 1% but the incidence is increasing, in part due to increased numbers of patients who are directly immunocompromised secondary to a transplant, immunosuppression for connective tissue and autoimmune disorders, and patients with HIV. The prevalence of AIN in HIV ranges from 25–90%. There is also a rising incidence of anal cancer in patients with AIDS. The prevalence of AIN in renal transplant patients is around 5%.

A number of factors have been identified that increase the risk of AIN/SIL. These include acquired or iatrogenic immunosuppression, concurrent HPV-related diseases, number of sexual partners, and history or presence of other sexually transmitted infections (STI). Certain HPV serotypes are associated with specific phenotypes. HPV types 6, 11, and 39 tend to be associated with AIN Grade 1 (LSIL) whereas high-risk HPV serotypes 16, 18, 58, and 45 are associated with high grade AIN (anal HSIL) and anal cancer.

Patients with AIN may present with perianal symptoms of skin irritation. However, many lesions are asymptomatic and only diagnosed after careful inspection where it may present as a slightly raised, flat, scaly, erythematous, pigmented, eczematous, or fissured lesion. The presence of ulceration is concerning for invasion.

Although patients with HIV are at increased risk of AIN, the current position in the United Kingdom is that there is probably no place for screening for AIN, even in high-risk groups. Some specialist centres in the United States have started screening for AIN in HIV patients using anal cytology (EXPLORE study). However, there is debate over the accuracy of this screening test and within the United Kingdom it is not currently felt that there is a role for either one-off or regular screening for AIN through cytology/anal smear tests in asymptomatic individuals. Additionally, in the absence of both symptoms and an identifiable abnormality, it would be inappropriate to subject the patient in this scenario to general anaesthetic and invasive biopsies.

Scholefield JH et al. Guidelines for management of anal intraepithelial neoplasia. *Colorectal Disease* 2011; 13(suppl 1):3–10.

Pineda CE and Welton ML. Management of anal squamous intraepithelial lesions. *Clinics in Colon and Rectal Surgery* 2009; 22(2):94–101.

26. C. Review at six months and discharge

AIN grade I/II (also referred to as low grade squamous intraepithelial lesion LSIL) tend to behave differently compared to AIN grade III (HSIL). It is felt that AIN grade I probably does not require long-term follow-up whereas AIN grade III and multifocal disease should be managed by clinicians with a special interest in this condition. Unfortunately, there are no clear guidelines as to how patients with AIN should be followed up. In general terms patients with AIN grades 1–2 are not felt to be at high risk of progression to invasive cancer. High-risk lesions such as AIN grade 3 (HSIL), the presence of multifocal disease and disease in immunocompromised individuals require much closer follow-up and management. In the immunocompetent patient, one can either review at 6 months with a view to discharge or alternatively 12 monthly. Immunocompromised patients may require somewhat closer review six monthly. See Figure 4.7.

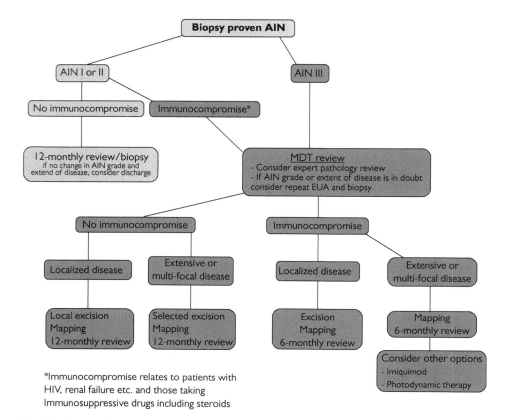

Fig. 4.7 Suggested protocol for management of AIN

27. H. Imiquimod 5% cream

The finding of AIN III is a significant cause for concern, particularly in HIV-positive patients. Some studies have suggested that up to 60% of HIV-positive patients will progress from low-grade to high-grade AIN III within 2 years of diagnosis. AIN III rarely regresses.

The risk of progression of AIN to invasive anal cancer is approximately 10% at 5 years. AIN III is found in 80% of cases of anal squamous cell carcinoma. Those most at risk of invasive cancer are patients with multifocal disease or those with immunocompromise. One study reported that 50% of immunocompromised patients (e.g. post-transplant, SLE (systemic lupus erythematosus)) with AIN III progressed to invasive cancer within 5 years of diagnosis, compared with no patients progressing to anal cancer in the immunocompetent group.

Localized areas of AIN III can be excised. However, wide local excision can be associated with significant morbidity and although some authors have suggested wide local excision and flap reconstruction, such procedures carry significant morbidity and may represent over-treatment. Local ablative therapy with cryotherapy, diathermy, or CO_2 laser has also been tried. Many studies have shown significant morbidity and high recurrence rates with such an approach. They may also be associated with significant post-operative pain. Immunomodulation therapies including imiquimod 5% cream have been shown to be quite effective. In one uncontrolled study, 77% of patients with AIN resolved after 16 weeks of treatment. Total lesion clearance was obtained in 46% of HIV-positive men who were treated for 20 weeks. With extensive multifocal change, immunomodulation therapy is a reasonable first-line therapy rather than subjecting patients to destructive surgery which can be associated with complications such as anal stenosis.

Scholefield JH et al. Guidelines for management of anal intraepithelial neoplasia. *Colorectal Disease* 2011; 13(suppl 1):3–10.

Side-effects of chemotherapy for colorectal cancer

28. I. Capecitabine *like 5-FU. hand-foot*

This scenario is typical of hand-foot syndrome which affects up to 50% of patients receiving capecitabine (Xeloda). Grade 3 toxicity can occur in 10–20% of patients. Development of the condition is thought to be a surrogate marker for capecitabine efficiency and there is a correlation between capecitabine-induced hand–foot syndrome and the efficacy of biomarkers in patients with metastatic breast cancer.

Typical symptoms include redness and swelling of the palms and soles, which can progress to dryness, scaling, pain, itching, and occasionally blisters and ulceration. The condition, which is also called palmar-plantar erythrodysesthesia, affects the palms more than the soles.

Patients should be advised to avoid excessive trauma or friction to the hands and feet and should use protective gloves and socks. High-dose steroid creams and keratolytic moisturizers, such as lactic acid or salicylic acid, can also be helpful.

29. C. Cetuximab

Up to 80% of patients receiving cetuximab will develop some sort of skin reaction. Typically, this is an acne-type rash affecting the face, neck, and trunk. The skin may also be dry and itchy. Up to 15% of patients will have a severe rash. Other side effects include tiredness, fatigue, sore throat, stomatitis, and infection or inflammation around nail folds. Less common side effects include neutropenia, diarrhoea, anorexia, nausea, and thrombocytopenia. Around 2% of patients develop a severe allergic reaction which normally develops within an hour of therapy.

30. E. Oxaliplatin *i.e. DNA crosslinking like cyclophos + cisplatin.*

Oxaliplatin is an alkylating chemotherapeutic drug that is used in patients who have metastatic colorectal cancer. It is the only platinum derivative with activity against advanced colorectal cancer. Its mode of action is to bind and cross-link strands of DNA. This leads to selective inhibition of DNA synthesis and activation of repair processes that ultimately lead to cell death.

It is frequently given in combination with fluoropyrimidines including 5-fluorouracil and capecitabine. Typically, it might be used for FOLFOX (oxaliplatin in combination with 5-fluorouracil and folinic acid) or XELOX (oxaliplatin in combination with capecitabine) regimens.

Up to 30% of patients receiving oxaliplatin will develop a peripheral neuropathy. Neurotoxicity is the dose-limiting side effect with this drug. This side effect can manifest as two distinct forms: the acute, reversible sensory neuropathy and a chronic, cumulative neuropathy. The acute form occurs with infusion or in the ensuing hours. The chronic toxicity does not become apparent until cycles 8–10 in the commonly used FOLFOX dosing regimen, making it more predictable.

NICE Colorectal Cancer Guidelines: <https://www.nice.org.uk/guidance/cg131/documents/colorectal-cancer-full-guideline2>.

[handwritten: 1-3% have the FOB's   10% = Cancer @ colonoscopy]

Bowel cancer screening programme

31. F. 10–25%

Males tend to be more likely to have a colorectal cancer, which was identified in 11.6% of males and 7.8% of females who underwent colonoscopy following a positive result during the first round of screening in England. The most recent Scottish data reported cancer in 7.1% of males and 5.5% of females who underwent colonoscopy following a positive result. Around 70% of cancers will be so-called early Dukes A (30%) or B cancers (30%) or polyp cancers (10%). In Scotland the 2010–12 figures report that 24% of cancers were polyp cancers.

Logan RFA et al. Outcomes of the Bowel Cancer Screening Programme (BCSP) in England after the first 1 million tests. *Gut* 2012; 61:1439–46.

Scottish Bowel Screening Programme. Key Performance Indicators Report 2010–2012. <http://www.isdscotland.org/Health-Topics/Cancer/Publications/2013-08-27/KPI_Report.pdf>.

32. H. 50%

The initial figures from England suggested that uptake was 49.6% for men and 54.4% for women. Uptake in Scotland is a little better at 52% for males and 58% for females.

33. D. 1–3%

The bowel cancer screening programme in England started in 2006. Subjects aged 60–69 years were invited to submit 3 FOB tests every two years. Rollout for the Scottish programme was completed in 2009. The Scottish programme invites people aged 50–74 years to attend for bowel screening. Patients aged 75 years and older can also request a screening kit.

In England, 2.5% of males and 1.5% of females had a positive test in the initial round of screening. Similar figures were seen in Scotland. The most recent figures from Scotland report a positive result in 3.4% of males and 2.1% of females.

Rectal cancer

34. A. Low Hartmann's procedure

This man has got a mid- to lower-third rectal cancer with clear margins and should therefore be able to proceed directly to resection. Of significant concern here, however, is his poor anal tone and inability to retain gas. He will require a TME (total mesorectal excision) and if one were to consider a restorative procedure, this would mean a low anterior resection. In the best circumstances this can be associated with faecal urgency and occasional incontinence. In an elderly patient with impaired sphincter tone, one has to be concerned that he would have major problems with continence and will develop low anterior resection syndrome. A low Hartmann's resection may offer a better alternative. These issues should be discussed with the patient and although an anterior resection (plus temporary defunctioning stoma) would be technically possible, it is unlikely to be the best option for this gentleman.

Low anterior resection syndrome (LARS) is a well-recognized phenomenon. The severity of LARS can be scored and patients divided into those with no LARS, minor LARS, or major LARS based on their score. Risk factors include the extent of operation (tumour height more or less than 5cm and total mesorectal excision/partial mesorectal excision), with or without preoperative chemoradiation. Some authors have also identified other risk factors including the use of a temporary defunctioning stoma, the presence of pain with defaecation, difficulty holding onto the bowel motion, and the need to use pads.

[handwritten in left margin: Sung can't see he will bleed no where.]

Emmertsen KJ and Laurberg S. Low anterior resection syndrome score: development and validation of a symptom-based scoring system for bowel dysfunction after low anterior resection for rectal cancer. *Annals of Surgery* 2012; 255(5):922–8.

35. G. Palliative radiotherapy

In ideal circumstances this gentleman should be treated with down-staging preoperative chemoradiation and then resection. It is likely that he would need an extra-levator abdomino–perineal resection of the rectum. However, it is clear that he would not be fit for this intervention given the need for home nebulisers and severe COPD. Palliative radiotherapy should help with symptoms. Were he to develop intractable symptoms, one might need to consider a defunctioning stoma. This would be a high-risk procedure given his medical comorbidity. A colonic stent would not be possible given the low-lying nature of the tumour.

36. E. Pelvic exenteration

In this scenario the patient has already received neoadjuvant chemoradiation. There is no evidence of metastatic disease so the tumour should be approached with curative intent. Given the invasion into the prostate and bladder neck, pelvic exenteration should be considered. Ideally this should be performed by a surgeon with experience in performing this operation, either alone or in conjunction with a urologist who also has regular experience of total cystectomy.

Yang TX et al. Pelvic exenteration for rectal cancer: a systematic review. *Diseases of the Colon & Rectum* 2013; 56(4):519–31.

Polyp cancers

37. F. Anterior resection

This is a Kukuchi level 2 polyp as it penetrates to the middle third of the submucosa. It has several poor prognostic factors—poor differentiation and lymphovascular invasion. The risk of lymph node metastasis is significant, so this patient should be offered an anterior resection.

38. B. Colonoscopy and tattoo

The lesion described is large and the fact that it was not possible to easily raise this lesion for EMR suggests that there is an underlying carcinoma. If EMR is not possible, a formal resection should be considered. In order to identify the site at laparoscopic surgery correctly, the lesion should be tattooed at the distal margin. The endoscopist should clearly state where the tattoo has been placed in relation to the polyp. This has not been performed at the first colonoscopy and therefore a colonoscopy should be repeated by the person performing the surgery.

Pelvic tumours

39. E. Chordoma

Chordomas are rare slow-growing malignant tumours that arise from the notochord (extends from the base of the occiput to the caudal limit of the embryo). They are the most common malignancy in the retrorectal space and may occur anywhere along the embryologic notochord. Up to 50% occur around the saccrococcyx.

Chordomas occur more commonly in males and tend to present in the fourth and fifth decade of life. Because they are slow growing and produce vague symptoms, there may be a delay in diagnosis and tumours may become quite large in size. They have tendency to invade bone and symptoms may relate to bone and nerve invasion. Around 20% of patients demonstrate metastatic disease (lung, liver, and bone) at presentation.

Patients may be asymptomatic or complain of vague symptoms such as positional buttock, pelvic, or lower back pain. Invasion of nerves may give rise to neuropathic pain or impotence and incontinence. Local recurrence rates are high, even with radical resection, and long-term survival rates of around 10–30% have been reported.

Neale JA. Retrorectal tumors. *Clinics in Colon and Rectal Surgery.* 2011; 24(3):149–60.

40. G. Meningocoele

Anterior meningocoeles and myelomeningocoeles develop because of a congenital defect in the anterior sacrum. This leads to herniation of the dural sac. The sacral bone defect has a rounded concave border (typically the edge is smooth, well calcified, and without bony destruction). This is pathognomonic of anterior sacral myelomeningocoeles and is called the 'scimitar sign'.

Meningocoeles may occur in combination with other congenital abnormalities including the presence of presacral cysts or lipomas, urinary tract or anal malformations, uterine or vaginal duplication, spina bifida, and a tethered spinal cord.

Patients are often young at presentation so may not give a typical history. However, some patients complain of headache associated with defaecation. This is thought to be due to a compression-induced increase in cerebrospinal fluid pressure during defaecation. Others may have symptoms secondary to pressure and a mass effect. These might include constipation, urinary symptoms, and lower back pain. If suspected, biopsy or aspiration is contraindicated as it might introduce infection leading to meningitis. These lesions are managed by ligation of the dural defect.

41. D. Rectal duplication cyst

Duplication cysts are developmental lesions that arise secondary to sequestration of embryogenesis of the developing hindgut. They develop from endodermal tissue so may contain squamous, cuboidal, columnar, or transitional epithelium. These lesions frequently have a multi-lobular appearance with a single dominant lesion/cyst and several satellite lesions. They are more common in women. They are usually benign although malignant transformation has been described. They may become infected and simulate a pilonidal or ischiorectal fossa abscess or fistula which does not respond to standard therapy.

Single Best Answers

1. **A 33 year old male with a long history of dry eyes presents with a 1-month history of obstructive jaundice and abdominal pain. Which blood test may be helpful in reaching a diagnosis?**
   a) CA 19-9
   b) ASMA
   c) Ki-67
   d) IgG4
   e) IL-17

2. **Which of the following is an absolute contraindication to resection of liver metastases from a colorectal primary?**
   a) The presence of pulmonary metastases
   b) Multiple bilobar metastases
   c) The resection margin is likely to be less than 1cm
   d) *KRAS* mutant-type colorectal cancer
   e) Only two adjacent liver segments would remain after resection
   f) None of the above

3. **Which of the following statements is accurate when considering the hepatic arterial blood supply?**
   a) The hepatic artery is the main blood supply to the liver
   b) The cystic artery is usually a branch from the hepatic artery proper
   c) Division of an accessory left hepatic artery is likely to increase the risk of leakage from a bilioenteric anastomosis
   d) A 'replaced' right hepatic artery arises from the superior mesenteric artery
   e) An accessory hepatic artery should never be ligated

4. **Which of the following hepatic resections involves resection of segments II, III, and IV?**
   a) Left bisectionectomy
   b) Right lobectomy
   c) Right trisegmentectomy
   d) Left lateral segmentectomy
   e) Extended left hepatectomy

5. **Which cells in the liver form part of the reticuloendothelial system?**
   a) Histiocytes
   b) Hepatocytes
   c) Kupffer cells
   d) Hepatic stellate cells
   e) All of the above

6. **You are asked to review a 9 year old male who has been admitted to A&E with a short history of being unwell with general malaise and then a sudden deterioration. On examination, the child is febrile, hypotensive, tachycardic, and obtunded. He previously underwent a splenectomy six months earlier for hereditary spherocytosis. Which of the following statements is true about his current condition?**
   a) The incidence is lower when splenectomy is performed for haematologic disease
   b) The incidence is highest within six months of splenectomy
   c) Patients require lifelong antibiotic prophylaxis, usually with penicillin, especially those older than five years
   d) Mortality rate approaches 90%
   e) Complications include peripheral gangrene, deafness, and endocarditis

7. **A 49 year old woman with idiopathic thrombocytopenic purpura (ITP) undergoes a successful splenectomy. Which of the following would be an expected finding five years after her surgery?**
   a) Absent Pappenheimer bodies in red cells
   b) Acanthocytes on blood film
   c) Immature spherocytes on blood film
   d) High levels of serum properdin and tuftsin
   e) More rapid maturation of red blood cells

8. **Which of the following statements regarding splenic anatomy is correct?**
   a) The average weight of an adult spleen is 500g
   b) The short gastric arteries (5–7 branches) are the first branches of the splenic artery
   c) The gastrosplenic ligament is avascular
   d) The splenorenal ligament often contains the tail of the pancreas
   e) Accessory spleens are most commonly located in the mesentery

9. **Which of the following clinical conditions is indicated by the presence of serum antibodies against hepatitis B surface antigen (anti-HBs) and anti-HBc in the absence of HBsAg (hepatitis B surface antigens)?**
   a) Asymptomatic chronic carrier of HBV
   b) Recovery from acute hepatitis B with subsequent immunity
   c) Normal response to vaccination with hepatitis B vaccine
   d) Active, acute infection with HBV
   e) Chronic active hepatitis secondary to HBV

10. **Which of the following is *not* associated with the development of hepatocellular carcinoma?**
    a) Alcoholic cirrhosis
    b) Haemochromatosis
    c) Hepatitis A virus
    d) Hepatitis B virus
    e) Non-alcoholic steatohepatitis (NASH)

11. **A 55 year old man with a long-standing hepatitis B infection is reviewed by gastroenterology because of mild abdominal pain. His serum alpha-fetoprotein (AFP) is 1250ng/ml. A CT scan identifies a cirrhotic liver with a 6cm enhancing lesion in the left lobe of the liver. What is the most appropriate management?**
    a) Radiofrequency ablation
    b) Selective internal radiotherapy (SIRT)
    c) Trans-arterial chemoembolization (TACE)
    d) Liver transplantation
    e) Surgical resection
    f) Oral sorafenib
    g) None of the above

12. **Which of the following proteins is *not* primarily synthesized within the liver?**
    a) C-reactive protein
    b) Transferrin
    c) Factor II
    d) Von Willebrand factor
    e) Albumin

13. A 35 year old man has previously undergone an ileo-caecal resection for terminal ileal Crohn's disease. He recently developed right upper quadrant (RUQ) pain secondary to gallstones. What is the mostly likely composition of the gallstones?

a) Cholesterol-rich
b) Calcium bilirubinate-rich
c) Calcium phosphate
d) Calcium oxalate
e) Pigment-rich

14. When considering the aetiology of acute pancreatitis, which of the following statements is *not* accurate?

a) L-asparaginase has been shown to cause acute pancreatitis
b) CMV, Coxsackie B, and mumps virus have been associated with acute pancreatitis
c) A malignant tumour in the head of the pancreas or ampulla can result in acute pancreatitis
d) Gallstones account for between 35% and 65% of cases of acute pancreatitis
e) Therapeutic ERCP is associated with a 3% risk of acute pancreatitis
f) The risk of developing gallstone pancreatitis following a diagnosis of cholelithiasis is <1%

15. Which of the following is the most appropriate indication to arrange a CT scan in the first 24 hours following admission with acute pancreatitis?

a) Staging the severity of pancreatitis
b) To confirm infected pancreatic necrosis
c) To predict disease severity
d) To confirm/clarify the diagnosis
e) To identify choledocholithiasis
f) All of the above

16. When considering the complications of acute pancreatitis, which of the following statements is not correct?

a) Acute peri-pancreatic fluid collections (APFC) have a well-defined wall and often contain solid components
b) Pancreatic pseudocyst refers to a fluid collection surrounded by a well-defined wall, containing essentially no solid material, that persists for more than four weeks
c) Acute necrotic collection (ANC) applies to a mixed collection of fluid and necrotic material during the first four weeks
d) Walled-off necrosis (WON) describes a collection contained within a mature enhancing wall of reactive tissue, occurring after four weeks of necrotizing pancreatitis.
e) Infected necrosis is often indicated by a clinical deterioration in the patient or by the presence of gas within the collection on CT

17. **A 30 year old female is admitted with right upper quadrant pain. Her LFTs are normal. An ultrasound suggests acute cholecystitis with multiple calculi in the gallbladder. Following a straightforward laparoscopic cholecystectomy, what is the most appropriate antimicrobial strategy for the post-operative period?**
    a) Five days of oral co-amoxiclav
    b) Three days of oral co-amoxiclav
    c) No antibiotics
    d) Three doses of broad spectrum intravenous antibiotics with gram-negative cover
    e) A single dose of broad spectrum intravenous antibiotics with gram-negative cover

18. **Cholecystectomy for acute cholecystitis during pregnancy is contraindicated in which of the following circumstances?**
    a) The patient has previously undergone abdominal surgery
    b) Cholecystitis during the first trimester
    c) Cholecystitis during the second trimester
    d) Cholecystitis during the third trimester
    e) None of the above

19. **You are consenting a 34 year old female for an elective laparoscopic cholecystectomy. The patient has no specific risk factors to suggest a difficult cholecystectomy. What figure should you quote regarding the risk of common bile duct injury?**
    a) 9%
    b) 0.03%
    c) 0.5%
    d) 1%
    e) 3%

20. **What is the optimal time to perform cholecystectomy for acute cholecystitis?**
    a) Within 48 hours of presentation
    b) Seven days after presentation
    c) Two weeks after presentation
    d) Six weeks after presentation
    e) Delay until a further more serious complication develops

21. An 85 year old previously healthy man is taken to theatre following a CT diagnosis of a gallstone ileus. What is the most appropriate management option for him?

a) Wedge excision of the small bowel segment containing the gallstone

b) Advance the stone into the colon without performing an enterotomy

c) Advance the stone into the colon and perform a small caecotomy to remove the gallstone

d) Milk the stone proximally, remove the gallstone through a small enterotomy, and ensure no more gallstones are present proximally

e) Milk the stone proximally, remove the gallstone through a small enterotomy, ensure no more gallstones are present proximally, and perform a cholecystectomy with repair of the choleduodenal fistula

22. A 25 year old man presents with obstructive jaundice. Imaging reveals that the cause is most likely to be a cholangiocarcinoma against a background of a choledochal cyst. Which pattern of disease is most common?

a) Choledochocele

b) Multiple cysts in the left hepatic duct

c) Diverticulum of the distal common bile duct

d) Single fusiform cystic dilatation of the common bile duct

e) Combination of proximal intra-hepatic duct dilatation with diffuse saccular dilatation of the entire common bile duct

23. A 64 year old fit male undergoes a laparoscopic distal pancreatectomy for a cystic tumour. On day 4 post-op, he is noted to have 500ml of fluid in his abdominal drain. This has an amylase level of 2500IU/L. What is the most appropriate next step in his management?

a) ERCP and stent placement

b) Re-operation and operative repair of the pancreatic duct

c) Total parental nutrition via a central line

d) Enteral feeding via jejunostomy

e) Leave the drain in place and consider starting octreotide

24. A 64 year old woman presents with obstructive jaundice. An ultrasound reveals a dilated CBD. An MRCP is requested; however, the patient states she has claustrophobia. Which of the following should be viewed as an absolute contraindication to MRI?

a) Recent laparoscopic cholecystectomy with the use of metallic clips

b) High BMI

c) Previous reaction to Gadolinium contrast

d) Suspected previous retinal eye injury with metal fragments

e) Claustrophobia

25. **What volume of bile is generated per day?**
    a) 100–150ml
    b) 200–300ml
    c) 300–500ml
    d) 500–1000ml
    e) 1000–2000ml

26. **You are asked to review a 71 year old diabetic man who is currently on a ventilator in ICU. He was admitted with a severe pneumonia. A CT scan has been performed because he has deteriorated. This has revealed gas within the gallbladder wall. What organism is most likely to be responsible?**
    a) *Staphylococcus aureus*
    b) *Escherichia coli*
    c) *Salmonella typhi*
    d) *Streptococcus pneumonia*
    e) *Clostridium perfringens*

27. **A 62 year old man has a cholangiocarcinoma occluding the common hepatic duct and extending into the right hepatic duct. How is this categorized in the Bismuth–Corlette classification?**
    a) Type I
    b) Type II
    c) Type IIIa
    d) Type IIIb
    e) Type IV

28. **Which of the following statements is true regarding cholangiocarcinoma?**
    a) Survival rates are better for distal cholangiocarcinoma compared to intra-hepatic cholangiocarcinoma
    b) Ductal margin status is not an independent prognostic indicator for survival
    c) Parenchymal liver disease such as primary sclerosing cholangitis is a contraindication to liver transplantation
    d) Adjuvant chemotherapy improves survival following resection
    e) None of the above

29. **Several genetic abnormalities have been linked with the carcinogenesis of pancreatic cancer. Which is the most common genetic abnormality?**
    a) *BRAF*
    b) *LKB1*
    c) *KRAS*
    d) *BRCA1*
    e) *SMAD4*

30. **A 20 year old male presents with a 2-year history of severe upper abdominal pain, weight loss, and steatorrhoea. A CT scan shows heavy calcification throughout his pancreas. He denies smoking or any significant alcohol intake. Which of the following is unlikely to be associated with the underlying diagnosis?**
    a) *CTFR* gene mutation
    b) *PRSS1* gene mutation
    c) Elevated calcium levels
    d) Elevated anti-transglutaminase antibodies
    e) *SPINK1* gene mutation

31. **Which regimen is associated with the best survival outcome for a fit 62 year old male with metastatic pancreatic cancer?**
    a) 5-FU/folinic acid, oxaliplatin, and irinotecan
    b) Nab-paclitaxel
    c) Gemcitabine
    d) 5-FU
    e) Gemcitabine/capecitabine

32. **What is the most appropriate post-operative adjuvant strategy following resection of pancreatic cancer?**
    a) Radiotherapy alone
    b) Chemoradiotherapy
    c) Gemcitabine
    d) 5-FU/folinic acid
    e) No adjuvant therapy required (no benefit)

33. **Which of the following is a risk factor for the development of a post-operative pancreatic fistula following pancreatico-duodenectomy?**
    a) Small pancreatic duct diameter
    b) Soft pancreatic texture
    c) High intraoperative blood loss
    d) High BMI
    e) All of the above

34. **Which of the following factors has been shown to minimize morbidity following resection of pancreatic cancer?**
    a) The use of prophylactic somatostatin analogue
    b) Pancreaticogastrostomy anastomosis
    c) Preoperative biliary drainage
    d) Avoidance of prolonged intra-abdominal drain placement
    e) Pylorus preserving pancreatico-duodenectomy

35. **What factors are associated with prolonged survival following resection of pancreatic ductal adenocarcinoma?**
    a) Extended lymphadenectomy
    b) Pancreaticogastrostomy anastomosis
    c) An R0 (>1mm) resection margin clearance
    d) Minimally invasive resection
    e) Extended vascular resection

36. **Which of the following is not a sinister feature in relation to a branch-duct IPMN (intraductal papillary mucinous neoplasm), visualized on CT scan, in a 79 year old male?**
    a) Size greater than 3cm
    b) Development of obstructive jaundice
    c) Mural nodules
    d) Central scar
    e) Associated main pancreatic duct dilatation greater than 6mm

37. **There is a clear role for the resection of hepatic metastases in which of the following situations?**
    a) Pancreatic adenocarcinoma
    b) Lung adenocarcinoma
    c) Breast cancer
    d) Pancreatic neuroendocrine tumour
    e) Oesophageal cancer
    f) None of the above

38. **A previously healthy 28 year old female undergoes a CT scan following a minor RTA. She is found to have an incidental 3.5cm hypervascular lesion with a central scar in the right lobe of her liver. Delayed sequences show increased contrast uptake in the scar in comparison with the surrounding liver parenchyma. Her LFTs and alpha-fetoprotein levels are within normal limits. Which of the following is the most appropriate management for this patient?**
    a) Chemoembolization
    b) Open surgical biopsy
    c) Observation
    d) Hepatic artery embolization
    e) Open liver resection

Extended Matching Items

Liver lesion

A. Focal nodular hyperplasia
B. Cavernous haemangioma
C. Hydatid cyst
D. Hamartoma
E. Amoebic cyst
F. Hepatic cystadenoma
G. Hepatic adenoma
H. Hepatocellular carcinoma

Select the most likely diagnosis for each of the following scenarios. Each option may be used once, more than once, or not at all.

1. A 34 year old female presents with right upper quadrant pain. She has no other symptoms and her only medication is the oral contraceptive pill. Clinical examination is unremarkable. US shows a single well-demarcated hyper-echoic mass on USS. A CT confirms this as a well-circumscribed vascular solid lesion.

2. A previously healthy 34 year old female presents with vague RUQ pain. Her only medication is the oral contraceptive pill. Her LFTs are unremarkable. An abdominal US is reported as showing a clearly defined 11cm lesion in right lobe of the liver. A subsequent triple-phase CT scan reveals a pre-contrast hypodense lesion that enhances peripherally during the arterial phase, with the centre only enhancing in delayed images.

3. A 40 year old female undergoes an abdominal US to investigate symptoms of RUQ pain. The biliary tree is reported as being normal. However, a solid lesion is noted in the liver. A subsequent MRI scan shows this lesion to be vascular with a central scar.

4. A 46 year old woman has a 3cm multi-loculated anaechoic lesion with internal septations in the right lobe of her liver on CT imaging. Surgical resection has been recommended.

Pancreatic cyst

A. Solid pseudopapillary neoplasms
B. Pancreatic pseudocyst
C. Cystic variant of a solid tumour (PNET (primitive neuroectodermal tumour), ductal adenocarcinoma)
D. Intrapapillary mucinous neoplasm (IPMN)
E. Mucinous cystic neoplasm
F. Serous cystadenoma
G. Pancreaticoblastoma
H. Lymphangioma

Select the most likely lesion for each of the following scenarios. Each option may be used once, more than once, or not at all.

5. A 40 year old female undergoes a CT of chest and upper abdomen because of a recent history of right-sided pleuritic pain. The chest component of the scan is unremarkable but

she is noted to have a solitary 7cm septated cystic lesion in the tail of the pancreas. It has a thick fibrotic wall.

6. A 60 year old female presents with non-specific upper abdominal pain. A CT scan is reported as showing a 5cm lobulated multi-cystic well-demarcated lesion in the neck of the pancreas. The lesion has a central scar.

7. A 15 year old female is involved in an RTA and undergoes a CT of chest, abdomen, and pelvis. She is noted to have a 7cm mass in the head of the pancreas. This shows a mixture of solid and cystic components with focal calcification in the wall of the cyst.

Complications of gallstones

A. Cholangiocarcinoma
B. Charcot's triad
C. Cholecystitis
D. Biliary colic
E. Gallbladder mucocele
F. Reynolds' pentad
G. Acute pancreatitis
H. Gallbladder carcinoma
I. Biliary peritonitis
J. Gallstone ileus
K. Empyema of gallbladder

Select the most likely diagnosis for each of the following scenarios. Each option may be used once, more than once, or not at all.

8. A 65 year old male with a recent past history of cholecystitis is referred by his GP with a mass in his abdomen. On examination, he has a smooth, non-tender mass in the right upper quadrant which moves with respiration. He is systemically well.

9. A 60 year old male presents with intermittent right-sided abdominal pain, jaundice, and rigors. He becomes increasingly confused and hypotensive.

10. A 55 year old male presents with acute onset of severe epigastric pain radiating to his back. There is associated vomiting. He is generally tender throughout the abdomen, is cool to the touch, hypotensive, and is tachycardic.

11. An 85 year old female with known gallstones has a 2-week history of intermittent crampy abdominal pain and vomiting. On examination, she is generally tender, distended, and with high-pitched bowel sounds.

12. A 24 year old obese female presents with a brief episode of crampy RUQ pain. The pain has radiated to her right shoulder. She remains afebrile with very minimal discomfort on abdominal examination. Inflammatory markers are within normal limits.

13. A 78 year old man with known gallstones and incomplete calcification of the gallbladder has been losing weight and experiencing vague right-sided abdominal pain for a number of months. He has become jaundiced in the last week.

Pancreatic trauma

A. Placement of drains and closure of the abdomen
B. Distal pancreatectomy with ligation of the proximal duct
C. Pancreaticojejunostomy to the distal pancreas with ligation of the proximal duct
D. Pancreaticojejunostomy to both the proximal and distal segments of the pancreas
E. Pancreatico-duodenectomy with pancreaticojejunostomy to the distal duct
F. Pancreatico-duodenectomy with delayed pancreaticojejunostomy at second look laparotomy
G. Conservative management with CT-guided percutaneous placement of drains if a collection develops

Select the most appropriate management for each of the following scenarios. Each option may be used once, more than once, or not at all.

14. A 12 year old male is admitted with blunt upper abdominal trauma following a bicycle handlebar injury. A CT scan suggests complete transection of the pancreatic neck to the left of the superior mesenteric vein. There are no other organ or vascular injuries.

15. A 25 year old male sustains several stab wounds to the anterior abdominal wall. At laparotomy there is a 2cm laceration to the anterior aspect of the head of pancreas.

16. A 30 year old male has been shot in the abdomen. A trauma laparotomy reveals extensive damage to the pancreatico-duodenal complex.

Biliary treatment options

A. Diagnostic ERCP
B. ERCP and sphincterotomy
C. ERCP and insertion of self expanding metallic stent (SEMS)
D. ERCP and insertion of plastic stent
E. Laparoscopic cholecystectomy
F. Laparoscopic cholecystectomy and intraoperative cholangiogram
G. Open cholecystectomy
H. Endoscopic ultrasound (EUS)
I. Endoscopic ultrasound (EUS) and FNA of pancreas
J. Percutaneous transhepatic cholangiogram and biliary drainage

Select the most appropriate treatment option for each of the following scenarios. Each option may be used once, more than once, or not at all.

17. A 54 year old male presents with painless obstructive jaundice (bilirubin 320μmol/L). A CT scan reveals a borderline resectable mass in the head of the pancreas. The mass is narrowing the portal vein/splenic vein confluence. An EUS–FNA confirms adenocarcinoma. Prior to undergoing neoadjuvant chemotherapy what management step is required?

18. A 40 year old female with known gallstones presents with abdominal pain. Her serum amylase is 1200U/L. An urgent MRCP reveals normal biliary anatomy with no evidence of choledocholithiasis. She has a past medical history of a sigmoid colon resection for diverticular disease.

19. An 81 year old female patient, with a history of congestive cardiac failure, presents with acute abdominal pain. Her serum amylase is elevated at 650U/L along with a bilirubin of 60μmol/L. An MRCP reveals an 8mm CBD and multiple small stones in the gallbladder. Her LFTs return to normal and her abdominal pain resolves.

20. A 65 year male has an episode of acute pancreatitis. No gallstones are present on USS or MCRP. He returns to the clinic 3 months later having lost 5kg in weight. A CT scan reveals a 2cm mass in the head of the pancreas close to the ampulla of Vater.

Jaundice

A. Head of pancreas adenocarcinoma
B. Ampullary adenocarcinoma
C. Cholangiocarcinoma
D. Primary sclerosing cholangitis
E. Primary biliary cirrhosis
F. Duodenal adenocarcinoma

Select the most likely diagnosis for each of the following scenarios. Each option may be used once, more than once, or not at all.

21. A 37 year old male patient is admitted with new-onset jaundice and weight loss. He has previously undergone a subtotal colectomy for ulcerative colitis. His bilirubin is 200µmol/ L and ALT 105IU/L. An MRCP reveals multiple intrahepatic strictures with a dominant stricture at the hilum.

22. A 47 year old male presents with painless jaundice. A CT shows double duct dilatation. However, no gallstones or mass in the head of the pancreas is seen.

23. A 42 year old male presents with painless jaundice. As an 18 year old, he underwent a total colectomy and end ileostomy for 'polyps'. He has not attended for follow-up for at least the last ten years.

Neuroendocrine tumours

A. Glugaconoma
B. Phaeochromocytoma
C. MEN 2
D. VIPoma
E. Insulinoma
F. Somatostatinoma
G. Zollinger–Ellison syndrome
H. Carcinoid syndrome

Select the most likely option for each of the following scenarios. Each option may be used once, more than once, or not at all.

24. A 61 year old male presents with abdominal pain and diarrhoea. On examination, he is noted to be cachectic and has facial flushing. His past medical history includes an appendicectomy and subsequent right hemicolectomy ten years previously.

25. A slim 55 year old female is referred from the diabetologist with new onset diabetes and a painful blistering rash around her mouth and on her hands. A CT scan reveals multiple small liver lesions.

26. A 47 year old male presents with recurrent episodes of hypoglycaemia that are relieved by ingestion of food. Biochemical investigation reveals high insulin levels and high C-peptide levels. The pancreas is unremarkable on CT scan.

27. A 23 year old female has previously undergone a parathyroidectomy for primary hyperparathyroidism and has a known pituitary adenoma. She has been diagnosed with diabetes, has troublesome diarrhoea, and a USS for RUQ pain has revealed gallstones.

Gallbladder

A. Gallbladder polyp
B. Adenomyomatosis
C. Cholesterolosis
D. Gallbladder cancer
E. Mirrizi syndrome
F. Porcelain gallbladder

Select the most likely option for each of the following scenarios. Each option may be used once, more than once, or not at all.

28. A pathology report states that there is significant degenerative change of the gallbladder with histological features of Rokitansky–Aschoff sinuses.

29. A 63 year old patient undergoes a US of the gallbladder which reveals two discrete, elevated mucosal lesions which appear to have a smooth surface. The largest of these is 20mm.

30. Following a routine cholecystectomy the pathology report states that the gallbladder wall was intact, but a polyp was identified with extension into the subserosal connective tissue.

31. Following cholecystectomy of a very abnormal gallbladder, the pathology report describes features of chronic cholecystitis, with widespread intramural calcification of the gallbladder wall.

[handwritten notes: IgG4 — Male 50's. — obstructive jaundice — Steroid responsive]

Single Best Answers

[handwritten note: — may rule out malignancy]

1. d) IgG4

Autoimmune pancreatitis (AIP) is a rare cause of chronic pancreatitis. It has recently been recognized as a distinct clinical entity. It is characterized as follows:

- Clinical presentation with obstructive jaundice
- Histology reveals a dense lymphoplasmacytic infiltrate with fibrosis
- Dramatic response to corticosteroid therapy   *[handwritten: autoimmune.]*

Multiple organs, including the bile duct, salivary glands, lacrimal glands, orbit, thyroid, kidneys, and lymph nodes can be involved either synchronously or metachronously. It is one of the few autoimmune conditions that predominantly affects male subjects, commonly in the fifth and sixth decades of life. AIP is part of a generalized autoimmune condition called IgG4-related disease, a relapsing–remitting condition with a tendency to form tissue-destructive mass lesions in multiple sites. The condition causes characteristic histological appearances in involved tissue.

[handwritten: B-plasma cells.]

The disease is mediated by plasma cells which produce IgG4 antibody, which is deposited in involved tissues. Elevated serum IgG4 may be seen in up to 70% of patients during the acute phase of inflammation. In addition to AIP, it is now thought that IgG4-related disease manifests as Riedel's thyroiditis, sclerosing sialadenitis, inflammatory pseudotumours (in various sites of the body), mediastinal fibrosis, and some cases of retroperitoneal fibrosis.

Obstructive jaundice is the most common presenting symptom of AIP. However, the presentation can be non-specific. There are established diagnostic criteria for AIP, most of which rely on a combination of clinical presentation, imaging of the pancreas and other organs (CT scan, MRI, and ERCP), serology, pancreatic histology, and response to steroids. It is imperative to differentiate AIP from pancreatic cancer.

The condition can be separated into two distinct steroid-responsive pancreatitides, defined by their histopathology, called type 1 AIP (lymphoplasmacytic sclerosing pancreatitis) and type 2 AIP (idiopathic duct-centric pancreatitis (IDCP)) as outlined in Table 5.1.

AIP responds dramatically to steroid treatment but relapses are common. A pancreatic mass that persists following a course of steroids is suspicious for pancreatic cancer. Both AIP and IDCP are corticosteroid-responsive; however, relapses are common in AIP and rare in IDCP. Maintenance therapy with either an immunomodulator (e.g. azathioprine, 6-mercaptopurine, or mycophenolate mofetil) or rituximab is often necessary for patients with AIP. Long-term survival is excellent for both patients with AIP and patients with IDCP. Persistence of a mass lesion following a trial of steroids must raise suspicion of an underlying pancreatic cancer.

Hart PA et al. Recent advances in autoimmune pancreatitis. *Gastroenterology* 2015; 149(1):39–51.

Table 5.1 Comparison between type I autoimmune pancreatitis (AIP) and idiopathic duct-centric pancreatitis (IDCP)

	AIP	**IDCP**
Mean age of diagnosis	7th decade	5th decade
Male sex	75%	50%
Elevation of serum IgG4 level	66%	25%
Other organ involvement	50%	No*
Histology		
Lymphoplasmacytic infiltration	++	++
Obliterative phlebitis	++	+
Periductal inflammation	++	++
IgG4 tissue staining	Abundant	Scant
Response to steroids	~100%	~100%
Risk of relapse	High (20–60%)	Low (<10%)
Associated with IgG4-RD	Yes	No

* *Inflammatory bowel disease is seen in approximately 10%–20% of patients with IDCP but may also occur in patients with AIP.*

2. f) None of the above

Colorectal cancer metastasizes to the liver in approximately 50% of patients and 20% will have evidence of metastatic liver disease at the time of presentation. Hepatic resection with or without chemotherapy is the standard of care for patients with resectable colorectal liver metastases (CRLM). Resection offers the best chance of cure. Modern multimodal therapy, including surgery, has resulted in 5-year survival of approximately 50% and 10-year survival of greater than 20%. Approximately two-thirds of patients will recur within five years of resection and one-third of patients who survive five years will eventually die of their disease. Patients who are disease-free at ten years from liver resection can be considered cured.

The criteria for resectability are based on whether an R0 resection is possible and the size of the future liver remnant. The American Hepatobiliary Association guidelines suggest metastatic liver disease from a colorectal primary should be considered for resection in the following circumstances:

- The metastatic liver disease can be completely resected
- At least two adjacent liver segments can be spared with adequate vascular inflow, outflow, and biliary drainage
- The remaining liver remnant will be at least 20% of the volume of the original liver

If a 70–80% resection is necessary then potential strategies to increase the size of the remnant should be considered. These include:

- Percutaneous portal vein embolization (PVE) of the right branch of the portal vein to induce hypertrophy of the contralateral left hemi-liver, enabling safer right hemi-hepatectomy
- Two-stage hepatectomy with sequential removal of different parts of the liver to enable regeneration between the two procedures
- Combination of staged hepatectomy and PVE/portal vein ligation

Long-term survival is possible after resection of liver metastases and concurrent extrahepatic disease. Resectable lung metastases, isolated extrahepatic metastasis to adrenal, spleen, peritoneum, and portal retroperitoneal nodes can all be resected. *Oligometastatic concept.*

The width of the resection margin is an important independent variable that can influence long-term survival. A wide margin should be attempted whenever possible. However, an anticipated close margin of 1–2mm should not preclude a resection as even sub-millimetre margin clearance is associated with improved survival compared to R1 resections.

Leung U et al. Colorectal cancer liver metastases and concurrent extrahepatic disease treated with resection. *Annals of Surgery* 2017; 255(1):158–65.

Sadot E et al. Resection margin and survival in 2368 patients undergoing hepatic resection for metastatic colorectal cancer: surgical technique or biologic surrogate? *Annals of Surgery* 2015; 262(3):476–85.

3. d) A 'replaced' right hepatic artery arises from the superior mesenteric artery

The hepatic arterial supply is normally derived from the coeliac axis by way of the common hepatic artery. This becomes the proper hepatic artery after giving off the gastroduodenal artery with subsequent bifurcation into right and left hepatic arteries. The hepatic artery lies anterior to the portal vein. The middle hepatic artery is usually a branch from the left hepatic artery, and the cystic artery is usually a branch from the right hepatic artery. *Mirrors drainage c middle (b)left vein. (e) IVC.*

There is, however, significant variability in hepatic arterial anatomy in up to 50% of patients. In approximately 15%, the right hepatic artery arises from the SMA (replaced right hepatic artery) and is found in the right dorsal border of the hepatoduodenal ligament. This region should always be checked for a pulsation prior to transection of the periductal tissue. In roughly 10% of individuals, the left hepatic artery originates from the left gastric artery and is located within the gastrohepatic ligament. These commonly encountered variants can have important surgical implications during upper abdominal operations. The most common variants of the hepatic artery are to find it arising from the abdominal aorta or SMA.

The arterial blood supply accounts for only 25% of hepatic blood flow, with the remainder being supplied by the portal vein. An accessory hepatic artery can be ligated if necessary.

The conventional description of the origin of the cystic artery is that its origin is from the right hepatic artery in more than 70% of cases.

Michel NA. *Blood Supply and Anatomy of the Upper Abdominal Organs, with a Descriptive Atlas.* Philadelphia, PA: Lippincott, 1955, pp. 64–9.

Stauffer JA et al. Aberrant right hepatic arterial anatomy and pancreaticoduodenectomy: recognition, prevalence and management. *HPB* 2009; 11(2):161–5.

4. a) Left bisectionectomy

Liver resections can be considered as anatomic resections, non-anatomic resections (wedge), or enucleation procedures. Anatomic resections are based on the French segmental system. The terminology may be confusing as a formal right hepatectomy may also be referred to as a right lobectomy and a right bisectionectomy, all of which remove V, VI, VII, and VIII. An extended right hepatectomy (also termed a right trisegmentectomy) also includes segment IV. A left lobectomy (also referred to as a left bisectionectomy or left hepatectomy) includes segments II, III, and IV. A left lateral segmentectomy includes only segments II and III.

The ligamentum teres and umbilical fissure is the line of true anatomic division between the right and left lobes of the liver. However, the middle hepatic vein is the line of functional

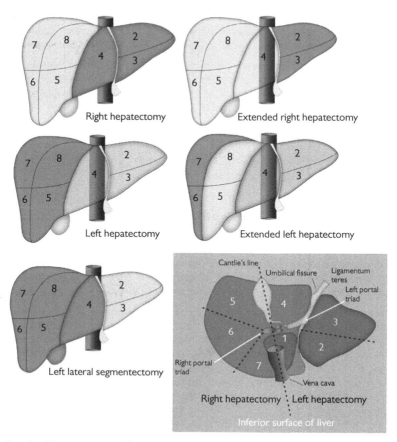

Fig. 5.1 Standard liver resections (anterior and inferior views)

demarcation between the right and left lobes of the liver. This functional separation (Cantlie's line) can be imagined as a plane running from the left side of the gallbladder fossa posteriorly to the left side of the inferior vena cava posteriorly. The left lobe therefore has three functional segments and the umbilical fissure is the segmental plane between the medial (IV) and lateral (II and III) segments of the left lobe of liver. A portion of the left branch of the portal vein, known as the pars umbilicus, runs in the inferior portion of the umbilical fissure. In a left lateral segmentectomy, the plane of the parenchymal dissection is to the left of the fissure, whereas in a right trisegmentectomy the parenchyma is divided to the right of the fissure. Both right and left lobectomies involve dissection well to the right of this plane along Cantlie's line. See Figure 5.1.

5. c) Kupffer cells

The reticuloendothelial system within the liver is primarily composed of Kupffer cells, which phagocytose and process gut antigens from the splanchnic and systemic circulation. These fixed phagocytic cells are located along the lining of the hepatic sinusoids. Along with macrophages, these cells also produce and regulate cytokines and inflammatory modulators forming part of the innate immune system.

Hepatocytes are the main functional cell of the liver and make up approximately 80% of the liver mass. They perform a wide range of metabolic, synthetic, and secretory functions. This includes: regulation of blood levels of cholesterol and glucose; synthesis of clotting factors, cholesterol, transport proteins, and bile constituents; and storage of glucose, vitamins, and minerals.

Ito cells (hepatic stellate cells) are presinusoidal cells that have a role in collagen and vitamin A metabolism. Ito cells are the major cell type involved in liver fibrosis, the formation of scar tissue in response to liver damage.

6. e) Complications include peripheral gangrene, deafness, and endocarditis

Overwhelming post-splenectomy infection (OPSI) is a rare but life-threatening disorder that must be recognized promptly and treated aggressively. Typically, it manifests as a prodromal phase of one to two days of non-specific symptoms such as sore throat, malaise, myalgias, diarrhoea, vomiting, fevers, and chills. This situation can progress rapidly to hypotension, disseminated intravascular coagulation, respiratory distress, and death. Mortality rates may exceed 50% and it may be complicated by severe sequelae such as peripheral gangrene, deafness, and endocarditis.

The infections are caused by encapsulated organisms and can give rise to overwhelming meningitis or disseminated sepsis. Patients are prone to infections with pathogens with polysaccharide capsules such as *Streptococcus pneumoniae*, *Salmonella typhi*, *Neisseria meningitidis*, *E. coli*, *Hemophilus influenzae*, and *Klebsiella pneumonia*.

The incidence of OPSI is higher following splenectomy performed for haematologic disorders and in younger patients. OPSI may occur at any time following splenectomy, although the incidence is highest within the first two years. Daily prophylactic penicillin therapy for asplenic patients remains controversial. The main reason for prophylaxis is to decrease the incidence of OPSI. The duration of, and need for, therapy is uncertain, although many advocate prophylaxis for three to five years, especially in younger children.

7. b) Acanthocytes on blood film

The granulocyte and platelet count are the first to be affected following splenectomy. Then reticulocytes increase. Although a lymphocytosis and monocytosis can occur, these take several weeks to develop. The loss of splenic tissue results in the inability to remove immature or abnormal red blood cells readily from the circulation. Acanthocytes (spur cells) are red blood cells with a spiked cell membrane. Acanthocytes or acanthocyte-like cells are seen with in conditions with altered membrane lipid metabolism, liver dysfunction and after splenectomy.

Pappenheimer bodies are abnormal granules of iron found inside red blood cells. They are an inclusion body formed by phagosomes. Howell–Jolly bodies are abnormal cytoplasmic inclusions of basophilic nuclear remnants within red blood cells. They are seen in individuals who have undergone splenectomy because normally they are removed by a functioning spleen. The absence of Pappenheimer bodies or Howell–Jolly bodies would suggest treatment failure usually due to a splenic remnant or splenosis. Stippling, spur cells, and target cells are all functionally altered erythrocytes that are normally cleared from the circulation by the spleen and thus are commonly seen following splenectomy.

Properdin and tuftsin are important opsonins manufactured in the spleen. Properdin helps initiate the alternative pathway of complement activation, which is particularly useful for fighting encapsulated organisms. Tuftsin enhances the phagocytic activity of granulocytes. Asplenic individuals lack the ability to produce these substances.

The spleen is the initial site of IgM synthesis in response to bacteria. Without this primary defence mechanism, asplenic individuals require increased levels of antibodies to clear organisms relative to the pre-splenectomy state.

Erythrocytes do not undergo maturation more quickly after splenectomy. As part of its 'pitting' function, the spleen removes cytoplasmic inclusions (particles such as nuclear remnants (Howell–Jolly bodies), insoluble globin precipitates (Heinz bodies), and endocytic vacuoles) from within circulating red blood cells.

8. b) The splenorenal ligament often contains the tail of the pancreas

Although the majority of the splenic ligaments are indeed avascular, the gastrosplenic ligament contains the short gastric vessels. Additionally, following the development of portal hypertension, other splenic ligaments may become vascularized.

The tail of the pancreas may be injured during splenectomy because it often lies within the splenorenal ligament.

The average weight of the adult spleen is 150g (range, 75–300g).

The first branches of the splenic artery are the pancreatic branches and then the short gastrics, the left gastroepiploic (which may also give rise to the short gastric arteries), and the terminal splenic branches. The splenic artery divides into segmental branches that enter the trabeculae of the spleen. The terminal branches of the splenic artery may be a distributive or magistral configuration. The distributive subtype is much more common (70% of individuals) and is characterized by a short splenic artery trunk and multiple branches that enter the hilum broadly over its surface. Conversely, the magistral configuration has one dominant long trunk that enters the hilum over a narrow/compact area.

Accessory spleens are common, especially in patients with haematological disorders, and are found in 15–35% of patients. In decreasing order of frequency, they are found in the splenic hilum, the gastrosplenic ligament, the splenocolic ligament, the splenorenal ligament, the greater omentum and mesentery, and the left pelvis along the left ureter or by the left testis or ovary. They have also been identified anywhere within the peritoneal cavity.

9. b) Recovery from acute hepatitis B with subsequent immunity

The pattern of negative HBsAg, positive anti-HBs, and positive anti-HBc assays is seen during the recovery phase following acute hepatitis B and clearance of HBsAg from the liver. This antibody pattern may persist for years and is not associated with liver disease or infectivity.

Vaccination with the hepatitis B vaccine (genetically manufactured HBsAg particles without HBcAg or HBV DNA) is associated with the development of anti-HBs antibody alone.

An acutely infected patient will have antigens (HBsAg and HBeAg) and antibodies (HBsAb and IgM HBcAb). The infected patient will then go on to recover or develop chronic active infection.

A patient who is chronically infected will have HBsAb and HBcAb (IgG) but will also have ongoing HBsAg and HBeAg. These patients are at the highest risk of developing structural liver disease, including HCC.

10. c) Hepatitis A virus

Primary hepatocellular carcinoma is the most common malignant neoplasm worldwide. The primary risk factors are chronic liver disease with cirrhosis (from any cause), chronic infection with HBV or HCV, and various hepatotoxins. 70–90% of HCCs develop within a background of chronic liver disease. Hepatocellular carcinoma can develop in patients with liver disease related to alcohol abuse, hemochromatosis, α1-antitrypsin deficiency, Wilson's disease, and other conditions. Exogenous risk factors include dietary alfatoxins, oral contraceptives, anabolic steroids, vinyl chloride, and certain pesticides. Non-alcoholic steatohepatitis has also recently emerged as a relevant risk factor. Smoking increases the risk but coffee may diminish it. Hepatitis A virus infections not associated with hepatocellular cancer. The mortality rate in most countries almost equals the incidence rate, indicating the lack of effective therapies at time of diagnosis

Forner A et al. Hepatocellular carcinoma. *Lancet* 2012; 379(9822):1245–55.

11. d) Liver transplantation

Extremely deadly.

Hepatocellular carcinoma (HCC) is the sixth most prevalent cancer and the third most frequent cause of cancer-related death. Cirrhosis from any cause is the most important risk factor. Patients with established cirrhotic liver disease should undergo ultrasound assessment six monthly in *Surveillance* order to identify HCC in the early stages when the tumour might be curable by resection, liver transplantation, or ablation. Five-year survival rates of >50% can be achieved if HCC is identified and treated early in its evolution. Patients with small solitary tumours and well-preserved liver function are the best candidates for surgical resection. Tumour recurrence develops in up to 70% of patients within 5 years. In part, this is secondary to recurrence of the primary tumour (usually within the first two years after resection) or due to the development of new HCC in the remaining liver.

Unfortunately, many patients are not good surgical candidates for resection either because of the size or number of lesions or due to the severity of the concomitant cirrhosis and portal hypertension. In these patients, liver transplantation offers the prospect of removal of the tumour and restoration of hepatic function. This is particularly so for patients with tumours which fit the Milan criteria which are as follows:

Tx → Single (solid) encircled Cirrhosis = transplant.

- Solitary tumour ≤5cm, or
- No more than 3 lesions, all less than 3cm *→ >5cm – TACE*
- No vascular invasion *– e.g. portal vein / hepatic artery.*
- No metastases[1] *→ multiple small = RFA*

Although HCC is the only solid cancer that can be treated by liver transplantation, the shortage of donor livers greatly limits the usefulness of this technique in managing patients with cirrhosis and HCC.

RFA solitary *TACE*

Tumour ablation by injection of chemicals (ethanol, acetic acid), heating (radio-frequency ablation *multiple* (RFA), microwave), or freezing (cryoablation) has been used at open and laparoscopic surgery and also using percutaneous techniques. However, the effectiveness of tumour ablation is limited by tumour size and location. Both ethanol injection and RFA achieve total tumour necrosis in almost 100% of HCC tumours <2cm and survival is almost identical after resection or ablation in this setting. Ablative techniques are much less successful when treating lesions greater than 5cm in size.

Trans-arterial chemoembolization (TACE) has also gained acceptance, particularly when used to treat patients with multifocal disease who are not amenable to curative treatments. HCC tends to have a dominant arterial vascular supply, which provides the rationale to treat these cancers through selective delivery of anticancer agents via TACE. Median survival exceeds four years when used in patients with multifocal disease but who do not have evidence of metastatic disease or vascular invasion.

Selective internal radiotherapy (SIRT) is a form of brachytherapy in which small glass beads (30µm) coated in radioactive yttrium are injected into the tumour. The procedure is performed under

[1] Source data from Mazzaferro V et al. Liver transplantation for the treatment of small hepatocellular carcinomas in patients with cirrhosis, *New England Journal of Medicine* 1996; 334(11):693–700.

angiography guidance via the hepatic artery. SIRT has been used in the palliative setting and as a bridge to surgery, potentially being more effective than TACE. The National Institute for Health and Care Excellence (NICE) therefore recommends that SIRT be offered following MDT discussion and that with all patients treated with this technique should be entered into national trials/audit to monitor results.

No conventional, systemically administered chemotherapeutic drug had been shown to improve patient survival with HCC. The introduction of sorafenib, an oral multi-kinase inhibitor with anti-angiogenic and anti-proliferative action, was much anticipated. Two RCTs have demonstrated a significant 30% improvement in survival (from 3 months to almost 6 months). The drug has an adequate safety profile and suggests that molecular-targeted therapies could be effective in this chemo-resistant cancer. However, it is not currently recommended for use by NICE.

In the current scenario, the presence of cirrhosis would be a relative contraindication to resection. Hepatitis B virus-related cirrhosis is not a contraindication to transplantation, which would also treat the HCC and remove the risk of the patient developing a metachronous HCC. Previously hepatitis B infection was a relative contraindication to transplantation because of the high risk of getting recurrent infection in the transplanted liver. However, with the introduction of hepatitis B immunoglobulin and oral nucleoside/nucleotide therapy, it is usually possible to prevent re-infection of the transplanted liver. RFA of the tumour is unlikely to work, given the size. In any event, ablation and resection are associated with recurrence rates of up to 70% over 5 years. Given his young age, he certainly should be considered for transplantation, recognizing that this might not be possible due to a shortage of donor livers, and alternative strategies may need to be considered.

Forner A et al. Hepatocellular carcinoma. *Lancet* 2012; 379(9822): 1245–55.

12. d) Von Willebrand factor

The liver is the principal source of plasma proteins including albumin, globins, and multiple transport proteins including transferrin, hepatoglobin, ferritin, and ceruloplasmin. Eleven proteins involved in haemostasis originate in the liver, including fibrinogen (Factor I), the vitamin K-dependent factors (II, VII, IX, and X), and procoagulation factors, except for von Willebrand factor which is synthesized in the vascular endothelium. The short half-life of factor VII (5–7hrs) enables utility for determining liver failure.

13. a) Cholesterol-rich

Terminal ileal resection is associated with impaired enterohepatic recycling and development of cholesterol stones. The reduced absorption of bile salts results in the cholesterol supersaturation of bile with subsequent cholesterol-rich stone formation.

Bile is composed of bile salts, bicarbonate, cholesterol, steroids, and water. Gallstones are found in 15% of the population over 60 years of age, but only 15% are symptomatic. There are three main factors regulating bile flow: hepatic secretion; gall bladder contraction; and sphincter of Oddi resistance. Bile salts are absorbed in the terminal ileum (and recycled to the liver). Over 90% of all bile salts are recycled in this way, such that the total pool of bile salts is recycled up to six times each day.

Primary bile salts include cholate and chenodeoxycholate. Secondary bile salts are formed by bacterial action on primary bile salts. These are deoxycholate and lithocholate. Of these, deoxycholate is reabsorbed, whilst lithocholate is insoluble and excreted. Bile salts have a detergent action. They aggregate to form micelles with a lipid centre in which fats may be transported. Excessive quantities of cholesterol cannot be transported in this way and will tend to precipitate, resulting in the formation of cholesterol-rich gallstones.

∴ Ileal resection → loss deoxycholate.

Cholesterol stones (15%) often form a single large stone (solitaire) but can form multiple mulberry stones. Pigment stones (5%) are usually small, black, irregular, fragile, and multiple. They are associated with bile stasis and haemolysis. Mixed stones (80%) appear laminated in cross-section. 15% of these are radio-opaque.

14. f) The risk of developing gallstone pancreatitis following a diagnosis of cholelithiasis is <1%

While gallstones account for 35–65% of episodes of acute pancreatitis, around 5% of patients with stones will subsequently develop episodes of acute pancreatitis. Alcohol is the second most common factor and may predominate in certain populations.

The most common drugs that have been implicated in the development of acute pancreatitis include valproic acid, azathioprine, L-asparaginase, and corticosteroids. However, unless gallstone disease is excluded (MRCP, EUS) it is unwise to ascribe acute pancreatitis to a drug cause. *↙ hy percalcaemia*

More unusual aetiologies include metabolic factors including hyperparathyroidism and hyperlipoproteinaemia (types I and V). Hyperlipidaemia is more commonly a secondary phenomenon. Benign pancreatic duct strictures can result in recurrent attacks of pancreatitis. Congenital or developmental abnormalities can rarely present with pancreatitis, for example choledochal cyst, duodenal duplication, anomalous pancreaticobiliary junction (the role of pancreatic divisum is unlikely to be significant). Genetic defects of the trypsinogen gene (*NS9I, RII7H*) and the cystic fibrosis gene (*CFTR*) may also be associated with acute pancreatitis.

Hyperamylasaemia may follow surgical or endoscopic procedures on the pancreas and is usually self-limiting. The risk increases with therapeutic ERCP (3%), particularly sphincterotomy. If there are significant symptoms or signs, then iatrogenic duodenal perforation should be excluded by CT.

Nitsche C et al. Drug-induced pancreatitis. *Current Gastroenterology Reports.* 2001; 2(2):131–8.

15. d) To confirm/clarify the diagnosis

In the United Kingdom it is not current practice to perform early CT for the detection and staging of severe cases of acute pancreatitis. It is unclear how soon the full extent of the necrotic process will occur in acute pancreatitis, but it is thought that it takes at least four days after the onset of symptoms and early CT may therefore underestimate the final severity of the disease.

The British Society of Gastroenterologists advise CT imaging in acute pancreatitis if patients have persisting organ failure, signs of sepsis, or deterioration in clinical status 6–10 days after admission.

The main role of CT in the early phase of acute pancreatitis is to clarify the diagnosis in cases where there is diagnostic uncertainty. In patients with severe acute pancreatitis, particularly when complicated by multi-organ dysfunction syndrome, CT imaging can exclude other pathologies, including intestinal perforation, colonic ischaemia, or a dissecting aortic aneurysm.

Dynamic contrast-enhanced CT can also be used to assess disease severity, predict the potential for complications, and enable clinical trial stratification.

Balthazar EJ et al. Acute pancreatitis: value of CT in establishing prognosis. *Radiology* 1990; 174(2):331–6.

Working Party of the British Society of Gastroenterology; Association of Surgeons of Great Britain and Ireland; Pancreatic Society of Great Britain and Ireland; Association of Upper GI Surgeons of Great Britain and Ireland. UK guidelines for the management of acute pancreatitis. *Gut* 2005; 54 (suppl 3):iii1–9.

Table 5.2 Radiological definition of local complications of acute pancreatitis according to the Atlanta classification

	Acute (<4 weeks, with no defined wall)		**Chronic (>4 weeks, with defined wall)**	
Content	No infection	Infection	No Infection	Infection
Fluid only	Acute peripancreatic fluid collection (APFC)	Infected APFC	Pseudocyst	Infected pseudocyst
Solid ± Fluid	Acute necrotic collection (ANC)	Infected ANC	Walled-off necrosis (WON)	Infected WON

Source data from *Gut*, 62, 1, Banks PA, Bollen TL Dervenis C et al. Classification of acute pancreatitis-2012: revision of the Atlanta classification and definitions by international consensus. Acute Pancreatitis Classification Working Group, pp. 102–11, 2003.

16. a) Acute peri-pancreatic fluid collections (APFC) have a well-defined wall and often contain solid components

The accurate description of local complications, including the presence of fluid or necrosis in or around the pancreas, the time course of progression, and the presence or absence of infection, will improve the stratification of patients with acute pancreatitis, both for clinical care in specialized centres and for reporting of clinical research. In the present classification (see Table 5.2), an important distinction is made between collections that are composed of fluid alone versus those that arise from necrosis and contain a solid component (and which may also contain varying amounts of fluid). Acute peri-pancreatic fluid collections by definition will not have a defined wall.

Banks PA et al. Classification of acute pancreatitis—2012: revision of the Atlanta classification and definitions by international consensus. Acute Pancreatitis Classification Working Group. *Gut* 2013; 62(1):102–11.

17. c) No antibiotics

There is controversy regarding the need for antibiotics in mild acute cholecystitis. In a RCT of 84 patients with mild acute cholecystitis undergoing delayed cholecystectomy randomized to antibiotics versus no antibiotics, there were no significant differences in the rates of cholecystostomy tube placement, readmissions, or perioperative course between the groups.

There is no current evidence to support the use of antibiotics post-cholecystectomy. Both the guidelines of the Infectious Diseases Society of America and the Tokyo guidelines recommend antibiotics in patients diagnosed with acute cholecystitis, with discontinuation of therapy within 24 hours of cholecystectomy, unless there is evidence of infection outside the gallbladder wall. Two trials have evaluated this approach. Regimbeau and colleagues, in a multicentre French study, randomized 400 patients to co-amoxiclav versus no antibiotic and found no significant differences in wound infection rates between the two groups. In another study, Rodriguez-Sanjuan and colleagues randomized 287 patients into three groups, administering antibiotics for different time frames. There was no difference in wound infection rates between the three groups. In complicated cases of acute cholecystitis, appropriate use of antibiotics should be based on clinical judgment.

Mazeh H et al. Role of antibiotic therapy in mild acute calculus cholecystitis: a prospective randomized controlled trial. *World Journal of Surgery* 2012; 36(8):1750–9.

Regimbeau JM et al. Effect of postoperative antibiotic administration on postoperative infection following cholecystectomy for acute calculous cholecystitis: a randomized clinical trial. *Journal of the American Medical Association* 2014; 312(2):145–5.

Rodriguez-Sanjuan JC et al. How long is antibiotic therapy necessary after urgent cholecystectomy for acute cholecystitis? *Journal of Gastrointestinal Surgery* 2013; 17(11):1947–52.

Pathway for the management of acute gallstone diseases, October 2015. <http://www.augis.org/wp-content/uploads/2014/05/Acute-Gallstones-Pathway-Final-Sept-2015.pdf>.

18. e) None of the above

Acute cholecystitis affects 0.1% of pregnant women and, along with acute appendicitis, is the most common causes of an acute abdomen during pregnancy. It is not clear if acute cholecystitis is more common in pregnancy although it clearly represents a surgical challenge because of concerns that surgical intervention (or the lack of it) may compromise the health of both the mother and the unborn child. *High level relapse.*

Relapse rates of 40–70% have been reported with conservative treatment of acute biliary diseases during pregnancy. Conversely, laparoscopic cholecystectomy has been safely performed during all trimesters of pregnancy, but may require a specific strategy for patient and port positioning. The SAGES guidelines recommend laparoscopic cholecystectomy for all patients with symptomatic gallstones presenting during pregnancy irrespective of the trimester. Patients who do not undergo cholecystectomy have increased rates of hospitalization, spontaneous abortions, pre-term labour, and pre-term delivery compared to those who undergo cholecystectomy. There are no published RCTs of cholecystectomy versus no cholecystectomy for acute cholecystitis in pregnancy. Pregnant patients undergoing laparoscopic cholecystectomy should be fully informed of the potential risks, however small, of foetal harm, and only surgeons experienced in difficult cholecystectomies should undertake laparoscopic cholecystectomy for acute cholecystitis in pregnant patients.

Pearl J et al. Guidelines for diagnosis, treatment, and use of laparoscopy for surgical problems during pregnancy. *Surgical Endoscopy* 2011; 25(11):3479–92.

19. c) 0.5%

Cholecystectomy remains the commonest cause of bile duct injury. Reported incidences range from 0.3–0.7% for laparoscopic cholecystectomy and 0.13% for an open procedure. The most common cause of bile duct injury is misinterpretation of the biliary anatomy—most often the CBD is confused with the cystic duct. Similarly, the right hepatic artery can also be confused with the cystic artery. Risk factors include an inexperienced operator, aberrant anatomy, and inflammation. Partial injury may result from a traction injury or diathermy burn.

The concept of the critical view of safety (CVS), pioneered by Stephen Strasberg, facilitates accurate and safe identification of the cystic duct and cystic artery during laparoscopic cholecystectomy.

Three criteria are required to achieve the CVS:

- The hepatocystic triangle is cleared of fat and fibrous tissue. The hepatocystic triangle is defined as the triangle formed by the cystic duct, the common hepatic duct, and inferior edge of the liver. The common bile duct and common hepatic duct do not have to be exposed.
- The lower one-third of the gallbladder is separated from the liver to expose the cystic plate. The cystic plate is also known as the liver bed of the gallbladder and lies in the gallbladder fossa.
- Two and only two structures should be seen entering the gallbladder.[2]

[2] Source data from Strasberg SM and Brunt LM. Rationale and use of the critical view of safety in laparoscopic cholecystectomy. *Journal of the American College of Surgeons* 2010; 211:132–8.

Blind clipping of arterial bleeding should also be avoided.

Some units advocate routine intraoperative cholangiography (IOC) or routine intraoperative USS to avoid bile duct injury. This strategy has been shown to reduce the incidence of injury in operations performed by inexperienced surgeons. However, images can be misinterpreted and injuries may be missed or may occur even before the surgeon performs the cholangiogram. If the anatomy is unclear consider alternative strategies, including fundus first dissection, laparoscopic subtotal cholecystectomy, or cholecystostomy tube placement, with a low threshold for conversion to an open procedure. Where a bile duct injury occurs, and if the operating surgeon does not regularly practice biliary tree reconstruction, then the area should be drained and the patient transferred to an HPB unit. A recent large retrospective cohort study did not demonstrate IOC to be effective as a preventive strategy against common duct injury during cholecystectomy. See Figure 5.2. *Identifying injury – not preventative.*

Shea JA et al. Mortality and complications associated with laparoscopic cholecystectomy. A meta-analysis. *Annals of Surgery* 1996; 224(5):609–20.

Ishizaki Y et al. Conversion of elective laparoscopic to open cholecystectomy between 1993 and 2004. *British Journal of Surgery* 2006; 93(8):987–91.

Strasberg SM and Brunt LM. Rationale and use of the critical view of safety in laparoscopic cholecystectomy. *Journal of the American College of Surgeons* 2010; 211:132–8.

Sheffield KM et al. Association between cholecystectomy with vs without intraoperative cholangiography and risk of common duct injury. *Journal of the American Medical Association* 2013; 310(8):812–20.

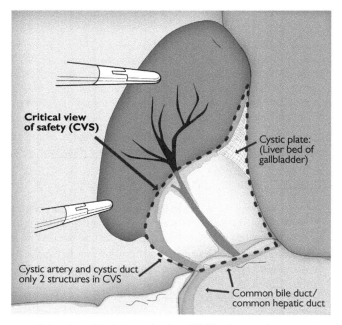

Fig. 5.2 Diagram outlining the critical view of safety (CVS) when performing a laparoscopic cholecystectomy

20. a) Within 48 hours of presentation

In patients with acute cholecystitis early laparoscopic cholecystectomy (ELC) is the standard of care and many studies have demonstrated benefit. A recent large randomized trial has shown that ELC within 24 hours of presentation is associated with significantly lower morbidity (11.8 vs 34.4%), shorter mean hospital stay (5.4 vs 10.0 days, p<0.001), and lower hospital costs (€2919 vs €4262, p<0.001) compared with delayed laparoscopic cholecystectomy (performed between 7 and 45 days after presentation). The 2014 NICE guidance also endorses early cholecystectomy for symptomatic gallstones and acute cholecystectomy for acute cholecystitis.

Where patients with symptomatic gallstones and acute cholecystitis do not undergo surgery, a subgroup of patients will fail to improve or settle and will ultimately require surgery before their planned elective, interval procedure. These patients have a high complication rate and the conversion rate to open surgery in such circumstances may be as great as 45%.

Percutaneous cholecystomy should be considered in patients who are either too unwell or are not fit enough to be considered for acute cholecystectomy. A percutaneous trans-peritoneal or trans-hepatic drain may be potential options. The former carries the risk of intra-peritoneal leakage of bile when the drain is displaced. The latter carries the risk of bleeding.

Gutt CN et al. Acute cholecystitis: early versus delayed cholecystectomy, a multicenter randomized trial (ACDC study, NCT00447304). *Annals of Surgery* 2013; 258(3):385–93.

National Institute for Health and Care Excellence. Gallstone disease: diagnosis and initial management (CG188), London: National Institute for Health and Care Excellence, 2013.

Gurusamy KS et al. Early versus delayed laparoscopic cholecystectomy for people with acute cholecystitis. *Cochrane Database of Systematic Reviews* 2013; 6:CD005440.

21. d) Milk the stone proximally, remove the gallstone through a small enterotomy, and ensure no more gallstones are present proximally

Gallstone ileus is mechanical obstruction caused by a gallstone that has entered the intestine via an acquired biliary enteric fistula. Although gallstone ileus accounts for only 1–3% of all small bowel obstructions, it is associated with a higher mortality rate than other non-malignant causes of bowel obstruction. This is because it tends to occur in elderly patients, often with diagnostic delay as a result of waxing and waning symptoms ('tumbling obstruction'). Pathognomonic radiologic features include a gas pattern of small bowel obstruction with pneumobilia and an opaque stone outside the gallbladder. Rarely are all of these radiologic features present however. The most common site of obstruction is the terminal ileum. Infrequently, sigmoid obstruction occurs in an area narrowed by intrinsic colonic disease or, rarer still, obstruction at the pylorus (Bouveret's syndrome).

Management includes appropriate resuscitation followed by surgery. Spontaneous passage of the gallstone is a rare phenomenon and non-operative management is associated with a prohibitive mortality rate. Stone removal is best accomplished with an enterotomy placed proximal to the site of obstruction. Care must be taken to search for additional intestinal stones, which are present in 10% of patients. Attempts to crush the stone inside the bowel lumen or to milk it distally are contraindicated because they may cause bowel injury. In rare instances, small bowel resection is necessary if there is ischaemic compromise or bleeding at the site of impaction. The main controversy regarding surgical treatment of gallstone ileus is whether a definitive biliary tract operation with cholecystectomy, fistula repair, and possible common duct exploration should be performed at the time of stone removal. This decision must be based on sound surgical judgment and consideration of the underlying physiologic status of the patient and the anatomic status of the right upper quadrant. Up to one-third of patients who do not undergo definitive biliary surgery experience recurrent biliary symptoms, including cholecystitis, cholangitis, and recurrent gallstone ileus. However, only 10% of these patients will require surgery. Furthermore, the rate of spontaneous fistula closure is open to question. While a definitive one-stage procedure could be considered in physiologically fit patients, one meta-analysis has shown a mortality rate of 16.9% for the one-stage procedure, compared to 11.7% for enterotomy alone. Because most of these patients are elderly, as in this scenario, surgical therapy is limited to stone removal in most instances. Interval cholecystectomy should be considered for patients with post-operative biliary symptoms who are physiologically fit. In practice this is an uncommon procedure for the reasons already stated.

Reisner RM and Cohen JR. Gallstone ileus: a review of 1001 reported cases. *American Journal of Surgery* 1994; 60:441–6.

22. d) Single fusiform cystic dilatation of the common bile duct

Choledochal cysts most commonly present in the first 12 months of life. The classical triad (in 50%) consists of right upper quadrant pain and jaundice with a right upper quadrant mass. While rare in a Western population (incidence of 1 in 200,000), the incidence in some Asian countries approaches 1 in 1000. The Todani classification is commonly used to describe type and location of the cysts. Type I are commonest (70–80%) and type IV accounts for around 20%.

A major concern in relation to choledochal cysts is the increased risk of malignancy. For this reason, the usual treatment of choledochal cysts is complete excision of the cyst, rather than simple drainage procedures. Reconstruction of the biliary system with hepaticojejunostomy is usually required. Formal liver resection is occasionally necessary in cases of intra-hepatic disease. Other possible complications include cholelithiasis, pancreatitis, cirrhosis, and portal hypertension. See Figure 5.3.

Todani T et al. Congenital bile duct cysts: classification, operative procedures, and review of thirty-seven cases including cancer arising from choledochal cyst. *American Journal of Surgery* 1977; 134:263–9.

Takeshita N et al. Forty-year experience with flow-diversion surgery for patients with congenital choledochal cysts with pancreaticobiliary maljunction at a single institution. *Annals of Surgery* 2011; 254(6):1050–3.

Ouaïssi M et al. Todani type II congenital bile duct cyst: European multicenter study of the French Surgical Association and literature review. *Annals of Surgery* 2015; 262(1):130–8.

23. e) Leave the drain in place and consider starting octreotide

A pancreatic fistula is characterized by leakage of pancreatic fluid as a result of disruption of pancreatic ducts. Disruption of pancreatic ducts can occur following acute or chronic pancreatitis, pancreatic resection, or trauma. Leakage of pancreatic secretions can cause significant morbidity due to malnutrition, skin excoriation, and infection.

A post-operative PF (as defined by the International Study Group for Pancreatic Fistulas) may be defined as an external fistula with a drain output of any measurable volume after post-operative day 3 with an amylase level greater than three times the upper limit of the normal serum value. Based on the clinical impact of the fistula on the patient's hospital course and outcome, post-operative PFs are separated into two categories (biochemical and clinically relevant) and three grades (A, B, and C). Biochemical (grade A) fistulas, also known as 'transient' fistulas, are characterized by a threshold of elevated serum amylase (>3 times the upper limit of normal serum amylase concentration). These fistulas cause little, if any, deviation from the normal clinical pathway.

Conversely, clinically relevant fistulas (grades B and C) are more morbid and demonstrate deviation from the expected recovery course. Grade B fistulas are typically characterized by any

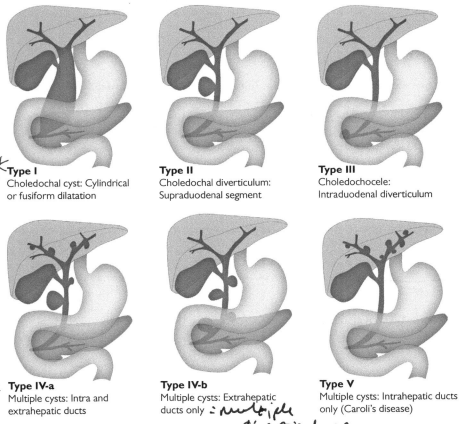

Type I
Choledochal cyst: Cylindrical
or fusiform dilatation

Type II
Choledochal diverticulum:
Supraduodenal segment

Type III
Choledochocele:
Intraduodenal diverticulum

Type IV-a
Multiple cysts: Intra and
extrahepatic ducts

Type IV-b
Multiple cysts: Extrahepatic
ducts only *= multiple*

Type V
Multiple cysts: Intrahepatic ducts
only (Caroli's disease)

Fig. 5.3 Todani classification of choledochal cysts *diverticulums.*

Source data from *American Journal of Surgery*, 134, Todani T, Watanabe Y, Narusue M, Tabuchi K, Okajima K., Congenital bile
duct cysts: classification, operative procedures, and review of thirty-seven cases including cancer arising from choledochal cyst,
pp. 263–9, 1977

or all of the following management strategies: antibiotic therapy, supplemental nutrition (TPN),
therapeutic octreotide, transfusions, maintenance of drains for a prolonged period (>21 days),
and/or percutaneous drainage. The more severe grade C fistulas require a major change in clinical
management and require aggressive treatment. They are characterized by at least one of three
qualifiers: an operative intervention under general anaesthesia, organ failure, or death (attributed to
the fistula).

Conservative management is the key strategy. Intra-abdominal drains are left *in situ* until daily *cloudy*
drainage volumes reduce. Empiric antibiotics can be given if signs of infection are present and *Sepsis*
adjusted depending on information from Gram stains or cultures. Therapeutic octreotide can also
be administered to reduce pancreatic secretions, typically until oral intake resumes. CT-guided
drainage is indicated if a conservative approach fails and the collection is amenable to drainage.
Surgical exploration is seldom required but is indicated when anastomotic dehiscence is suspected
and for patients who deteriorate clinically, often in the setting of a non-drainable abscess, sepsis, or
multi-organ dysfunction.

Type C = anastomotic dehiscence
= peritonitis + sepsis

Bassi C et al. Postoperative pancreatic fistula: an international study group (ISGPF) definition. *Surgery* 2005; 138:8.

Callery MP et al. Prevention and management of pancreatic fistula. *Journal of Gastrointestinal Surgery* 2009; 13(1):163–73.

24. d) Suspected previous retinal eye injury with metal fragments

Absolute contraindications to MRI, including MRCP, include cardiac pacemakers, retinal metal fragments, and subarachnoid aneurysm ferromagnetic surgical clips. A suspicion that there is a retained metal eye fragment should be viewed as an absolute contra-indication to MRI. Relative contraindications include those with severe claustrophobia, massive ascites, or haemodynamic instability.

In comparison to iodinated contrast media, reaction to gadolinium occurs at a much lower frequency. Severe, life-threatening, anaphylactoid, or non-allergic anaphylactic reactions are exceedingly rare (0.001–0.01%)

A very high BMI may compromise MRCP images and prevent the patient from entering the scanner. Claustrophobia and emotional distress prevents acquisition of the scan in up to 5% of patients.

Almost all modern surgical clips are non-ferrous and made from titanium alloys and are not a contraindication to MRI. If there is any doubt, the same type of clip can be easily tested to ensure it does not respond a test magnetic field.

25. d) 500–1000ml

An adult human will produce between 500–1000ml of bile daily. The volume is influenced by the amount of food consumed.

26. e) Clostridium perfringens

Emphysematous cholecystitis is a rare form of cholecystitis characterized by the development of a severe and life-threatening infection of the gallbladder with a gas-forming organism. It is considered a surgical emergency that can rapidly progress without appropriate management.

Typically, it occurs in males aged 50–70 years who may be unwell for other reasons (as for the patient in this scenario) or have another cause of immunocompromise (e.g. diabetes). Not infrequently, the condition occurs in the absence of gallstones. It is also thought that thrombosis of the cystic artery may play a role in some patients. This leads to ischaemia which facilitates proliferation of gas-forming organisms and bacterial translocation in the devitalized tissue with low oxygen saturation. Emphysematous cholecystitis has also been reported in association with the use of Sunitinib, which is used in the treatment of gastrointestinal stromal tumours (GIST). This is likely to be secondary a thromboembolic event which can occur with this class of drugs (vascular endothelial growth factor (VEGF) receptor inhibitors).

It accounts for 1–3% of cases of acute cholecystitis. Radiologically, gas is seen in the gallbladder lumen, gallbladder wall, and surrounding tissues. Rarely, it can lead to gas spreading into the retroperitoneum or even free intraperitoneal gas. Is tends to progress rapidly to gangrene and perforation and without urgent treatment can be associated with high mortality rates of 15–25%.

Clostridia, Escherichia coli, and *Klebsiella* species have all been implicated in its pathophysiology although *Clostridium perfringens* has been implicated in almost 50% of all cases where an organism has been identified. *Clostridia* produce several different exotoxins, the most prevalent being oxygen-stable lecithinase-C, an alpha-toxin which is haemolytic, tissue-necrotizing, and lethal.

The treatment is emergency cholecystectomy and although conversion rates may be high there is no reason not to consider a laparoscopic approach.

Chiu HH et al. Emphysematous cholecystitis. *American Journal of Surgery* 2004; 188(3):325–6.

27. c) Type IIIa

Cholangiocarcinoma is an epithelial cell malignancy arising from within the biliary tree. Immunocytochemistry suggests that most tumours display cholangiocyte differentiation. Tumours may be classified anatomically into intrahepatic (10%), perihilar (50%), and distal cholangiocarcinoma (40%). Tumours occurring at the junction of the left and right hepatic ducts (the most common location) are eponymously referred to as Klatskin tumours. Perihilar disease may be further sub-classified into four different groups according to the Bismuth–Corlette classification system. This is based on perihilar longitudinal extension. Although this is helpful for surgeons who are considering a radical resection, it does not describe the radial extension of the tumour which may also influence decision-making regarding resectability.

Most cholangiocarcinomas can be classified as well, moderate, or poorly differentiated adenocarcinomas. Mixed hepatocellular–cholangiocellular carcinomas have only recently been accepted as a distinct subtype of cholangiocarcinoma.

The majority of patients present with painless jaundice. Most cholangiocarcinomas are sporadic tumours occurring in patients with no obvious risk factors. That said, there are a number of established risk factors including chronic inflammatory bowel disease leading to primary sclerosing cholangitis which has a lifetime risk of 5–10%. Other risk factors include congenital cystic disease of the biliary tree including choledochal cysts, Caroli's disease — *e bruntally* (15% risk of malignancy), congenital hepatic fibrosis, and infection with *Clonorchis sinensis*. *type IV/V* Gallstones themselves do not increase the risk of cholangiocarcinoma. However, long-standing *Todeni'* choledocholithiasis, particularly in the context of parasitic infection, may be associated with *chdedxled* increased risk. Up to 7% of patients with hepatolithiasis will go on to develop an intrahepatic *cyr.* cholangiocarcinoma. Biliary-enteric drainage also predisposes patients to cholangiocarcinoma through bile duct colonization and infection with enteric bacteria. Recently, cirrhosis and viral hepatitis B and C have been recognized as risk factors for cholangiocarcinoma, especially intrahepatic disease. See Figure 5.4 and Figure 5.5.

Razumilava N and Gores GJ. Cholangiocarcinoma. *Lancet* 2014; 383(9935):2168–79.

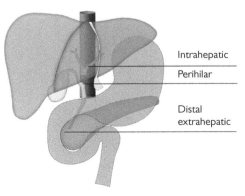

Intrahepatic

Perihilar

Distal
extrahepatic

Fig. 5.4 Classification of cholangiocarcinoma based on anatomical location of the tumour

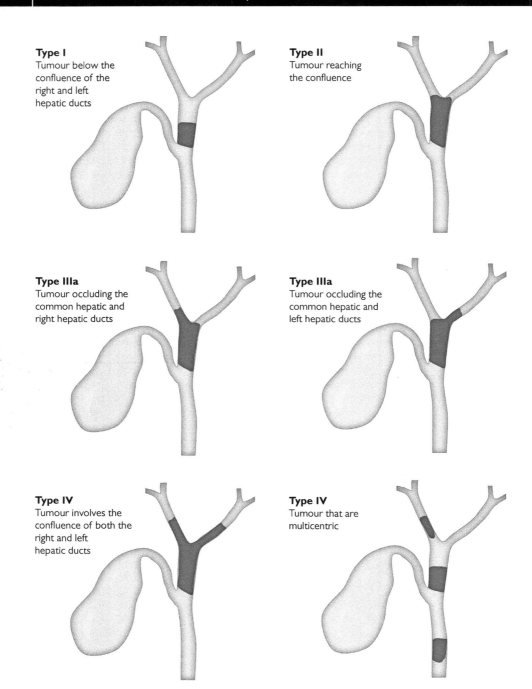

Type I
Tumour below the confluence of the right and left hepatic ducts

Type II
Tumour reaching the confluence

Type IIIa
Tumour occluding the common hepatic and right hepatic ducts

Type IIIa
Tumour occluding the common hepatic and left hepatic ducts

Type IV
Tumour involves the confluence of both the right and left hepatic ducts

Type IV
Tumour that are multicentric

Fig 5.5 The Bismuth–Corlette sub-classification of perihilar cholangiocarcinomas

28. a) Survival rates are better for distal cholangiocarcinoma compared to intra-hepatic cholangiocarcinoma

Surgical resection of cholangiocarcinoma is the only therapy that offers the prospect of long-term cure. However, most patients present with advanced disease and cannot be considered for resection. Of the 10% of patients who present with early-stage disease, those with distal tumours have the best prognosis as these are the group who are most likely to undergo resection (resection rates of up to 50%), whereas only 15–30% of patients with perihilar/intrahepatic disease are candidates for complete resection or transplantation.

Distal tumours can be resected via a pancreatico-duodenectomy (Whipple procedure) and periampullary region tumours have a uniformly better prognosis. Long-term survival rates of up to 30–40% have been reported.

Surgical resection rates for perihilar cholangiocarcinoma are improved by extended resection, portal vein embolization, and associating liver partition and portal vein ligation for staged hepatectomy. However, orthotopic liver transplantation with neoadjuvant chemoradiation is the treatment of choice and is associated with the best outcomes in the select few who are suitable for this intervention. Unfortunately, many patients present late or have concomitant disease that precludes a liver transplantation. Transplantation is only considered in patients who:

- Do not have a locally resectable perihilar tumour
- Tumours ≤3cm in radial diameter
- No evidence of intrahepatic or extrahepatic metastases.

Five-year recurrence-free survival rates of 50–80% have been recorded with liver transplantation. Liver transplantation in patients with perihilar cholangiocarcinoma associated with primary sclerosing cholangitis benefit from removal of both the tumour and the diseased liver as the entire biliary tree will have undergone a field change. Such an approach may also reduce the risk of complications from the underlying advanced parenchymal liver disease (e.g. portal hypertension).

Palliative decompression can be achieved by surgical bypass, or endoscopic or percutaneous drainage and placement of stents.

Gemcitabine and cisplatin combination therapy may be of some benefit when given with palliative intent to patients with advanced intrahepatic cholangiocarcinoma. However, the benefit in advanced perihilar disease is less certain.

Razumilava N and Gores GJ. Cholangiocarcinoma. *Lancet* 2014; 383(9935):2168–79.

29. c) *KRAS*

Recent genomics analysis of pancreatic cancer tumours has confirmed that more than 50% of cases show *KRAS* activation along with inactivation of *TP53*, *CDKN2A*, and *SMAD4*. The frequency of other genes harboring mutations with potential functional consequences dropped rapidly with most <5%.

In addition to increased risk of breast and ovarian cancer, approximately 10% of pancreatic cancers have *BRCA1/2* mutations.

LKB1 mutation is associated with Peutz–Jeghers syndrome, an autosomal dominant disorder characterized by hamartomatous polyps in the gastrointestinal tract and pigmented macules of the lips, buccal mucosa, and digits. Carriers have been shown to have an 11–32% lifetime risk of pancreatic cancer. Mutations in the *LKB1* gene explain more than 80% of Peutz–Jeghers cases.

BRAF mutation is not associated with pancreatic cancer.

Wolfgang CL et al. Recent progress in pancreatic cancer. *CA: A Cancer Journal for Clinicians* 2013; 63(5):318–48.

30. d) Elevated anti-transglutaminase antibodies

Chronic pancreatitis is a benign inflammatory disease characterized by an irreversible loss of pancreatic parenchyma, leading to exocrine insufficiency with maldigestion and ultimately endocrine insufficiency.

Chronic pancreatitis is a highly complex process that begins with episodes of acute pancreatitis and progresses to end-stage fibrosis at different rates in different people due to different mechanisms. Frequent causes include long-term excess alcohol consumption (70–90%), cholelithiasis, autoimmune or individual genetic predisposition, and anatomical variants such as pancreas divisum. Cigarette smoking probably has an equivalent impact to alcohol. In up to 20% of patients it is not possible to identify a predisposing factors or likely cause. The peak presentation of the disease occurs in patients between 35 and 55 years of age.

Normally, if trypsinogen becomes prematurely activated within the pancreas, it is inhibited by *SPINK1* (serine protease inhibitor Kazal-type 1) and then self-destructs or is degraded by trypsin-activated proteases. Hereditary pancreatitis is a rare condition that is caused by a gain-of-function mutation (autosomal dominant, 80% penetrance) in the cationic trypsinogen gene (*PRSS1*), which produces a degradation-resistant form of trypsin. Idiopathic chronic pancreatitis is associated with a mutation in the CFTR gene. Patients can have one abnormal recessive allele, but possession of two confers a 40 times increased risk of developing idiopathic chronic pancreatitis. This rises to 500 times in patients who also have a *SPINK1* mutation. Some patients with apparent idiopathic chronic pancreatitis who have *CFTR* mutations have an atypical form of cystic fibrosis. Causative factors for chronic pancreatitis are as follows:

- Exogenous: alcohol; cigarette smoke; occupational volatile hydrocarbons; drugs (valproate, phenacitin, thiazide, oestrogen, and azathioprine)
- Endogenous: hypercalcaemia; hyperparathyroidism; hyperlipidaemia; lipoprotein lipase deficiency; chronic renal failure
- Infections or infestations: HIV; mumps virus; Coxsackie virus; *Echinococcus*; *Cryptosporidium*
- Genetic: *CFTR* mutation; *PRSS1* mutation; *SPINK1* mutation
- Obstruction of main pancreatic duct: cancer; post-traumatic scarring; post-duct destruction in severe attack
- Recurrent acute pancreatitis
- Autoimmune
- Miscellaneous: gallstones; after transplant; after irradiation; vascular disease
- Idiopathic: early or late onset
- Tropical pancreatitis

Braganza JM et al. Chronic pancreatitis. *Lancet.* 2011; 377(9772):1184–97.

31. a) 5-FU/folinic acid, oxaliplatin, and irinotecan

The standard combination of gemcitabine/capecitabine has been shown to prolong survival in comparison to either single-agent chemotherapy or best supportive care.

Patients with metastatic cancer with adequate performance status should be considered for palliative chemotherapy ideally with FOLFIRINOX, a combination of folinic acid (FOL), 5-FU (F), irinotecan (IRIN), and oxaliplatin (OX), demonstrated by the PRODIGE4/ACCORD11 study. This regimen resulted in prolonged survival when compared to gemcitabine (overall median survival 11.1

vs 6.8 months, p<0.001). While it is associated with significant toxicity it has been better tolerated than expected.

The Phase III MPACT (Metastatic Pancreatic Adenocarcinoma Clinical Trial) RCT compared gemcitabine versus gemcitabine plus nab-paclitaxel (nanoparticle albumin-bound paclitaxel sold under the trade name of Abraxane®). It demonstrated the addition of nab-paclitaxel conferred significant survival benefit over gemcitabine alone in patients with metastatic pancreatic cancer (median overall survival 8.5 vs 6.7 months, p<0.001).

A tissue diagnosis is necessary prior to commencement of chemotherapy. This is increasingly achieved by EUS–FNA or at the time of stent insertion via ERCP brushings.

Conroy T et al. FOLFIRINOX versus gemcitabine for metastatic pancreatic cancer. *New England Journal of Medicine* 2011; 364(19):1817–25.

Von Hoff DD et al. Increased survival in pancreatic cancer with nab-paclitaxel plus gemcitabine. *New England Journal of Medicine*. 2013; 369(18):1691–703.

32. c) Gemcitabine

The ESPAC-1 study randomized patients in the adjuvant setting to receive either chemoradiation (20Gy over 2 weeks plus 5FU) or chemotherapy alone (5-FU/folinic acid). While there was no advantage associated with chemoradiation, chemotherapy alone was associated with a six-month improvement in median survival when compared to observation alone.

The ESPAC-3 study randomized patients to receive treatment with either 5-FU/folinic acid or gemcitabine. While there was no difference in survival between the groups, gemcitabine was associated with a better side-effect profile. This trial also demonstrated benefit of gemcitabine in periampullary malignancies.

Further analysis of ESPAC-3 data revealed that completion of all six cycles of planned adjuvant chemotherapy, rather than early initiation, was an independent prognostic factor after resection for pancreatic adenocarcinoma.

Recently the ESPAC-4 trial has reported that combination gemcitabine/capecitabine is superior to single-agent gemcitabine in the adjuvant setting. The median overall survival was 28.0 months with the combination regimen vs 25.5 months with gemcitabine alone.

Neoptolemos JP et al. Adjuvant chemoradiotherapy and chemotherapy in resectable pancreatic cancer: a randomised controlled trial. *Lancet* 2001; 358(9293):1576–85.

Neoptolemos JP et al. Adjuvant chemotherapy with fluorouracil plus folinic acid vs gemcitabine following pancreatic cancer resection: a randomized controlled trial. *Journal of the American Medical Association* 2010; 304(10):1073–81.

Valle JW et al. Optimal duration and timing of adjuvant chemotherapy after definitive surgery for ductal adenocarcinoma of the pancreas: ongoing lessons from the ESPAC-3 study. *Journal of Clinical Oncology* 2014; 32(6):504–12.

Neoptolemos JP. ESPAC-4: A multicenter, international, open-label randomized controlled phase III trial of adjuvant combination chemotherapy of gemcitabine (GEM) and capecitabine (CAP) versus monotherapy gemcitabine in patients with resected pancreatic ductal adenocarcinoma. *Journal of Clinical Oncology* 34, 2016 (suppl; abstr LBA4006).

33. e) All of the above

The development of a pancreatic fistula from either the pancreato-enteric anastomosis in pancreatic head resections and from pancreatic stump leakage in distal pancreatectomies is one of the most significant causes of morbidity in pancreatic surgery. Leakage increases the risk of subsequent intra-abdominal abscesses, post-pancreatectomy haemorrhage, or delayed gastric emptying. Soft pancreatic texture with a small pancreatic duct diameter is one of the most relevant risk factors for leakage. Other risk factors include older age, obesity, and pulmonary or renal comorbidity. Procedure related factors include prolonged operating time, high blood loss, and the need for blood transfusion, vascular or multi-visceral resections, type of anastomosis, or pancreatic stump closure and stent use.

McMillan MT and Vollmer CM Jr. Predictive factors for pancreatic fistula following pancreatectomy. *Langenbecks Archives of Surgery* 2014; 399(7):811–24.

34. d) Avoidance of prolonged intra-abdominal drain placement

Pancreatico-duodenectomy (PD) remains the preferred resectional procedure for malignant and benign disorders of the pancreatic head and the peri-ampullary region. Although previously associated with high post-operative mortality, service centralization, innovations in surgical technique, and advances in perioperative management have successfully reduced this to 5% or less in high-volume centres. Despite these measures, morbidity rates of 40–50% are not uncommon.

Synthetic analogues of somatostatin, with their inhibitory effects on pancreatic enzyme secretion, have been well studied in patients undergoing pancreatic surgery. Theoretically, somatostatin analogues could reduce pancreatic fistula rate and thereby overall morbidity and mortality. With more than 2200 randomly assigned patients, a Cochrane review identified a significantly lower pancreatic fistula rate and a lower overall number of patients with post-operative complications in the somatostatin analogue group. However, the evidence that these drugs lead to a reduction in clinically relevant pancreatic fistulas is not clear as many of the studies were performed prior to the establishment of consensus definitions of pancreatic fistula. That said, a recent RCT of a new somatostatin analogue (Paresotide) demonstrated a significant reduction in pancreatic fistula rate across all pancreatic resection types.

The pylorus-preserving PD was introduced with the aim of reducing the extent of the gastric resection without constraining lymph node clearance or long-term survival. Several meta-analyses including a Cochrane review have shown no significant differences in major complication rates, long-term survival, or death due to complications. In addition, it does not appear that the pylorus-preserving technique is associated with delayed gastric emptying compared to a classic Whipple operation. The main benefit of the pylorus preserving technique may relate to a faster operative time and a significant reduction in intraoperative blood loss.

Preoperative biliary drainage for pancreatic head cancer might alter perioperative morbidity. A Dutch RCT, which assigned 202 patients to undergo early surgery or preoperative biliary drainage followed by surgery, showed a significantly higher rate of serious complications in the drainage group. No effect was observed on perioperative mortality, length of hospital stay, or median survival. Likewise, a Cochrane review including five randomized studies (one trial with endoscopic drainage and four with percutaneous transhepatic biliary drainage) showed no evidence of benefit of biliary drainage before surgery in patients with obstructive jaundice. On the basis of these results, preoperative biliary drainage should be reserved for patients with extraordinarily high bilirubin concentrations, associated with coagulation disorders, or for patients for whom neoadjuvant therapy is intended.

Controversy exists regarding drain management of patients undergoing PD. Although it seems clear that prolonged drainage is associated with an increased complication rate, length of hospital stay, and economic resource utilization, adopting a standard no-drain policy may be associated with an increased risk of mortality. A recent randomized multicentre trial concluded that elimination of drainage increases severity and frequency of complications, and may have contributed to increased mortality.

Many centres now adopt a compromise position of routine use of drains in all patients undergoing PD, followed by selective, early drain removal in order to minimize drain-associated morbidity. Some centres have adopted a selective drain placement as an alternative strategy.

Because of its clinical relevance, much effort has been made to reduce the risk of pancreatic leakage. Pancreaticogastrostomy has been suggested as a promising alternative to pancreaticojejunostomy. The technique seems to be particularly favoured by smaller centres for patients with soft pancreatic texture and small duct size. Although the subject of a number of randomized controlled trials, it is still unclear if this is a superior technique. Although pancreaticogastrostomy may reduce the risk of pancreatic fistulas, the overall post-operative complication rate and mortality rates are similar for the two operations.

Gurusamy KS et al. Somatostatin analogues for pancreatic surgery. *Cochrane Database of Systematic Reviews* 2012; 6:CD008370.

Allen PJ et al. Pasireotide for postoperative pancreatic fistula. *New England Journal of Medicine* 2014; 370(21):2014–22.

Topal B et al. Pancreaticojejunostomy versus pancreaticogastrostomy reconstruction after pancreaticoduodenectomy for pancreatic or periampullary tumours: a multicentre randomised trial. *Lancet Oncology* 2013; 14:655–62.

van der Gaag NA et al. Preoperative biliary drainage for cancer of the head of the pancreas. *New England Journal of Medicine* 2010; 362:129–37.

Fang Y et al. Pre-operative biliary drainage for obstructive jaundice. *Cochrane Database of Systematic Reviews* 2012; 9:CD005444.

Correa-Gallego C et al. Operative drainage following pancreatic resection: analysis of 1122 patients resected over 5 years at a single institution. *Annals of Surgery* 2013; 258(6):1051–8.

Witzigmann H et al. No need for routine drainage after pancreatic head resection: the Dual-Center, randomized, controlled PANDRA trial (ISRCTN04937707). *Annals of Surgery* 2016; 264(3):528–37.

Van Buren G 2nd et al. A randomized prospective multicenter trial of pancreaticoduodenectomy with and without routine intraperitoneal drainage. *Annals of Surgery* 2014; 259(4):605–12.

35. c) An R0 (>1mm) resection margin clearance

Historically, the lack of a standardized pathological examination has made it difficult to compare outcomes between centres. However, the recent adoption of standardized reporting techniques has clearly identified a margin clearance >1mm as an independent prognostic factor.

Pancreatico-duodenectomy (PD) with major vascular resection has been performed by some centres in recent years. Acceptable outcomes have been reported, despite the technical difficulties in performing this type of resection. However, the survival benefits are marginal and the technique requires further assessment.

A number of comparative studies and randomized trials have assessed the benefit of extended lymphadenectomy including retroperitoneal soft-tissue clearance in PD. A recent meta-analysis suggested that extended lymphadenectomy did not significantly improve survival but patients undergoing this more extensive surgery were perhaps more likely to suffer from delayed gastric emptying. Standard lymphadenectomy should therefore be regarded as the procedure of choice in PD. Similarly, there is no good evidence to support the adoption of extended lymphadenectomy and soft-tissue clearance in distal pancreatectomy.

Grade III to IV evidence exists to show that laparoscopic distal pancreatectomy is a feasible and safe technique associated with lower morbidity and shorter hospital stay compared to the open technique. However, many of the reported case series consist of patients with benign or borderline malignant disease and there is little hard evidence to support its adoption in malignant disease. Despite this paucity of supportive data, laparoscopic distal pancreatectomy is increasingly performed in malignant disease. There is little on the role laparoscopic resection of cancer of the head of the pancreas.

Al-Haddad M et al. Vascular resection and reconstruction for pancreatic malignancy: a single center survival study. *Journal of Gastrointestinal Surgery* 2007; 11:1168–74.

Verbeke CS et al. Redefining resection margin status in pancreatic cancer. *HPB* 2009; 11(4):282–9.

Iqbal N et al. A comparison of pancreaticoduodenectomy with extended pancreaticoduodenectomy: a meta-analysis of 1909 patients. *European Journal of Surgery Oncology* 2009; 35:79–86.

Jamieson NB et al. Positive mobilization margins alone do not influence survival following pancreaticoduodenectomy for pancreatic ductal adenocarcinoma. *Annals of Surgery* 2010; 251(6):1003–10.

36. d) Central scar

An intraductal papillary mucinous neoplasm (IPMN) of the pancreas is a premalignant condition characterized by papillary projections of mucin-secreting epithelial cells, excessive mucin production, and cystic dilation of the pancreatic duct. IPMNs are divided radiologically into main duct-type and branch duct-types, depending on the extent of the pancreatic ducts that are involved. The goals of evaluation are to identify factors associated with a higher risk for malignancy and to determine the anatomic extent of disease. There are four subtypes with differing malignant potential (pancreaticobiliary, intestinal, gastric, and oncocytic).

Progression of IPMN through the adenoma–carcinoma sequence is most likely a slow process, requiring 10 to 20 years. Therefore, patient comorbidity and life expectancy must be considered prior to resection. Main duct-type tumours have a much greater risk for malignant transformation (40–50%) than the branch duct-type. The Sendai Consensus Guidelines identified the following features as risk factors for cancer and as general indicators for resection

- Main pancreatic duct dilation >10mm
- Cyst size >3cm
- Mural nodules
- Atypical cytology

Additional risk factors include high-grade dysplasia, multifocal or synchronous tumours, and increasing cyst size during follow-up. In branch duct-type tumours, mural nodularity or atypical cytology may be more important determinants than size. More recently the IAP Fukuoka Guidelines (2012) introduced 'high-risk stigmata' (recommend resection) and 'worrisome features' (recommending further investigations). See Table 5.3.

A central scar is associated with serous cystadenoma, a benign tumour of pancreas. It is usually found in the head of the pancreas and may be associated with von Hippel–Lindau syndrome.

Tanaka M et al. International consensus guidelines for management of intraductal papillary mucinous neoplasms and mucinous cystic neoplasms of the pancreas. *Pancreatology* 2006; 6:17–32.

Tanaka M et al. International consensus guidelines 2012 for the management of IPMN and MCN of the pancreas. *Pancreatology* 2012; 12(3):183–97.

Table 5.3 The Sendai and Fukuoka guidelines for managing patients presumed to have BD-IPMN

Sendai Guidelines, 2006*	Fukuoka Guidelines	
	High-risk stigmata*	Worrisome features#
Symptomatic cyst < 3cm	Obstructive jaundice	Cyst ≥3cm
Asymptomatic cyst >3cm	Enhancing solid component within cyst	Thickened/enhancing cyst walls
Main pancreatic duct >6mm	Main pancreatic duct >10mm	Main pancreatic duct 5–9mm
Presence of mural nodule		Non-enhancing mural nodule
		Abrupt tapering of pancreatic duct with distal pancreatic atrophy

*Surgical resection should be considered if clinically appropriate.

#An EUS should be performed for further investigation. If mural nodule, main duct features suspicious for involvement or cytology suspicious/positive for malignancy present, surgical resection should be considered is clinically appropriate.

Adapted from *Annals of Surgery*, 263, 5, Fong ZV et al., Intraductal Papillary mucinous neoplasm of the pancreas: current state of the art and ongoing controversies, pp. 908–17. Copyright (2016) with permission from Wolters Kluwer Health, Inc.

Fong ZV et al. Intraductal papillary mucinous neoplasm of the pancreas: current state of the art and ongoing controversies. *Annals of Surgery* 2016; 263(5):908–17.

37. d) Pancreatic neuroendocrine tumour

Resection of hepatic metastases from colorectal cancer provides a clear survival advantage over any other treatments and should be considered whenever possible. The 5-year survival rate is approximately 25% and is as high as 40% in favourable subgroups. This remains the case even when recurrent hepatic metastases are resected.

Resection of metastatic neuroendocrine tumours (e.g. carcinoid, insulinoma, and gastrinoma) can be valuable for controlling the symptoms of excessive endocrine secretion. Experience with hepatic resection for metastases from other GI primaries (e.g. stomach, pancreas, and biliary) or non-GI sites (e.g. lung, breast, melanoma, gynaecologic, head and neck, and renal) is limited, and the results have not generally been encouraging.

Although resection of an isolated liver metastases in a patient with a non-colorectal primary occasionally results in long-term cure, the natural history of most such tumours is such that isolated liver metastases rarely develop. Hepatic resection for direct, contiguous growth of the primary tumour (e.g. stomach and biliary) into the liver occasionally produces long-term survivors.

Tan MC et al. Surgical management of non-colorectal hepatic metastasis. *Journal of Surgical Oncology* 2014; 109(1):8–13.

Hoffmann K et al. Is hepatic resection for non-colorectal, non-neuroendocrine liver metastases justified? *Annals of Surgical Oncology* 2015; 22 suppl 3:S1083–92.

38. c) Observation

This patient has focal nodular hyperplasia (FNH), which is often found incidentally on imaging or during laparotomy. FNH is a benign liver tumour that predominantly occurs in women in the third to fifth decades of life. It is similar to hepatic adenoma (HA), but with important differentiating clinical and histologic features and therapeutic implications. Both occur most commonly in women of child-bearing age; however, HA is associated with the use of oral contraceptives and anabolic steroids and is also seen in certain glycogen storage diseases. HA is usually symptomatic (80% of cases) and is associated with rupture and bleeding in a substantial proportion of patients, whereas FNH is usually asymptomatic and an incidental finding. Furthermore, HA has potential for malignant transformation, whereas the risk for malignancy in FNH is uncertain but probably unlikely. Histologically, HA consists of hepatocytes without bile ducts or Kupffer cells. FNH contains Kupffer cells along with a central stellate scar surrounded by fibrous tissue. Scanning for Kupffer cell activity with technetium-99m (^{99m}Tc)-labelled sulfur colloid is thus useful in differentiating the lesions. Because of the asymptomatic nature of this patient, small size of the lesion, and negligible risk for malignant transformation, observation is appropriate. Surgical resection is reserved for symptomatic patients or when the diagnosis is uncertain.

MRI gadolinium scan → only taken up by functional hepatocytes (handwritten)

Extended Matching Items

Liver lesion

1. G. Hepatic adenoma *0.04%* (handwritten)

Men = resect adenoma (handwritten)
♀ < 5cm : observe X>5cm : resect (handwritten)

Hepatic adenomas (HA) are rare benign tumours, causatively linked to the oral contraceptive pill (OCP). Up to 90% of patients with a HA are using or have used the OCP. Imaging typically shows a mixed or hyper-echoic lesion with a heterogenous texture. Biopsy is contraindicated if HA is suspected due to the increased risk of haemorrhage. The imaging characteristics described in this scenario are typical of HA. Because these lesions do not contain Kupffer cells, they do not take up radioisotope. This helps to differentiate it from focal nodular hyperplasia but not necessarily from other mass lesions of the liver. *Do not gad enhance.* (handwritten)

Hepatic adenomas associated with use of the OCP tend to be larger and have a higher risk for bleeding. Regression does not reliably occur with cessation of the OCP. However, a trial of cessation of the OCP +/− concomitant steroids can be considered for lesions <4cm. Resection may need to be considered in larger or symptomatic lesions or where the diagnosis cannot be made with confidence on imaging alone. Embolization may be useful for treating haemorrhage in a patient who has an inoperable HA.

Cristiano A et al. Focal nodular hyperplasia and hepatic adenoma: current diagnosis and management. *Updates in Surgery* 2014; 66(1):9–21.

2. B. Cavernous haemangioma *4%* (handwritten)

True centripetal filling. *FNH = centrifugal filling.* (handwritten)

Cavernous haemangiomas are the most common benign liver tumour. These lesions can grow to a considerable size. However, they are frequently found as an incidental finding or present with vague symptoms and signs.

Despite their size, the LFTs usually remain normal. US assessment is usually suggestive of the diagnosis and reveals a well-defined and hyper-echoic lesion. Triple-phase CT is usually diagnostic, revealing peripheral enhancement of the lesion during the arterial phase with very delayed central filling. A similar pattern is seen on MRI, which is highly sensitive and specific in the diagnosis of hepatic haemangioma. There is no definite association with OCP use. Clinically they are reddish-purple hypervascular lesions. They are usually separated from normal liver by a ring of fibrous tissue.

Bajenaru N et al. Hepatic hemangioma—review. *Journal of Medicine & Life* 2015; 8:4–11.

FNH liver = Central Scar ; Cystadenoma in
pancreas = Central Scar.

3. A. Focal nodular hyperplasia *o. 4%*

Focal nodular hyperplasia (FNH) is the second most common benign liver lesion after haemangiomas. The term describes lobular proliferation of normally differentiated hepatocytes. Typically, the lesion is centred on a fibrous scar which is seen on MRI imaging in up to 70% of cases.

Lesions are usually asymptomatic and the condition does not have malignant potential. MRI can usually distinguished FNH from hepatic adenomas. It is thought that the lesion develops as a response to an underlying congenital arteriorvenous malformation which may show central necrosis (and hence a central scar) as it increases in size. Once the diagnosis is confirmed, no specific treatment is required and patients do not require follow-up.

Navarro AP et al. Focal nodular hyperplasia: a review of current indications for and outcomes of hepatic resection. *HPB* 2014; 16(6):503–11.

4. F. Hepatic cystadenoma

Hepatic cystadenomas are rare, multilocular, mucinous tumours. Although derived from biliary epithelium, most tumours develop within the liver parenchyma (85%) where they most commonly affect the right lobe. They are more common in females. CT scan typically shows low-attenuation areas within the lesion. Focal enhancement following contrast is also seen. The multilocular/ septated structure is usually visible. They are often diagnosed incidentally on US. Up to 10% of cystadenomas are malignant and distinguishing between benign and malignant disease (even on biopsy) is difficult. Surgical resection is therefore recommended. Treatment of benign lesions is surgical excision (usually enucleation) or lobectomy. The differential diagnoses include focal nodular hyperplasia, adenoma, angiomyolipoma, and hepatic cystadenocarcinoma.

Marrero JA et al. ACG clinical guideline: the diagnosis and management of focal liver lesions. *American Journal of Gastroenterology* 2014; 109(9):1328–47.

Pancreatic cyst

5. E. Mucinous cystic neoplasm *= unifocal*

Cystic lesions of the pancreas are not uncommon may occur for a number of reasons. They can be broadly categorized in pancreatic cystic tumours (10–15%) and pancreatic pseudocysts (90%). Once a pseudocyst has been excluded, it is important to try and confirm the underlying pathology using a combination of imaging +/– cyst fluid analysis.

Mucinous cystic neoplasms (MCN) typically are mucin-producing, septated, cyst-forming epithelial tumours of the pancreas. They have a distinctive ovarian-type stroma. They predominantly occur in women (95%) and in the distal pancreas (97%). Most lesions are slow growing and asymptomatic. Not infrequently, they are identified as an incidental lesion in patients undergoing imaging for unrelated pathology. Symptoms such as anorexia, weight loss, nausea, and vomiting raise concern about the possibility of malignant transformation. Malignancy is more common in older patients and in tumours localized to the head of the pancreas, where there is an increased likelihood that the underlying diagnosis is mucinous cysadenocarcinoma.

There is a significant risk (5–35%) of malignant transformation in lesions with high-grade dysplasia. Surgical resection is therefore usually recommended provided that the patient has no precluding comorbidities. A distal pancreatectomy (laparoscopic or open) is most commonly performed as the majority of these lesions originate in the tail of pancreas.

Multifocality is not a feature and 5-year survival following complete resection of benign lesions is 100%. The 5-year disease specific survival for invasive cancer is 20–60%, which is better than pancreatic ductal adenocarcinoma. Occasionally, MCNs may be associated with an anaplastic carcinoma, which has an extremely poor prognosis.

Testini M et al. Management of mucinous cystic neoplasms of the pancreas. *World Journal of Gastroenterology* 2010; 16(45):5682–92.

Crippa S et al. Mucinous cystic neoplasm of the pancreas is not an aggressive entity. Lessons from 163 resected patients. *Annals of Surgery* 2008; 247(4):571–9.

6. F. Serous cystadenoma

Serous cystadenomas (SCA) are uncommon tumours, accounting for 1–2% of all pancreatic tumours. Typically, they tend to be multi-cystic, well-demarcated lesions and the presence of a central stellate scar is pathognomic and seen in up to 30% of lesions. SCAs can be classified as macrocystic or microcystic (most common) and appear as a solid mass on CT, with EUS demonstrating the microcystic nature (honeycomb appearance). Larger macrocystic lesions can be difficult to differentiate from mucinous lesions and EUS–FNA is usually performed.

Typically, they occur in female patients (75%) with a peak incidence at 60–70 years. Most lesions are seen in the head and neck of the pancreas. They are more common than MCNs (ratio of 2:1). It is important to differentiate SCAs from both MCNs and IPMNs as malignant transformation is exceedingly rare in SCAs whereas the other lesions have a variable behaviour. Asymptomatic lesions do not require resection or follow-up. SCA may be associated with mutation in the von Hippel–Lindau (tumour suppressor) gene. In this case other lesions may be seen on CT including phaeochromocytoma or renal tumours.

Tseng JF et al. Serous cystadenoma of the pancreas. Tumor growth rates and recommendations for treatment. *Annals of Surgery* 2005; 242(3):413–21.

7. A. Solid pseudopapillary neoplasm

Solid pseudopapillary neoplasm (SPN) of the pancreas is a very rare tumour that typically presents in young women (female: male ratio 10:1) and up to one-quarter are seen in children. They are slow-growing tumours that give rise to non-specific symptoms of abdominal pain, nausea, vomiting, weight loss, or a palpable mass. Not infrequently, they are diagnosed as an incidental finding when patients are scanned for other symptoms.

Radiologically, these lesions present as a well-demarcated, heterogeneous mass with solid and cystic components and a peripheral capsule which may show some areas of calcification. The tail of the pancreas is the most common site. EUS-guided FNA or core biopsy is often diagnostic, showing uniform cells forming a mixture of solid, cystic, and pseudopapillary patterns.

They have a low but recognized malignant potential and should be considered for resection in most cases given the young age of patients at diagnosis. Around 10–15% of lesions are malignant at presentation. SPN is genetically distinct from ductal adenocarcinoma and is characterized by activation of the β-catenin pathway, with β-catenin mutations, alterations of the Wnt (wingless-type) pathway, and disorganization of E-cadherin detected in up to 90%.

Farrell JJ. Prevalence, diagnosis and management of pancreatic cystic neoplasms: current status and future directions. *Gut Liver* 2015; 9(5):571–89.

Complications of gallstones

8. E. Gallbladder mucocele

A mucocele of the gallbladder occurs due to obstruction of the outflow, commonly by an impacted stone in the gallbladder neck or the cystic duct. The obstruction causes the gallbladder to distend with clear mucoid fluid. The contents are often sterile as the initial condition is non-inflammatory but secondary bacterial overgrowth can lead to an empyema of the gallbladder. Perforation is also a possible complication of this condition. The following features are more suggestive of other conditions:

- Continuance of pain or persistence of tenderness for longer than six hours—acute cholecystitis
- Fever and chills—infected bile with possible gallbladder empyema
- Jaundice—coexisting obstruction of the common bile duct

As both mucocele and empyema of the gallbladder frequently present in elderly patients with comorbid disease, percutaneous or operative cholecystostomy may be considered. This is a temporary measure, usually performed when the patient is very sick or if the dissection is technically very difficult. This should be followed by a completion cholecystectomy where possible. Increasingly, endoscopic ultrasound drainage using a transluminal drainage system provides a further option.

9. F. Reynolds' pentad

This patient has clinical evidence of ascending cholangitis—jaundice, right-sided abdominal pain, and pyrexia. These symptoms constitute the classical description of Charcot's triad. However, deterioration associated with an obstructed biliary tree containing pus may lead to the development of septic shock with altered mental status (Reynolds' pentad). Urgent decompression via ERCP or PTC (percutaneous transhepatic cholangiography) is indicated.

Reynolds BM and Dargan EL. Acute obstructive cholangitis; a distinct clinical syndrome. *Annals of Surgery* 1959; 150 (2):299–303.

10. G. Acute pancreatitis

In approximately 80% of patients, acute pancreatitis is a rapidly resolving condition requiring little more than analgesia and a short period of intravenous fluid resuscitation. The remainder develop a multisystem illness characterized by a systemic inflammatory response with a variable degree of organ dysfunction. The development of severe pancreatitis should raise the possibility of underlying pancreatic necrosis, although some patients with oedematous pancreatitis may manifest clinical features of a severe attack. Infected pancreatic necrosis is the principal cause of death in severe acute pancreatitis.

The mortality rate of severe acute pancreatitis is around 15%, despite aggressive intravenous fluid replacement, enteral nutritional support, avoidance of prophylactic antibiotics (unless culture positivity), intensive organ support, and a 'step-up' approach to intervention for pancreatic necrosis.

van Santvoort HC et al. A step-up approach or open necrosectomy for necrotizing pancreatitis. *New England Journal of Medicine* 2010; 362(16):1491–502.

Bakker OJ et al. Early versus on-demand nasoenteric tube feeding in acute pancreatitis. *New England Journal of Medicine* 2014; 371(21):1983–93.

11. J. Gallstone ileus

Gallstone ileus is an infrequent cause of small bowel obstruction in general (1–4%). However, it is responsible for up to 25% of non-strangulated bowel obstructions in the elderly. As is the case with cholelithiasis, women are more frequently affected. The presentation is often preceded by a history of small bowel obstruction that partially resolves as the gallstone progresses down the GI tract until obstructing in the terminal ileum. Rigler's triad describes the findings of pneumobilia, small bowel obstruction, and a gallstone outside the gallbladder, usually in the right iliac fossa

Rigler's Triad.

(only 12.5% are calcified). At operation and enterotomy to remove the obstructing stone, it is important to check the proximal bowel for any additional stones that might cause a secondary obstruction.

12. D. Biliary colic

In this scenario with no evidence of systemic insult, pain represents biliary colic. An US scan should be performed. Cholelithiasis is generally indicated by the presence of mobile, hyperechoic, intraluminal objects with posterior shadowing. If these three criteria are not met, the diagnosis is less certain. Gallbladder distention, pericholecystic fluid, a sonographic Murphy sign, and gallstones can all be seen on a sonogram in the presence of cholecystitis. Gallbladder wall thickness is considered abnormal if it is greater than 3mm. The patient does not require antibiotics; however, they should be offered elective cholecystectomy.

13. H. Gallbladder carcinoma

Gallbladder cancer is more common than cholangiocarcinoma. This patient is most likely to have chronic cholecystitis and has subsequently developed a carcinoma on the background of a porcelain gallbladder. Patchy or incomplete calcification of the gallbladder is thought to represent an increased risk of gallbladder cancer compared to global calcification. Jaundice is most likely to be secondary to local invasion into the biliary tree.

Pancreatic trauma

14. B. Distal pancreatectomy with ligation of the proximal duct

Traumatic pancreatic injury is a rare event, occurring in less than 2% of cases of blunt trauma. Traffic accidents in adults and handlebar or direct blunt trauma in children are the most common causes. Given the severity of impact that is required to injure the pancreas, frequently there are associated vascular and organ injuries that require concomitant management. However, children may sustain isolated traumatic disruption of the pancreas from relatively minor blunt upper abdominal trauma. Whereas pancreatic injury is uncommon after blunt trauma, up to 30% of patients who present with penetrating abdominal trauma from gunshot wounds and stab wounds will have sustained a pancreatic injury.

It is important to consider the possibility of pancreatic injury in any abdominal trauma patient as a delay in diagnosis of a major pancreatic duct disruption is associated with significant and ongoing morbidity and mortality.

Although isolated pancreatic trauma may present with the classic features of acute pancreatitis, it is more usual that the symptoms of pancreatic injury are masked by associated visceral, organ, and vascular injuries. The pancreatic injury may therefore only become obvious sometime after the primary event. A CT scan will usually diagnose the most severe pancreatic injuries such as a fracture of the pancreas or diffuse enlargement of the pancreas which are pathognomonic of pancreatic injury, more subtle non-specific signs that should raise concern include the presence of a dilated pancreatic duct, fluid surrounding the superior mesenteric artery, fluid in the anterior and posterior pararenal spaces, and fluid in and around the transverse mesocolon and lesser sac.

Preoperative classification of the injury is helpful (see Table 5.4). Associated organ, intestinal, and vascular injuries will usually take priority and only then can the surgeon properly evaluate the pancreatic injury. Isolated contusions or lacerations that do not involve the main pancreatic duct may be treated conservatively. ERCP-guided stent placement has also been used in both early and delayed management of pancreatic duct injuries. However, if there is a complete pancreatic transection or a major ductal injury, early surgery should be considered.

Table 5.4 American Association for the Surgery of Trauma classification of pancreatic trauma

Grade	Injury	Description
I	Haematoma	Minor contusion without ductal injury
	Laceration	Superficial laceration without ductal injury
II	Haematoma	Major contusion without ductal injury or tissue loss
	Laceration	Major laceration without ductal injury or tissue loss
III	Laceration	Distal transection or pancreatic parenchymal injury with ductal injury*
IV	Laceration	Proximal transection or pancreatic parenchymal injury involving the ampulla
V	Laceration	Massive disruption of the pancreatic head

*Distal pancreas lies to the left of the superior mesenteric vein.

Surgical management options include duodenal diversion, pyloric exclusion, or simple drainage. On rare occasions a pancreatic resection may need to be considered. In the current scenario, the patient has a grade III pancreatic injury and early surgery and distal pancreatectomy is appropriate. Distal pancreatectomy with identification and closure of the proximal duct and drainage is safe and resections involving up to 80% of an otherwise normal gland can be accomplished without subsequent endocrine insufficiency.

It is very rare that a surgeon might need to consider a pancreatico-duodenectomy. In such circumstances, it is likely that priority will need to be given to the associated injuries and consideration should be given to initial damage control surgery followed by a second laparotomy where anastomoses can be completed.

Moore EE et al. Organ injury scaling, II: Pancreas, duodenum, small bowel, colon, and rectum. *Journal of Trauma* 1990; 30:1427–9.

Debi U et al. Pancreatic trauma: A concise review. *World Journal of Gastroenterology* 2013; 19(47):9003–11.

15. A. Placement of drains and closure of the abdomen

Pancreatic contusions or lacerations without ductal disruption are managed by drainage alone. Consideration should be given to early ERCP or MRCP with a view to recognizing occult duct disruption which can be treated with a pancreatic stent. See Figure 5.6.

16. F. Pancreatico-duodenectomy with delayed pancreaticojejunostomy at second look laparotomy

The pancreatic neck is a frequent site of pancreatic injury in association with blunt trauma. Theoretically, Roux-en-Y pancreaticojejunostomy may achieve pancreatic tissue preservation but it is not recommended for the management of acute injuries because of the risk associated with a pancreatic anastomosis and the need to open the bowel. Pancreatico-duodenectomy is indicated for patients with severe combined duodenal, pancreatic, and bile duct injuries. The vascular anatomy in and around the head of the pancreas also frequently precludes attempts at repair of injuries to the head of the pancreas. A Whipple's procedure is a major resection and requires specialist skills. Primary anastomosis of the bile duct, bowel, and pancreatic duct may not therefore be appropriate at the initial laparotomy, particularly in an unstable patient. Consideration should be given to performing a damage limitation laparotomy in the first instance with a view to a second-look laparotomy and performing definitive anastomoses at that time.

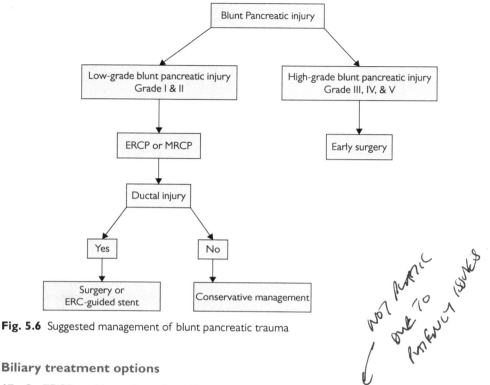

Fig. 5.6 Suggested management of blunt pancreatic trauma

Biliary treatment options

17. C. ERCP and insertion of a self expanding metallic stent (SEMS)

A metal, partially covered, SEMS is the optimal management for drainage of the biliary tree in the context of pancreatic malignancy that is not due to undergo immediate resection and will be managed with neoadjuvant chemotherapy. A plastic stent should not be used as the rate of complications, blockage, and subsequent need for repeat procedure is higher. The use of SEMS is also supported in the palliative setting.

18. E. Laparoscopic cholecystectomy

An urgent cholecystectomy should be performed to prevent further attacks of acute pancreatitis. This should ideally be attempted laparoscopically even in the context of previous abdominal surgery.

van Baal MC et al. Timing of cholecystectomy after mild biliary pancreatitis: a systematic review. *Annals of Surgery* 2012; 255(5):860–6.

19. B. ERCP and sphincterotomy

In patients with mild biliary pancreatitis who cannot undergo surgery, such as the frail elderly or those with severe comorbidity, ERCP and sphincterotomy alone may be an effective way to reduce further attacks of pancreatitis. The patient should be warned that further attacks of cholecystitis may still occur.

20. I. Endoscopic ultrasound (EUS) and FNA of pancreas

Although rare, acute pancreatitis can be the presenting feature of a pancreatic adenocarcinoma. In a patient aged >50yrs, where the aetiology of acute pancreatitis remains unclear, consideration should always be given to a malignant cause of pancreatic duct obstruction. This may require repeat cross-sectional imaging to be performed once the peri-pancreatic oedema has settled. Pancreatic EUS and FNA is often helpful in the context of post-inflammatory change.

Boulay BR and Parepally M. Managing malignant biliary obstruction in pancreas cancer: choosing the appropriate strategy. *World Journal of Gastroenterology* 2014; 20(28):9345–53.

Banks PA and Freeman ML. Practice guidelines in acute pancreatitis. *American Journal of Gastroenterology* 2006; 101:2379–400.

Jaundice

21. C. Cholangiocarcinoma

Epidemiologic studies suggest that the lifetime risk of cholangiocarcinoma for a person with primary sclerosing cholangitis (PSC) is 10–15%. Autopsy series have found rates as high as 30% in this population. The mechanism by which PSC increases the risk of cholangiocarcinoma is not clear, although other chronic inflammatory conditions, including congenital liver abnormalities (e.g. Caroli's syndrome and congenital hepatic fibrosis), have been associated with an approximately 15% lifetime risk. In the current scenario, the recent history of weight loss and a dominant stricture suggests a diagnosis of cholangiocarcinoma given the history of ulcerative colitis against a background of PSC.

22. B. Ampullary adenocarcinoma — *double duct up front... [handwritten]*

Although this patient might have a small stone impacted in the ampulla which might not be seen on *[handwritten: only]* CT, this patient should be considered to have an ampullary adenocarcinoma until proven otherwise. An endoscopic ultrasound and MR would be helpful in the first instance. It is important to try to establish the diagnosis in the first instance and although an ERC, sphincterotomy, and stent might relieve the jaundice, there is a risk that such an approach might preclude a definitive resection.

Adenocarcinoma of the ampulla of Vater is the second most common malignancy of the periampullary region and accounts for up to 30% of all pancreatico-duodenectomies. The broad range of outcomes for patients with adenocarcinoma of the ampulla of Vater impairs the interpretation of clinical trials and hampers clinical decision-making. This is not surprising as these tumours may arise from any one of the three epithelia (duodenal, biliary, or pancreatic) that converge at this location.

However, it is frequently not possible to distinguish a primary ampullary carcinoma from other periampullary tumours preoperatively. True ampullary cancers have an intestinal phenotype and have a better prognosis than periampullary malignancies of pancreatic or bile duct origin. Resectability rates are also higher and 5-year survival rates of 30–50% have been reported in patients with limited lymph node involvement. In contrast, <10% of patients with completely resected node-positive pancreatic cancer are alive at two years. Thus, an aggressive approach to diagnosis and treatment of true periampullary tumours is needed to ensure that patients with these comparatively favourable cancers are treated optimally.

23. F. Duodenal adenocarcinoma *[handwritten: ≥ FAP = colon + duodenum]*

It is likely that this patient has a diagnosis of familial adenomatous polyposis (FAP). The duodenum is the second most common site of malignancy in such patients (after colorectal cancer). Most patients with FAP will develop duodenal polyps and patients have a 100–300 fold increased risk of developing duodenal cancer. However, duodenal cancer is a rare condition in the general population with an incidence of 0.01–0.04%. Although estimates vary, a number of studies suggest that the cumulative risk of developing duodenal cancer in FAP is around 5% at 60 years of age with a median age of onset at 52 years of age.

In addition to FAP and Gardner syndrome, other risk factors for the development of duodenal cancer include Lynch syndrome, Muir–Torre syndrome, coeliac disease, Puetz–Jeghers, Crohn's disease, and juvenile polyposis syndrome.

The Spigelman system is the most commonly used classification to grade severity of duodenal polyposis. This classification describes five (0–IV) stages. Points are given for the number, size, histology, and severity of dysplasia of polyps. Stage I indicates mild disease whereas stages III–IV imply severe duodenal polyposis. Approximately 70–80% of FAP patients have stage II/III duodenal disease while the remainder have stage I or stage IV disease. The estimated cumulative likelihood of patients with FAP developing stage IV duodenal disease is 50% at age 70 years.

Given that it is such an infrequent cancer, evidence is limited on which to base treatment decisions. Among periampullary adenocarcinomas (pancreatic, ampullary, distal bile duct, and duodenal), the duodenum is the primary site for only 7% of cases. That said, duodenal cancer accounts for up to 50% of all small bowel cancers. Overall, small bowel cancer accounts for only 2% of GI malignancies.

The surgical approach to adenocarcinoma of the duodenum largely depends on the location of the tumour. Tumours arising in the first, second, or third part of the duodenum will usually require a pancreatico-duodenectomy, whereas it may be possible to consider a segmental resection in tumours arising from the fourth part. Unlike pancreatic adenocarcinoma, the majority of patients diagnosed with duodenal adenocarcinoma will be candidates for curative resection. See Table 5.5 and Table 5.6.

Table 5.5 Spigelman's score and classification of duodenal polyposis and an additional table of suggested management based on the stage

Findings at duodenoscopy	1 point	2 points	3 points
No. of polyps	1–4	5–20	>20
Polyp size (mm)	1–4	5–10	>10
Histology	Tubular	Tubulovillous	Villous
Dysplasia	Mild	Moderate	Severe

Reprinted from *The Lancet*, 334, Spigelman AD, Talbot IC, Williams P et al., Upper gastrointestinal cancer in patients with familial adenomatous polyposis, pp. 783–5. Copyright © 1989 Published by Elsevier Ltd.

Table 5.6 Suggested management based on the Spigelman's score and classification of duodenal polyposis

Stage	0	I	II	III	IV
Points	0	1–4	5–6	7–8	9–12
Risk of malignancy	0	0	2–3%	2–4%	35%
Endoscopic surveillance	4 yearly	2–3 yearly	2–3 yearly	6–12 monthly	6–12 monthly
Chemoprevention	No	No	+/−	+/−	+/−
Surgery	No	No	No	+/−	Yes

Brosens LAA et al. Prevention and management of duodenal polyps in familial adenomatous polyposis. *Gut* 2005; 54(7):1034–43.

Bulow S et al. Duodenal adenomatosis in familial adenomatous polyposis. *Gut* 2004; 53:381–6.

Solaini L et al. Outcome after surgical resection for duodenal adenocarcinoma in the UK. *British Journal of Surgery* 2015; 102(6):676–81.

Serrano PE et al. Progression and management of duodenal neoplasia in familial adenomatous polyposis: A cohort study. *Annals of Surgery* 2015; 261(6):1138–44.

Neuroendocrine tumours

24. H. Carcinoid syndrome

The incidence of carcinoid tumours is estimated to be 1–2 per 100,000. These tumours are usually slow-growing tumours and are diagnosed as an incidental finding at appendicectomy or autopsy (incidence approx. 8%). More than 90% of carcinoid tumours originate in the appendix or terminal ileum (the embryologic midgut), although they can arise from any cells of the amine precursor uptake and decarboxylation (APUD) endocrine system including sites in the colorectum and lung.

Around 30% of tumours produce hormones such as serotonin, histamine, dopamine, and prostaglandins. Serotonin is the most commonly produced hormone. It is inactivated in the liver and lungs and transformed to 5-hydroxyindoleacetic acid (5-HIAA) which can be measured in the urine to aid diagnosis. Serum chromogranin A can also be helpful. Tumours are staged using a combination of CT/MRI and octreoscan.

The release of serotonin and other vasoactive hormones is the reason patients may develop carcinoid syndrome (5% of cases) with facial flushing, diarrhoea, bronchospasm, and valvular heart disease. Carcinoid syndrome occurs only after the primary tumour has metastasized, as the liver breaks down the secretory products of tumours restricted to the portal system. Carcinoid syndrome is more common with tumours of the small bowel. The rule of thirds states that a third of tumours are multiple, a third may have a second malignancy, and a third will metastasize.

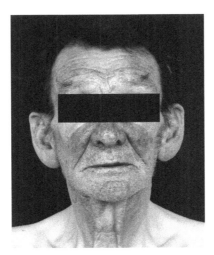

Fig. 5.7 Facial flushing and cachexia in a patient with Carcinoid syndrome.

25. A. Glugaconoma

A glucagonoma is a rare neuroendocrine tumour (1 in 20 million) arising from the alpha cells of the pancreas. Glucagon has the opposite action to insulin and raises blood glucose levels by increasing gluconeogenesis and lipolysis. Patients with glucagon-secreting tumours develop diabetes, anaemia, weight loss, venous thrombosis (especially pulmonary embolism), glossitis, and a characteristic cutaneous lesion known as necrolytic migratory erythema.

In the majority of cases (approx. 80%) the glucagonoma is malignant and in half of these cases metastases are present at diagnosis. Treatment is directed at achieving as complete a resection as possible. Post-operatively, chemotherapy with dacarbazine or streptozocin may be useful for residual or recurrent disease. Everolimus has been approved for progressive neuroendocrine tumours that are metastatic or unresectable, along with Sunitinib and Lanreotide (a long-acting octreotide depot).

26. E. Insulinoma

This patient presents with Whipple's triad of fasting or exercise-induced hypoglycaemia, symptoms of hypoglycaemia at the time of the low glucose level, and relief of symptoms following glucose administration. The presence of these three criteria raises the possibility of an insulinoma. The biochemical diagnosis of insulinoma is based on the findings of fasting hypoglycaemia (<2.8 mmol/L) and hyperinsulinaemia (>6μU/mL). The use of tolbutamide or leucine as a provocative test to release insulin may be dangerous and is not required. C-peptide is cleaved from insulin before its release and determining C-peptide levels may be useful to exclude factitious hyperinsulinaemia. In organic hyperinsulinism, serial blood sampling after giving oral glucose followed by a period of fasting will demonstrate persistent hypoglycaemia and hyperinsulinaemia. When reactive hypoglycaemia is present, insulin levels initially rise and glucose levels fall, but the levels become normal after several hours. Most insulinomas are small (<2cm) and usually benign (up to 90%). Arteriography or selective venous sampling may provide useful preoperative localization. EUS and intraoperative ultrasonography can also aid in identification. See Table 5.7.

Tucker ON et al. The management of insulinoma. *British Journal of Surgery* 2006; 93:264–75.

Okabayashi T et al. Diagnosis and management of insulinoma. *World Journal of Gastroenterology* 2013; 19(6):829–37.

Table 5.7 Comparison of traditional and current criteria for the diagnosis of insulinoma

Traditional diagnosis of insulinoma	Current consensus (following a 72hr fast)
Low plasma glucose (glucose <2.8mmol/L)	Low plasma glucose (glucose <2.8mmol/L)
Hypoglycaemic symptoms	Insulin >5mIU/L (36pmol/L)
Prompt relief of hypoglycaemic symptoms with IV glucose	C-peptide >0.6ng/ml (0.2nmol/L)
	Insulin/C-peptide ratio <1.0
	Proinsulin cut-off level: 20pmol/L
	Absence of sulphonylurea (metabolites) in plasma or urine

27. F. Somatostatinoma

Somatostatinoma is a rare neuroendocrine tumour (1 in 40 million) arising from either the pancreas or gastrointestinal tract. These tumours are characterized by excessive secretion of the hormone somatostatin. Somatostatin is normally secreted by delta cells present in the pyloric antrum, duodenum, and pancreatic islets. Its serves as the 'brake' on the GI tract, inhibiting the secretion of many hormones. The generalized inhibition of gastrointestinal hormones leads to a reduction in gallbladder contractility, reduced pancreatic exocrine function, and impaired intestinal secretion/motility. These tumours can cause:

- diabetes mellitus (by inhibiting insulin secretion)
- cholelithiasis (by inhibiting cholecystokinin (CCK) and reducing gallbladder contractility
- steatorrhoea and diarrhoea (inhibition of CCK and secretin)
- weight loss/malabsorption (combination of actions)
- hypochlorhydria/achlorhydria (inhibition of gastrin)

Somatostatin reduces insulin secretion resulting in diminished glucose use and overproduction of glucose in the liver. The associated inhibitory syndrome leads to the development of diabetes mellitus in the majority of patients. Cholelithiasis and biliary tract disease occurs in 25–70% of patients due to suppression of CCK, inhibition of biliary motility, and altered fat metabolism. Diarrhoea and steatorrheoa are common symptoms of pancreatic somatostatin tumours and contribute to weight loss. In most patients, hypochlorhydria or achlorhydria occurs because of inhibited gastric acid secretion.

Most somatostatinomas are sporadic although a small proportion occur in association with MEN 1 syndrome. MEN 1 leads to the development of tumours of the parathyroid, pituitary, and pancreas glands. Adenomas and hyperplasia of the thyroid and adrenal glands may also occur. Neurofibromatosis and phaeochromocytoma are associated with the duodenal form of somatostatinoma.

Most patients have evidence of metastatic disease at the time of presentation. Post-operative 5-year survival rates of 30–60% have been reported for such patients. However, 5-year survival rates approaching 100% have been reported following resection of localized tumours when there is no evidence of metastatic disease.

Williamson JM et al. Pancreatic and peripancreatic somatostatinomas. *Annals of the Royal College of Surgeons of England* 2011; 93(5):356–60.

Yao JC et al. Everolimus for advanced pancreatic neuroendocrine tumours. *New England Journal of Medicine* 2011; 364(6):514–23.

Raymond E et al. Sunitinib malate for the treatment of pancreatic neuroendocrine tumours. *New England Journal of Medicine* 2011; 364(6):501–13.

Caplin ME et al. Lanreotide in metastatic enteropancreatic neuroendocrine tumours. *New England Journal of Medicine* 2014; 371(3):224–33.

Gallbladder

28. B. Adenomyomatosis

Adenomyomatosis of the gallbladder is a benign, degenerative condition characterized by the development of hyperplastic proliferation of the mucosa of the gallbladder wall. The mucosa becomes invaginated and develops diverticulae, which may penetrate into a thickened muscular layer: the so-called Rokitansky–Aschoff sinuses. *see this also on pathology reports – Pathognomonic of*

It is not related to inflammation or neoplasia. Approximately 50% of patients with this condition also have cholelithiasis and cholecystitis but this does not appear to be a causal relationship. *adenomyomatosis* Both adenomyomatosis and cholesterolosis may be associated with abnormalities on functional imaging of the gallbladder, such as dysmotility or hyperconcentration. For the most part, however, adenomyomatosis does not cause any symptoms and it is usually identified as an incidental finding either on ultrasonography performed for suspected gallstones or after histologic examination of surgical gallbladder specimens.

29. A. Gallbladder polyp

Polypoid lesions of the gallbladder may be benign, premalignant, or malignant. Inflammatory polyps and cholesterol polyps are benign, non-neoplastic lesions. Benign adenomas have a malignant potential similar to adenomas arising in other areas of the GI tract. Polypoid lesions are typically diagnosed by US imaging or CT. Cholecystectomy should be considered for symptoms or due to the risk of malignancy. *GB polyp <1cm = 6/12 US ; >1cm or <1cm = PX*

Malignant transformation in gallbladder polyps occurs more commonly in patients aged >50 years. *lap. live* Solitary, sessile, hypoechogenic polyps also appear to be more likely to undergo malignant transformation. However, polyp size is the single most important risk factor. Polyps <1cm are felt to be low risk and can be monitored with 6–12-monthly US to detect growth. The risk of malignant transformation is not insignificant for lesions >15mm. Therefore, cholecystectomy is performed if the patient has biliary tract symptoms (regardless of polyp size or the presence or absence of gallstones) or if the lesion is >10mm. The threshold for intervention should also be lower in older patients given the increased risk.

30. D. Gallbladder cancer

Gallbladder cancer represents 2% of all cancers and is associated with gallstones in 90% of cases. 60% of tumours are located in the fundus. Complete surgical resection of the tumour with clear margins is the goal of surgery in these patients. Traditional teaching suggests that simple cholecystectomy is acceptable management for stage T1a disease that is confined to the lamina propria. Tumours of stage T1b or higher (in the absence of overt metastatic disease) require a partial hepatectomy, regional lymphadenectomy, and cystic duct resection (with frozen section of margins intra-operatively), as well as a common bile duct resection with biliary-enteric reconstruction if the tumour is directly invading the CBD.

A partial hepatectomy of the gallbladder fossa can range from a wedge resection to an extended right hepatectomy depending on the extent of disease and surgeon preference. The extent of lymphadenectomy can also vary. A lymphadenectomy will usually include resection of nodes in the hepatico-duodenal ligament, whereas resection of involved lymph nodes at the coeliac axis and retro-pancreatic areas may also be required. *5,8,17,19*

nodes 12 x 13

A 2010 paper from the Memorial Sloan Kettering Cancer Center group, which evaluated the extent of resection and benefit to patients, found that major hepatectomy and CBD resection were sometimes performed when the extent of disease did not necessitate this. They also reported that major hepatic and biliary resections are associated with significant morbidity, which did not seem to justify the marginal improvement in outcome with aggressive resection. They concluded that resection of segment IVb and V should be adequate in the majority of patients. Major hepatectomies should only be performed in fit patients with tumour involving inflow structures. Overall survival is less than 10% at 5 years although an R0 resection with negative nodes can be associated with prolonged disease-specific survival.

Rocha FG et al. Hilar cholangiocarcinoma: the Memorial Sloan Kettering Cancer Center experience. *Journal of Hepato–Biliary–Pancreatic Sciences* 2010; 17(4):490–6.

31. F. Porcelain gallbladder

An abdominal radiograph revealing an incidental calcified lesion in the region of the gallbladder usually suggests the diagnosis. Patients with a porcelain gallbladder are often asymptomatic but are at increased risk of developing gallbladder cancer, which has a poor prognosis.

The incidence of a calcified gallbladder at autopsy ranges from 0.06–0.08% and is more common in females (male:female ratio 1:5). The risk of gallbladder malignancy associated with a porcelain gallbladder remains unclear, with reports ranging from 0–62%. However, it has recently been suggested that the risk of cancer in a porcelain gallbladder has been overstated.

The pattern of calcification may be particularly important in predicting which patients are at increased risk for malignancy. Selective mucosal or incomplete calcification of the gallbladder wall appears to have a higher risk compared to complete gallbladder wall calcification.

D'Angelica M et al. Analysis of the Extent of Resection for Adenocarcinoma of the gallbladder. *Annals of Surgical Oncology* 2009; 16:806–16.

Stephen AE and Berger DL. Carcinoma in the porcelain gallbladder: a relationship revisited. *Surgery* 2001; 129(6):699–703.

Complete calcification = less likely to be truly dystrophic

Single Best Answers

1. Which microorganism is responsible for Chagas disease?

a) *Clostridium botulinum*
b) *Trypanosoma cruzi*
c) *Trypanosoma brucei*
d) *Onchocerca volvulus*
e) *Strongyloides stercoralis*

2. A 45 year old man presents with chest pain and shock after forceful vomiting. A chest X-ray shows a left-sided pleural effusion. What is the most likely diagnosis?

a) Myocardial infarction
b) Mallory–Weiss tear
c) Lower respiratory tract infection
d) Perforated peptic ulcer
e) Boerhaave's syndrome

3. A 70 year old lady complains of abdominal fullness and severe post-prandial pain which comes on 30 minutes after eating. Some hours later, she gets projectile bilious vomiting which relieves the pain. She had a gastrojejunostomy for peptic gastric outlet obstruction six months previously. What is the most likely diagnosis?

a) GORD
b) Stenosis of the gastrojejunostomy
c) Dumping syndrome
d) Chronic afferent loop syndrome
e) Bacterial overgrowth

4. **A 65 year old diabetic is admitted acutely to hospital with diabetic ketoacidosis, hypotension, and complaining of severe retrosternal chest pain and regurgitation of food. An OGD demonstrates black discolouration of the distal oesophageal mucosa. What is the most likely diagnosis?**
   a) Reflux oesophagitis
   b) Gurvit's syndrome
   c) Barrett's oesophagus
   d) Boerhaave's syndrome
   e) Oesophageal melanosis

5. **What is the most reliable predictor of good outcome following anti-reflux surgery?**
   a) DeMeester score <18
   b) Lower oesophageal sphincter competence
   c) Good clinical response to acid suppression therapy
   d) Normal manometry
   e) BMI <35
   f) None of the above

6. **What is the most appropriate next course of action following an unsuccessful endoscopic attempt to control an actively bleeding duodenal ulcer?**
   a) Laparotomy and under-running of ulcer
   b) Omeprazole infusion
   c) Angioembolization
   d) CT angiography
   e) Gastric lavage and repeat endoscopy

7. **Which of the following prognostic factors is the most important predictor of cancer-specific survival in cases of gastric GIST?**
   a) Lymph node status
   b) Size of tumour
   c) Tumour grade
   d) Lymphovascular invasion
   e) Perineural invasion

8. **A 58 year old male is diagnosed with a gastric GIST. Staging CT of the thorax, abdomen, and pelvis demonstrates multiple bilobar liver lesions consistent with metastatic disease. Which of the following is the most appropriate management?**
    a) Chemotherapy
    b) Radiotherapy
    c) Combined chemoradiotherapy
    d) Imatinib
    e) Bevacizumb
    f) Cetuximab

9. **A 60 year old female is diagnosed with a primary gastric MALT lymphoma. Staging confirms this as a single lesion confined to the stomach with no obvious serosal penetration or nodal involvement. What is the most appropriate treatment?**
    a) Eradication of *H. pylori* and repeat biopsies in six months
    b) Surgical resection by distal gastrectomy
    c) CHOP chemotherapy regimen
    d) CHOP chemotherapy regimen and rituximab
    e) Targeted radiotherapy to the lesion
    f) Total gastrectomy

10. **A 47 year old male with chronic GORD has a short segment of flat, circumferential Barrett's on OGD. Biopsies are reported as showing low-grade dysplasia. What is the most appropriate next step in management?**
    a) Repeat OGD and biopsies in three months
    b) Repeat OGD and biopsies in six months
    c) Endoscopic mucosal resection
    d) Radiofrequency ablation
    e) Daily omeprazole and aspirin then repeat OGD and biopsies in 12 months

11. **Hereditary diffuse gastric carcinoma syndrome (HDGC) is associated with a germline mutation in which of the following genes?**
    a) *APC*
    b) *STK11/LKB1*
    c) *PTEN*
    d) *SMAD4*
    e) *CDH1*

12. **A 65 year old lady undergoes an OGD for symptoms of dysphagia and weight loss. An exophytic, ulcerated lesion is noted immediately proximal to the oesophagogastric junction. What is the minimum number of biopsies required for diagnosis?**
    a) 2
    b) 4
    c) 6
    d) 12
    e) 16

13. **A 55 year old lady undergoes an OGD for persistent dyspeptic symptoms despite taking omeprazole for 2 years. At endoscopy a 4mm single polypoid lesion is noted within the gastric body. What is the most likely diagnosis?**
    a) Fundic gland polyp
    b) Hamartoma
    c) Hyperplastic polyp
    d) Adenomatous polyp
    e) Early gastric cancer
    f) None of the above

14. **Which of the following is *not* a recognized risk factor for the development of gastric adenocarcinoma?**
    a) *STK11/LKB1* gene germline mutation
    b) *Helicobacter pylori* infection
    c) EBV infection
    d) Smoking
    e) Alcohol consumption

15. **A 72 year old male undergoes an Ivor–Lewis oesophagectomy with 2-field lymphadenectomy for a lower-third oesophageal adenocarcinoma. Which of the following lymph-node groups will not be resected as a component of this procedure?**
    a) Splenic
    b) Subcarinal
    c) Brachiocephalic
    d) Coeliac
    e) Right paratracheal

16. **A 59 year old male undergoes an Ivor–Lewis oesophagectomy for a middle-third T3 N1 oesophageal adenocarcinoma. On the seventh post-operative day he develops a pyrexia and tachycardia following commencement of oral feeding the previous day. A gastrograffin swallow is performed which shows a leak of contrast from the oesophagogastric anastomosis into the right pleural cavity. He has a feeding jejunostomy *in situ*. What is the optimum management?**

    a) Insertion of a self-expanding oesophageal stent over the anastomosis

    b) Return to theatre for exploration and resuturing of anastomotic dehiscence

    c) Conservative management with pleural drainage, antibiotics, NG suction, and total parenteral nutrition

    d) Conservative management with pleural drainage, antibiotics, NG suction, and enteral nutrition through feeding jejunostomy

    e) OGD and application of an endoclip over the anastomotic dehiscence

17. **A 62 year old female undergoes an EMR of a gastric lesion. Pathology reveals a T1 gastric adenocarcinoma. The lesion is 35mm in diameter with lymphovascular invasion and an undifferentiated phenotype. What is the risk of lymphatic spread?**

    a) 1%

    b) 4%

    c) 7%

    d) 12%

    e) 15%

18. **A 60 year old man undergoes a D2 total gastrectomy and Roux-en-Y reconstruction for an adenocarcinoma of the gastric body. On the second post-operative day, he is noted to have 600ml of bile in a drain that was placed in front of the duodenal stump. He has a feeding jejunostomy *in situ*. What is the most appropriate management plan?**

    a) Stop enteral feeding through feeding jejunostomy and commence TPN

    b) Octreotide

    c) Immediate reoperation

    d) Continue enteral feeding and monitor output from drain over 48hr with a return to theatre if output remains >500ml/day

    e) Continue enteral feeding and commence broad-spectrum IV antibiotics

19. **A 67 year old male has been diagnosed with an adenocarcinoma of the oesophagogastric junction. Following staging investigations, the centre of the tumour is noted to be 1.5cm below the cardia. How would this tumour be classified?**
    a) Type I junctional tumour
    b) Type II junctional tumour
    c) Type III junctional tumour
    d) Type IV junctional tumour
    e) Not a junctional tumour

20. **A 74 year old male undergoes a transhiatal oesophagectomy for a lower-third oesophageal adenocarcinoma. Pathological analysis reports an R1 resection at the circumferential margin. At what distance will cancer cells be noted to the circumferential margin?**
    a) Involving margin
    b) Within 5mm
    c) Within 2mm
    d) Within 1mm
    e) Within 0.5mm

21. **A 60 year old man undergoes an OGD for dysphagia. An exophytic mass which is highly suspicious for an adenocarcinoma is seen just above the OG junction. It is not possible to pass the endoscope through the area. What is the most appropriate next step in his management?**
    a) Dilate the stricture using a balloon dilator to allow passage of the scope, biopsy the lesion and arrange staging investigations
    b) Dilate the stricture using a Savaray–Gilliard dilator to allow passage of the scope, biopsy the lesion, and arrange staging investigations
    c) Biopsy the lesion, remove the endoscope, and arrange staging investigations
    d) Stop the OGD, admit, and arrange for a gastrostomy tube to be placed
    e) Stop the OGD, admit, and re-scope the patient the following day with a planned balloon dilatation and passage of a nasoenteral tube

22. **A 78 year old woman presents with a history of acute onset of epigastric pain radiating through to her back and vomiting. She reports a long-standing history of post-prandial chest pain and occasional regurgitation of foodstuffs. CXR demonstrates a retrogastric air fluid level. What is the most likely diagnosis?**
    a) Paraoesophageal hernia
    b) Achalasia
    c) Boerhaave's syndrome
    d) Morgagni hernia
    e) Bochdalek hernia

23. **A 44 year old lady complains of a long-standing difficulty in swallowing which has become worse over the preceding few months. She also complains of severe halitosis and regurgitation of foodstuffs. Her weight is stable. A recent OGD was reported as being normal other than a comment on a 'slightly patulous oesophagus'. What is the next step in her management?**
    a) Repeat upper GI endoscopy
    b) Barium meal
    c) Gastric emptying study
    d) Oesophageal manometry
    e) CT abdomen

24. **A 38 year old woman complains of severe retrosternal chest pain, dysphagia, and occasional regurgitation. High-resolution manometry demonstrates a normal integrated relaxation pressure but with hyper-contractile premature contractions (DCI >8000mmHg-s-cm) in 30% of measured swallows. What is the diagnosis?**
    a) Pseudoachalasia
    b) Nutcracker oesophagus
    c) Jackhammer oesophagus
    d) Type II achalasia
    e) Diffuse oesophageal spasms

25. **A 50 year old male with alcoholic cirrhosis presents with an oesophageal variceal bleed. His GCS is 15 and he is orientated in time and place. His bilirubin is 72µmol/L and albumin 26g/L. The PT ratio is 1.8. He has no ascites. What is the Child–Pugh classification for this patient?**
    a) Child–Pugh class A
    b) Child–Pugh class B
    c) Child–Pugh class C
    d) Child–Pugh class D
    e) Child–Pugh class cannot be calculated accurately from these data

26. **What is the underlying pathological abnormality in achalasia?**
    a) Overabundance of excitatory ganglion cells
    b) Overproduction of acetylcholine by excitatory ganglion cells
    c) Overproduction of substance P by excitatory ganglion cells
    d) Absence of non-adrenergic, non-cholinergic inhibitory ganglion cells
    e) None of the above

27. **A 55 year old man undergoes a gastrectomy for a carcinoma of the gastric cardia. The right and left cardia lymph nodes, as well as nodes along the greater and lesser curvature, and the right and left gastroepiploic vessels are removed. How would this procedure be best described?**
    a) D0 lymphadenectomy
    b) D1 lymphadenectomy
    c) D2 lymphadenectomy
    d) D3 lymphadenectomy
    e) D4 lymphadenectomy

28. **Which of the following parameters does not form part of the Glasgow–Blatchford score to assess the likelihood that a patient with an upper GI haemorrhage will require intervention?**
    a) Blood urea
    b) Haemoglobin
    c) Age greater than 60 years
    d) Presentation with melaena
    e) Cardiac failure

29. **A 56 year old female with a history of coeliac disease presents with difficulty in swallowing, food impaction, regurgitation, and vomiting. An OGD shows white patches in the distal oesophagus and the impression of several rings in the lower oesophageal wall. What is the likely diagnosis?**
    a) Oesophageal candidiasis
    b) Multiple Schatzki rings
    c) Eosinophilic oesophagitis
    d) Achalasia
    e) Gastro-oesophageal reflux

30. **An 80 year old female with a past history of IDDM and two previous MIs, is admitted having collapsed with a haematemesis. Her BP is 110/60mmHg and pulse is 105bpm. She is known to have a gastric cancer. What is her Rockall score?**
    a) 2
    b) 5
    c) 6
    d) 7
    e) Score cannot be calculated from these data

31. Which of the following statements best describes a vagal-sparing oesophagectomy?

a) Another name for a trans-hiatal oesophagectomy

b) Equivalent morbidity to a trans-hiatal oesophagectomy

c) Considered for cancers invading into the submucosa but not beyond

d) Associated with less late morbidity such as weight loss, dumping, and diarrhoea

e) Considered for advanced cancers where a palliative resection is being considered

32. A 45 year old male is diagnosed as having a distal one-third squamous oesophageal cancer that invades into the muscularis mucosae. Which of the following statements describes the T stage of this lesion?

a) Tis

b) T1a

c) T1b

d) T2

e) Cannot be given a T stage with this information

33. Which of the following conditions is not a risk factor for the development of Barrett's oesophagus?

a) Female gender

b) Older age

c) History of reflux symptoms

d) Family history of Barrett's disease

e) Obesity

34. A 40 year old female with type 2 diabetes attends a bariatric clinic for a discussion about the surgical options for her obesity. According to the WHO classification, she is noted to be Obese Class II. Her BMI is within what range?

a) 25–29.9

b) 30–34.9

c) 35–39.9

d) 40–49.9

e) 50–59.9

35. Which of the following is a component of the NICE criteria for bariatric surgery?

a) BMI >30 and hypertension

b) BMI >35 and type 2 diabetes

c) Failure to achieve clinically beneficial weight loss using pharmacological intervention

d) Loss of weight of >2kg following an intensive management plan within a specialty obesity service

e) Failure of all dietary interventions

36. The most common cause of mortality following bariatric surgery is:

a) Anastomotic leak
b) Bleeding from suture line or anastomosis
c) Acute band slippage
d) Staple-line leak
e) DVT/PE

37. A 38 year old female, with a history of having had a gastric band inserted 2 years previously, presents with acute severe epigastric pain, vomiting, and an inability to eat or drink. The volume in the band has not been adjusted within the preceding year. What is the correct management plan?

a) Urgent CT scan
b) Urgent contrast swallow
c) Laparotomy and removal of band
d) Urgent decompression of the band using a Huber needle
e) Urgent decompression of the band using a Huber needle, contrast swallow, and laparoscopy

38. The risk of anastomotic leak following gastric bypass surgery for morbid obesity is:

a) 0.1%
b) 1%
c) 3%
d) 5%
e) 10%

Extended Matching Items

Therapeutic endoscopy

A. Enteric stent
B. Banding
C. Endoscopic mucosal resection
D. Radiofrequency ablation
E. YAG laser
F. Fully covered oesophageal stent
G. Partially covered oesophageal stent
H. Oesophageal balloon dilatation
I. Surveillance upper GI endoscopy
J. Pyloric balloon dilatation
K. Cyanoacrylate endoscopic injection

For each of the following scenarios, select the most appropriate therapeutic endoscopic intervention from the preceding list. Each option may be used once, more than once, or not at all.

1. You perform a planned repeat balloon dilatation of a peptic stricture in a 70 year old male with a history of COPD and ischaemic heart disease. After deflation of the balloon, you note modest bleeding and are concerned about a possible full-thickness tear. Your patient develops surgical emphysema. What is the most appropriate next step in his management?

2. A 64 year old male with congestive cardiac failure and stage III chronic renal failure is investigated for dysphagia. He has a modest hiatus hernia below a 6cm circumferential segment of Barrett's oesophagus. Seattle protocol biopsies demonstrate predominantly non-dysplastic Barrett's with a single focus of high-grade dysplasia. What is the most appropriate next step in his management?

3. A 72 year old woman complains of bloating and persistent vomiting. Two years previously she underwent a transhiatal oesophagectomy following a complete pathological response to a distal oesophageal adenocarcinoma. What is the most appropriate next step in her management?

4. An 80 year old man attends for radiofrequency ablation of Barrett's oesophagus. A raised slightly nodular area is noted within the Barrett's segment. What is the most appropriate next step in his management?

5. A 77 year old frail woman with metastatic gastric cancer complains of more frequent vomiting. At endoscopy there is gastric food and fluid residue and an established distal gastric carcinoma occluding the antrum and pylorus. What is the most appropriate next step in her management?

Treatment of upper gastrointestinal bleeding

A. Interventional radiology and embolization
B. Endoscopic band ligation
C. Laparotomy
D. Trans-jugular intra-hepatic portosystemic shunt
E. Sengstaken–Blakemore tube
F. CT angiogram
G. ERCP
H. YAG laser
I. Radiotherapy
J. Cyanoacrylate endoscopic injection
K. Endoscopic argon plasma coagulation

For each of the following scenarios, select the most appropriate intervention from the preceding list. Each option may be used once, more than once, or not at all.

6. A 65 year old gentleman with advanced gastric carcinoma requires ongoing weekly blood transfusion. He has an extensive linitus plastica and palliative laser has been unhelpful in reducing his transfusion requirements. What is the most appropriate next step in his management?

7. A 34 year old man undergoes ERCP with sphincterotomy and duct clearance for choledocholithiasis. He develops melaena overnight and his haemoglobin drops by 3g/dl. He is haemodynamically stable. What is the most appropriate next step in his management?

8. You are called to the emergency department resuscitation area where a deeply jaundiced male has had a fresh haematemesis. He is in extremis with an unrecordable blood pressure. His wife tells you he recently had an admission two weeks previously and underwent banding of oesophageal varices. What is the most appropriate next step in his management?

9. A 40 year old male with alcoholic cirrhosis has an upper GI bleed. An endoscopy reveals active bleeding in isolated gastric varices located in the fundus of the stomach. What is the most appropriate next step in his management?

Upper GI functional disorders

A. Gastrojejunostomy
B. Implantable gastric pacemaker
C. Injection of lower oesophageal sphincter with Botox™
D. Injection of pylorus with Botox™
E. Lower oesophageal pneumatic balloon dilatation
F. Calcium channel antagonists
G. Pyloric balloon dilatation
H. Laparoscopic Heller's myotomy with partial fundoplication

For each of the following scenarios, select the most appropriate management option from the preceding list. Each option may be used once, more than once, or not at all.

10. A 38 year old woman with type I diabetes presents with upper abdominal discomfort, vomiting and abdominal bloating. Upper GI endoscopy is unremarkable. She has not responded to a range of antiemetics and prokinetics resulting in poor glycaemic control. What is the most appropriate next step in her management?

11. A 54 year old woman has been investigated for chest pain and occasional dysphagia. Upper GI endoscopy is normal and manometry demonstrates vigorous distal oesophageal contractions in over 20% of swallows and normal OGJ relaxation. What is the most appropriate first-line treatment?

12. A 45 year old man with swallowing difficulties undergoes upper GI endoscopy and manometry. Oesophageal manometry reveals impaired oesophagogastric junction relaxation and pan-oesophageal pressurization in over 20% of swallows. What is the most appropriate treatment?

Management of oesophageal cancer

A. Two-phase subtotal (Ivor–Lewis) oesophagectomy
B. Neoadjuvant chemotherapy and Ivor–Lewis oesophagectomy
C. Ivor–Lewis oesophagectomy + adjuvant chemotherapy
D. Three-phase subtotal oesophagectomy
E. Neoadjuvant chemotherapy and three-phase subtotal oesophagectomy
F. Three-phase oesophagectomy and adjuvant chemotherapy
G. Transhiatal oesophagectomy
H. Neoadjuvant chemotherapy and transhiatal oesophagectomy
I. Transhiatal oesophagectomy and adjuvant chemotherapy
J. Chemotherapy alone
K. Radiotherapy alone
L. Chemoradiotherapy

For each of the following scenarios, select the most appropriate management option from the preceding list. Each option may be used once, more than once, or not at all.

13. An otherwise fit and well 72 year old male is diagnosed with a cT3 N1 M0 squamous cell carcinoma within the proximal third of the oesophagus. What is the best management option?

14. An otherwise fit and well, 67 year old female is diagnosed with a cT3 N1 M0 oesophageal adenocarcinoma of the middle third of the oesophagus (at 28cm).

15. An otherwise well, 45 year old male is diagnosed with a short segment of Barrett's with high-grade dysplasia. He declines endoscopic management and requests definitive intervention, as he plans to emigrate. Staging investigations show no nodal or metastatic disease.

Management of gastric cancer

A. Subtotal gastrectomy
B. Total gastrectomy
C. Segmental gastrectomy
D. No resection
E. Radiotherapy alone
F. Neoadjuvant chemotherapy, total gastrectomy, and adjuvant chemotherapy
G. Total gastrectomy and adjuvant chemotherapy
H. Neoadjuvant chemotherapy and total gastrectomy
I. Neoadjuvant chemotherapy, distal gastrectomy, and adjuvant chemotherapy
J. Distal gastrectomy and adjuvant chemotherapy
K. Neoadjuvant chemotherapy and distal gastrectomy

For each of the following scenarios, select the most appropriate management option from the preceding list. Each option may be used once, more than once, or not at all.

16. A 69 year old male is diagnosed with a cT3 N1 M0 gastric adenocarcinoma measuring 2cm arising just proximal to the pylorus.

17. A 55 year old female is diagnosed with a cT2 N2 M0 gastric adenocarcinoma arising from the middle third of the stomach. Histology from the biopsies shows a diffusely infiltrative pattern with multiple signet rings.

18. A 30 year old female is diagnosed with a CDH1 germline mutation (hereditary diffuse gastric carcinoma syndrome). Her father and grandfather both died of metastatic gastric cancer in their early 50s. Upper GI endoscopy and random biopsies show normal mucosa only.

Investigations and staging of oesophageal cancer

A. CT chest/abdomen
B. Barium swallow
C. Upper GI endoscopy
D. Laparoscopy and peritoneal cytology
E. PET–CT scan
F. EUS
G. PET–CT and EUS
H. MRI
I. Laparoscopic ultrasound
J. EBUS
K. CT-guided biopsy
L. No further staging investigations required

For each of the following scenarios, please select the most appropriate investigation plan from the preceding list. Each option may be used once, more than once, or not at all.

19. A 70 year old male is diagnosed with an oesophageal adenocarcinoma within the distal third of the oesophagus, 7cm proximal to the OG junction. There is concern from his initial staging CT regarding the presence of both local and regional nodal disease.

20. A 58 year old female is diagnosed with a Siewert Type III junctional adenocarcinoma. Initial staging with CT chest/abdomen and PET–CT suggests a cT2 N1 M0 cancer.

21. A 64 year old male is diagnosed with a cT4 N2 M0 distal third oesophageal adenocarcinoma. Although there is no overt metastatic disease on initial staging, you are concerned the tumour may be irresectable because of local advancement. He subsequently undergoes three cycles of neoadjuvant chemotherapy.

22. A previously fit and well 80 year old male is admitted with a 3-month history of progressive weakness, lethargy, and abdominal pain. He is anaemic (Hb 77g/dL). CT demonstrates a thickened irregular area on the lesser curve of the stomach with multiple peritoneal and liver lesions.

23. A 58 year old male is diagnosed with a gastric body GIST following an OGD for haematemesis.

Staging of oesophagogastric cancer

A. T4 N3 M1
B. T4 N3 M0
C. T3 N2 M1
D. T3 N2 M0
E. T2 N1 M0 R0
F. T2 N2 M0 R1
G. T3 N1 M0 R0
H. T3 N2 M0 R0
I. T4 N2 M0 R1
J. T3 N2 M0 R0

For each of the following scenarios, select the TNM stage of the cancer from the preceding list. Each option may be used once, more than once, or not at all.

24. A distal oesophageal adenocarcinoma invading the muscularis propria, but not through the adventitia. A total of 24 nodes are recovered and 2 of those taken from the left gastric artery are positive for adenocarcinoma. There is no radiological evidence of metastatic disease. Disease is noted microscopically at 3mm from the circumferential margin.

25. An adenocarcinoma of the gastric antrum which invades into the subserosa but not through to the visceral peritoneum. No obvious metastatic disease is identified on CT scanning. Twenty nodes are retrieved. Six taken from stations 7, 8, and 9 are positive for cancer cells. Disease is noted microscopically at 2mm from the circumferential margin.

26. There is a tumour located in the gastric body. Multiple lymph nodes (>6 nodes, >1cm in size) are noted in the peri-gastric region on CT. At laparoscopy the tumour is clearly seen invading through the serosa of the stomach and there are tumour cells present in the peritoneal cytology specimen.

Palliative management of oesophagogastric cancer

A. Insertion of duodenal stent
B. External beam radiotherapy
C. Single agent chemotherapy and trastuzumab
D. Combination chemotherapy and trastuzumab
E. Single agent chemotherapy
F. Combination chemotherapy
G. Laparoscopic gastrojejunostomy
H. Insertion of oesophageal stent
I. Laser treatment
J. Oesophageal balloon dilatation
K. Argon beam plasma coagulation
L. Photodynamic therapy

For each of the following scenarios, select the most appropriate management option from the preceding list. Each option may be used once, more than once, or not at all.

27. A 75 year old male with a cT3 N2 M1 distal oesophageal adenocarcinoma presents with progressive dysphagia and is now unable to swallow liquids.

28. A 58 year old female is diagnosed with a cT4 N1 M1 adenocarcinoma of the gastric antrum. She is otherwise fit and well and is being considered for entry into a trial of a new, targeted therapy alongside standard palliative therapy. She is admitted with persistent and intractable large-volume non-bilious vomiting.

29. A 72 year old male is diagnosed with a cT2 N2 M1 adenocarcinoma of the gastric body. He is otherwise fit and well and is currently asymptomatic. Molecular testing of the adenocarcinoma demonstrates a high degree of HER2 positivity

Causes of upper GI haemorrhage

A. Oesophageal varices
B. Oesophagitis
C. Oesophageal cancer
D. Mallory–Weiss tear
E. Gastric varices
F. Gastric ulcer
G. Gastritis
H. Gastric cancer
I. Dieulafoy's lesion
J. Duodenal ulcer
K. Stress ulcer
L. Haemobilia

For each of the following scenarios, select the most likely diagnosis from the preceding list. Each option may be used once, more than once, or not at all.

30. A 60 year old hypertensive, non-insulin dependent diabetic, male presents with a significant upper GI bleed. He has had two similar bleeds over the preceding three months and has undergone an OGD on two occasions which only showed blood in the stomach. What is the most likely diagnosis?

31. A 45 year old male with alcoholic cirrhosis presents with an upper GI bleed. An OGD reveals small varices that are not actively bleeding and have no stigmata of a recent bleed. What is the most likely cause for the bleed?

32. You are called to see a 22 year old male who was admitted 24 hours previously following a road traffic accident involving blunt trauma to the chest and abdomen. He now complains of a six-hour history of severe upper abdominal pain which was followed by a haematemesis of slightly altered blood. He has dropped his haemoglobin to 90g/dL and you also note that his liver function tests are deranged with a bilirubin of 90μmol/L. What is the most likely diagnosis?

Causes of dysphagia

A. Achalasia
B. Spastic motility disorder of the oesophageal body
C. Systemic sclerosis
D. Diffuse oesophageal spasm
E. Oesophageal stricture
F. Pharyngeal pouch
G. Oesophageal tumour
H. Foreign body
I. Nutcracker oesophagus
J. Non-specific oesophageal motility disorder
K. Oesophageal ring
L. Gastroesophageal reflux disease
M. Eosinophilic oesophagitis

For each of the following scenarios, select the most likely diagnosis from the preceding list. Each option may be used once, more than once, or not at all.

33. An 80 year old male presents with a 5-year history of a choking sensation when eating, dysphagia, halitosis, and a recent history of hoarseness. Food just eaten can be regurgitated. On examination, there is evidence of cachexia.

34. A 40 year old female presents with difficulty swallowing. An OGD shows no cause for concern. A barium swallow is reported as showing a 'bird's beak' appearance.

35. A 44 year old female undergoes an OGD and manometry because of dysphagia, chest pain, and reflux symptoms. She is noted to have severe erosive oesophagitis. Manometry shows reduced lower oesophageal sphincter pressure and a loss of distal oesophageal body peristalsis. She has also recently been referred to the dermatology clinic because she has developed brown hyperpigmented plaques over her upper chest wall.

Single Best Answers

1. b) Trypanosoma cruzi

Chagas disease, or trypanosomiasis, is a tropical parasitic disease caused by the protozoan *Trypanosoma cruzi*. It is usually spread by insects known as Triatominae or kissing bugs. The disease may also be spread through blood transfusion, organ transplantation, eating food contaminated with the parasites, and by vertical transmission (from a mother to her foetus).

Initial infection may be asymptomatic or associated with a mild fever, lymphadenopathy, headaches or local swelling at the site of the bite. After a quiescent period of 8–12 weeks, affected individuals enter a chronic phase of the disease. Most patients are asymptomatic (70%). However, the remainder will develop further symptoms 10–30 years after the initial infection. Up to 10% of patients will display chronic manifestations of infection, which include cardiomyopathy, heart failure, cardiac arrhythmias, and gastrointestinal dysmotility syndromes leading to megaoesophagus and megacolon. Early-stage disease is diagnosed by microscopic identification of the parasite in blood of infected individuals. Chronic disease is diagnosed by finding antibodies for *T. cruzi*.

Patients are managed with a combination of anti-parasitic treatment to kill the parasite and symptomatic treatment to manage symptoms and signs of infection. Much of the cardiovascular and gastrointestinal morbidity relates to failure of the parasympathetic nervous symptom. The mechanism whereby Chagas disease targets the parasympathetic autonomic nervous system and spares the sympathetic autonomic nervous system is poorly understood.

Bern C. Chagas' disease. *New England Journal of Medicine* 2015; 373:456–66.

2. e) Boerhaave's syndrome

This scenario is consistent with perforation of the oesophagus. Boerhaave first described spontaneous rupture of the oesophagus in 1924. The classic syndrome occurs after forceful vomiting. It is commonly associated with overindulgence of food and/or alcohol. The most common anatomical position is the lower one-third of the oesophagus in the left posterolateral wall just above the gastro-oesophageal junction. The condition is defined by the presence of a full-thickness perforation of the oesophagus and should be distinguished from Mallory–Weiss syndrome which is a non-full thickness oesophageal tear, also associated with vomiting.

Reported mortality is up to 35%. The best outcomes are obtained with early diagnosis and early definitive surgical management. If treatment is delayed or a conservative approach is undertaken, mortality rates of up to 90% have been recorded. Left untreated, the classic syndrome has a mortality rate of up to 100%. Mortality is usually due to infection including mediastinitis, pneumonia, empyema, and pericarditis.

Mackler's triad, consisting of a history of vomiting, sudden onset of thoracic pain and subcutaneous emphysema, is present in only 14% of patients with Boerhaave's syndrome. The diagnosis can usually be made with a simple chest X-ray, although a gastrograffin swallow or CT with contrast may be performed to identify the size and location of the perforation.

Teh E et al. Boerhaave's syndrome: a review of management and outcome. *Interactive CardioVascular and Thoracic Surgery* 2007; 6:640–3.

3. d) Chronic afferent loop syndrome

Delayed bilious vomiting associated with resolution of the pain suggests chronic afferent loop syndrome (ALS). ALS may present as an acute or chronic problem following a gastrojejunostomy. It may occur as a complication of distal or subtotal gastrectomy, Billroth II reconstruction, and simple gastrojejunostomy performed to bypass other foregut pathology.

The afferent limb, which usually contains duodenum and proximal jejunum, is out of direct circuit with food. However, pancreatic juices and bile will enter this limb and if it becomes obstructed, the limb will become distended on eating. The classic syndrome describes relief of the pain as the obstructed limb decompresses into the stomach, resulting in bilious vomiting (which may be projectile).

In the acute early post-operative setting, there is a real risk of blowout of the duodenal stump (if present) and acute ALS is treated as a surgical emergency. It may also be responsible for post-operative jaundice, ascending cholangitis, and pancreatitis due to high pressures within the obstructed afferent limb and back pressure on the pancreatic and biliary duct systems. It has also been associated with ischaemia and gangrene of the afferent limb, giving rise to subsequent perforation. Acute ALS usually occurs because of a complete obstruction whereas the chronic syndrome may be a partial obstruction, relieved when increased pressure within the limb leads to decompression of bile into the stomach (which may be associated with bilious vomiting). Long-standing stasis of secretions may give rise to bacterial overgrowth. The syndrome may be precipitated by compression or entrapment of the afferent limb by post-operative adhesions, internal herniation, volvulus or kinking of the afferent limb itself. An ante-colic gastrojejunostomy is also at increased risk, as is an afferent limb of more than 40cm in length.

The acute syndrome is a surgical emergency and requires immediate decompression. Mortality rates of up to 60% have been recorded. This is particularly the case where the diagnosis and management have been delayed, giving rise to stump blowout, bowel ischaemia, rupture, or peritonitis. The chronic syndrome will require elective revisional surgery. See Figure 6.1.

Delcore R and Cheung LY. Surgical options in postgastrectomy syndromes. *Surgical Oncology Clinics of North America* 1991; 71(1):57–75.

4. b) Gurvit's syndrome

Gurvit's syndrome or acute oesophageal necrosis (AEN) is associated with acute hypotension resulting in oesophageal hypoperfusion and necrosis of the mucosa. The condition is thought to arise as a combination of an ischaemic insult, because of haemodynamic compromise, and low-flow states. It may also be associated with corrosive injury from gastric contents due to vomiting or gastric outlet obstruction. The endoscopic appearance is of circumferential black discolouration of the distal oesophagus. There may be associated mucosal sloughing. The discolouration and mucosal changes stop abruptly at the gastro-oesophageal junction. Black discolouration is due to mucosal necrosis, which is confirmed on histology.

The mainstay of management is directed at correcting any coexisting medical conditions, restoration of haemodynamic stability, and acid suppression. The high mortality of over 30% is

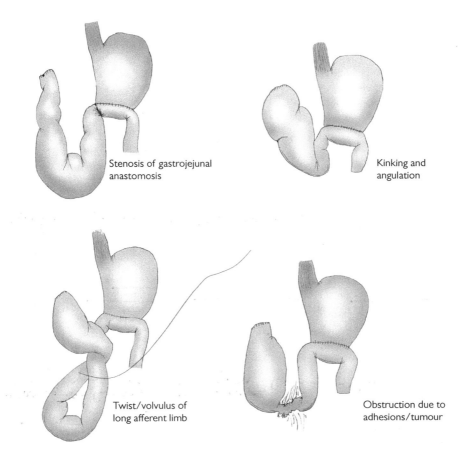

Fig. 6.1 Causes of afferent loop syndrome

usually attributed to the underlying cause of hypotension. Oesophageal strictures may develop as a complication of this condition.

Gurvits GE et al. Acute esophageal necrosis: a rare syndrome. *Journal of Gastroenterology* 2007; 42:29–38.

5. c) Good clinical response to acid suppression therapy

Most published studies have recorded success rates of 90% or better in patients undergoing laparoscopic anti-reflux surgery. A variety of preoperative factors have been assessed to determine if any can predict post-operative success. The single most important factor that has consistently been shown to be an excellent predictor of a good post-operative outcome is a good preoperative clinical response to acid suppression therapy.

Jackson PG et al. Predictors of outcome in 100 consecutive laparoscopic antireflux procedures. *American Journal of Surgery* 2001; 181:231–5.

Campos GMR et al. Multivariate analysis of factors predicting outcome after laparoscopic Nissen fundoplication. *Journal of Gastrointestinal Surgery* 1999; 3:292–300.

6. c) Angio-embolization

Acute haemorrhage from a peptic ulcer is a common medical emergency with an incidence of around 100 cases per 100,000 adults per year. Around 80% of patients who present with an upper GI bleed will stop spontaneously. Endoscopy and endotherapy is the gold standard treatment. However, endoscopic therapy is not successful in controlling bleeding in 5–25% of patients. Although surgery was the traditional next step in the management of such patients, there is increasing evidence that arterial embolization is an effective second-line management. Interventional radiologic embolization (when available) is minimally invasive, repeatable, and can be used even in very sick and unstable patients. It has a 70–90% success rate at 30 days and is associated with significantly lower morbidity when compared to surgery.

Wang YL et al. Emergency transcatheter arterial embolization for patients with acute massive duodenal ulcer hemorrhage. *World Journal of Gastroenterology* 2012; 18:4765–70.

7. b) Size of tumour   *NOT BIOLOGY AS 2 INTER-LINKED*

Gastrointestinal stromal tumours (GISTs) are the most common primary mesenchymal tumours of the GI tract, with the majority (70%) occurring within the stomach. They have malignant potential and their behaviour is related to several well-documented prognostic factors. These include tumour size, mitotic count, symptoms at diagnosis, and organ of origin. Tumours <2cm in size have an associated low mitotic index and are low risk for progression to metastatic disease. Conversely, those of 6–10cm with a high mitotic index, and all tumours >10cm, are classified as high risk for progression to metastatic disease. Lymphatic spread is rare in GISTs.

DeMatteo RP et al. Two hundred gastrointestinal stromal tumours: recurrence patterns and prognostic factors for survival. *Annals of Surgery* 2000; 231(1):51–8.

8. d) Imatinib   *Effectively GIST's are considered like solid organ malignancy e.g. breast/liver.*

Resection should be considered for non-metastatic GISTs >2cm in size (tumours <2cm may be managed conservatively with serial examination). GISTs are generally chemo- and radio-resistant so imatinib (Glivec®) forms the mainstay of management of metastatic disease. This is a receptor tyrosine kinase inhibitor with multiple targets including BCR–ABL, PDGFR, and KIT. GISTs with activating KIT mutations are generally imatinib-sensitive while conversely, those with activating PDGFR mutations are imatinib-resistant. For those with metastatic GIST, treatment with imatinib will result in >50% 5-year survival. Imatinib can also be used as adjuvant therapy following resection of high-risk tumours. *e.g. 6–10 cm & high mitoticity give as adjuvant.*

Van Oosterom AT et al. Safety and efficacy of imatinib (ST1571) in metastatic gastrointestinal stromal tumours: a phase I study. *Lancet* 2001; 358(9291):1421–3.

DeMatteo RP et al. Adjuvant imatinib mesylate after resection of localized, primary gastrointestinal stromal tumour: a randomized, double-blind, placebo-controlled trial. *Lancet* 2009; 373(9669):1097–104.

9. a) Eradication of H. pylori and repeat biopsies in six months

All lymphomas can affect the GI tract and up to 75% of these will occur in the stomach. Primary gastric lymphomas constitute 5% of all gastric tumours. The two most common primary gastric lymphomas are mucosa-associated lymphoid tissue (MALT) lymphomas and diffuse large B-cell lymphoma. MALT lymphomas are also known as extra-nodal marginal zone B-cell lymphomas and are associated with *H. pylori* infection. It is thought that the *H. pylori* infection causes chronic inflammation which initiates the lymphoma. They are staged by the modified Blackledge system and those deemed as low-grade (Blackledge stage 1—no nodal involvement and no serosal penetration

Resection NOT a treatment for primary gastric lymphoma.

of the primary lesion), as suggested in the current scenario, may be treated with *H. pylori* eradication. 50–95% of cases achieve complete response with *H. pylori* treatment. Patients should be followed up with six-monthly endoscopy and biopsy. Higher-stage MALT lymphomas and diffuse large B-cell lymphomas will generally require chemotherapy and rituximab. ← *CD20 ligand inhibitor*

Pinotti G et al. Clinical features, treatment and outcome in a series of 93 patients with low-grade gastric MALT lymphoma. *Leukemia & Lymphoma* 1997; 26(5–6):527–37.

10. d) Radiofrequency ablation   *or PDT equivalent.*

Barrett's oesophagus is the most important risk factor for the development of oesophageal adenocarcinoma. Current evidence suggests that those with any grade of dysplasia should be referred for endoscopic therapy rather than continued surveillance. Of these, radiofrequency ablation is the preferred endoscopic ablative therapy for those with flat dysplasia. Intra mucosal carcinoma and nodular lesions may need to be treated with EMR followed by endoscopic radiofrequency ablation. Patients with non-dysplastic Barrett's can undergo endoscopic surveillance with most guidelines recommending this in a three- to five-yearly cycle.

Phoa KN et al. Radiofrequency ablation vs endoscopic surveillance for patients with Barrett esophagus and low-grade dysplasia: a randomized clinical trial. *Journal of the American Medical Association* 2014; 311(12):1209–17.

11. e) CDH1   *– Emma @ work.*

Approximately 1–3% of gastric carcinomas are related to inherited gastric carcinoma predisposition syndromes. The hereditary diffuse gastric carcinoma syndrome (HDGC) is due to a germline mutation in the E-cadherin (*CDH1*) gene and is an autosomal dominant inherited syndrome. Patients also have an increased risk of lobular breast cancer and colonic cancer. The overall risk of gastric cancer is 67% in men and 83% in women who are identified as high-risk according to the International Gastric Cancer Linkage Consortium Criteria (IGCLC). For those with gastric cancer a total gastrectomy is advocated and this should also be considered as a prophylactic procedure in asymptomatic patients.

Fitzgerald RC et al. Hereditary diffuse gastric cancer: updated consensus guidelines for clinical management and directions for future research (International Gastric Cancer Linkage Consortium). *Journal of Medical Genetics* 2010; 47:436–44.

12. c) 6

It has been shown that the optimal number of endoscopic biopsies in oesophageal cancer needed to obtain a definitive tissue diagnosis is at least 6 with this number providing a diagnosis in 100% of cases.

Lal N et al. Optimal number of biopsy specimens in the diagnosis of carcinoma of the oesophagus. *Gut* 1992; 33:724–6.

13. a) Fundic gland polyp

The most common type of polyp encountered within the stomach is the fundic gland polyp. Fundic gland polyps are present in around 5% of patients undergoing upper GI endoscopy and account for around 75% of all gastric polyps. They are associated with proton pump inhibitors and therefore acid suppression is thought to play a role in their pathogenesis. The risk of dysplasia is low in sporadic cases although the presence of low-grade dysplasia is common in patients with familial adenomatous polyposis (FAP). Fundic gland polyps are usually diagnosed by their distribution and the history of PPI use, but representative biopsies should be taken when they are first diagnosed.

Sporadic = β-Catenin
dysplasia ↑ FAP?

Most fundic gland polyps are <1cm in size but polyps >1cm should be removed for histological analysis. Sporadic fundic gland polyps with dysplasias tend to follow an indolent course.

Carmack SW et al. The current spectrum of gastric polyps: a 1-year national study of over 120,000 patients. *American Journal of Gastroenterology* 2009; 104:1524–32.

14. e) Alcohol consumption   *Epstein - Barr is a risk factor !*

At the present, there is no definitive epidemiological evidence linking alcohol intake to risk of gastric adenocarcinoma. There is, however, strong evidence linking *H. pylori*, EBV, and smoking to gastric adenocarcinoma. The *STK11/LKB1* gene germline mutation is associated with Peutz–Jeghers syndrome and of all the polyposis syndromes this has the highest risk of the development of gastric adenocarcinoma. Patients with this syndrome develop hamartomatous polyps within the stomach.

Giardiello FM et al. Very high risk of cancer in familial Peutz–Jeghers syndrome. *Gastroenterology* 2000; 119:1447–53.   *adequate lymphadenectomy is not just for*

15. c) Brachiocephalic   *— cervical lymph node chain staging.*
— levels V, VI + VII neck lymph nodes.

Lymphadenectomy is an essential component of oesophageal cancer surgery and lymph node status is an <u>independent prognostic factor for cancer-specific and disease-free</u> survival. A radical lymphadenectomy potentially allows for optimal staging, locoregional control and improved cure. Lymphadenectomy is best described in terms of nodal tiers with one-, two-, and three-field lymphadenectomy possible in oesophageal cancer surgery. A one-field lymphadenectomy involves resection of the upper abdominal lymph nodes; a two-field lymphadenectomy involves resection of thoracic nodes and upper abdominal nodes; and a three-field lymphadenectomy involves resection of all of the above as well as cervical nodes. For adenocarcinomas of the lower and middle third, usual practice would be a two-field lymphadenectomy. In the current scenario, the <u>brachiocephalic</u> lymph nodes would not be included as these are incorporated within the cervical field and would only be resected in a three-field lymphadenectomy. Patients with cancer within the proximal third of the oesophagus may benefit from a dissection of the cervical field of lymph nodes.

Lerut T et al. Surgical strategies in esophageal carcinoma with emphasis on radical lymphadenectomy. *Annals of Surgery* 1992; 216(5):583–90.

16. d) **Conservative management with pleural drainage, antibiotics, NG suction, and enteral nutrition through feeding jejunostomy**

Late anastomotic leaks usually occur between the <u>fifth and tenth post-operative day</u>. These are usually best managed conservatively with NG tube placement, radiological-guided drainage, antibiotics, and enteral nutrition, ideally through a jejunostomy. In contrast, early anastomotic leaks (<u>up to the third post-operative day</u>) usually occur because of a technical failure and are best managed with surgical re-intervention. The use of covered stents in this context is <u>contraindicated</u>.

Moore FA et al. Early enteral feeding, compared with parenteral, reduces postoperative septic complications. The results of a meta-analysis. *Annals of Surgery* 1992; 216(2):172–83.

Griffin SM et al. Diagnosis and management of a mediastinal leak following radical oesophagectomy. *British Journal of Surgery* 2001; 88(10):1346–51.   *Late vs early leaks.*
< 3   dy. 5 -10.

17. c) 7%

Early gastric cancer is defined as tumour confined to the mucosa or submucosa and represents a T1 cancer. It may be treated by endoscopic mucosal resection (EMR) or endoscopic submucosal dissection (ESD). A local resection does not, however, provide any <u>pathological lymph node staging</u>. Lymph node metastasis is the most common mode of spread in gastric cancer and even T1 lesions have a risk of

Important point that lymph nodes cannot be staged + 10% harn met.

up to 10% for nodal metastases. Key features within an EMR/ESD specimen that predict the presence of nodal metastases include size >3cm, undifferentiated histological type and lymphovascular invasion. Lesions with any of the above features have a risk of 7% for nodal metastases.

Gotoda T et al. Incidence of lymph node metastasis from early gastric cancer: estimation with a large number of cases at two large centers. *Gastric Cancer* 2000; 3:219–25.

18. c) Immediate reoperation — *This is essentially acute afferent limb syndrome.*

The above scenario is consistent with a duodenal stump leak. Bilious discharge from a drain placed adjacent to a duodenal stump is an indication for immediate reoperation. Resuturing of the duodenal stump is often difficult and control of the leak may occur by placing a Foley catheter into the duodenum to create a controlled fistula, or placement of a suction drain close to the site of leakage. The duodenal stump may also be decompressed in a retrograde fashion from the jejunum. This may allow the continuation of enteral feeding through a feeding jejunostomy.

19. b) Type II junctional tumour

Siewert and Stein defined gastro-oesophageal junctional adenocarcinomas as those with their centre within 5cm of the anatomical cardia and are separated into Types I–III. They are classified on the basis of radiological, endoscopic, and intraoperative findings. Type IV does not exist. Type I, or Barrett carcinomas, infiltrate from above and have a centre within 1–5cm above the cardia. Type II, or junctional carcinomas, arise from the gastric cardia or gastro-oesophageal junction and have a centre within 1cm above to 2cm below the cardia. Type III, or proximal gastric carcinomas, infiltrate the oesophagogastric junction from below and have a centre within 2–5cm below the cardia. See Fig. 6.2.

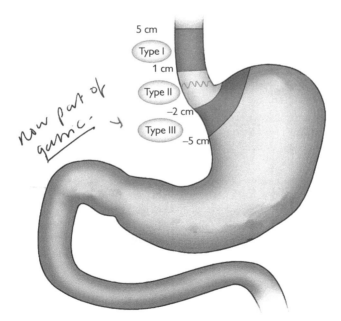

now part of gastric. →

5 cm

Type I

1 cm

Type II

−2 cm

Type III

−5 cm

Fig. 6.2 Siewert and Stein's classification of gastro-oesophageal junctional adenocarcinomas

Source data from *British Journal of Surgery*, 85, Siewert JR, Stein HJ, Classification of adenocarcinoma of the oesophagogastric junction. pp. 1457–9, 1998.

Siewert JR and Stein HJ. Classification of adenocarcinoma of the oesophagogastric junction. *British Journal of Surgery* 1998; 85:1457–9.

20. d) Within 1 mm

Disease present at or within 1mm of the circumferential margin in an oesophageal resection will be classified as an R1 resection. This occurs in up to 50% of stage III cancers and is an independent poor prognostic factor.

Dexter SP et al. Circumferential resection margin involvement: an independent predictor of survival following surgery for oesophageal cancer. *Gut* 2001; 48(5):667–70.

21. c) Biopsy the lesion, remove the endoscope, and arrange staging investigations

It is not an uncommon scenario to be unable to pass the endoscope through a stenotic tumour within the oesophagus at the time of the initial OGD. It is possible to dilate the stricture using a balloon dilatator although the risk of perforation ranges from 0–25%. This risks rendering a potentially operable tumour inoperable or significantly affecting prognosis. It is therefore usually safest to obtain a tissue diagnosis and stage the tumour in the first instance before considering dilatation. In the current scenario, the patient does not have total dysphagia and dilatation is not therefore immediately indicated.

It is possible that a further OGD and dilatation with placement of a nasoenteral feeding tube may be required for nutritional supplementation at a future date. Oral nutritional supplementation could be used in the interim time period as well as the use of a high calorie soft diet. The risk of perforation using a through-the-scope balloon dilator at endoscopic staging has been reported to be as low as 1%. Percutaneous endoscopic gastrostomy insertion would be contraindicated due to potential compromise of a future gastric conduit if oesophagectomy were planned.

Di-Franco F et al. Iatrogenic perforation of localized oesophageal cancer. *British Journal of Surgery* 2008; 95:837–40.

Jacobson BC et al. Through-the-scope balloon dilation for EUS staging of stenosing esophageal cancer. *Digestive Diseases and Sciences.* 2007; 52(3):817–22.

22. a) Paraoesophageal hernia

This scenario describes a paraoesophageal hernia presenting acutely with potential obstruction and strangulation. Contrast CT would be the most appropriate first-line investigation. Given her advanced age, it is unlikely to be secondary to a congenital diaphragmatic hernia such as a Bochdalek or Morgagni hernia.

Paraoesophageal hernia is an uncommon condition which accounts for around 5% of all hiatal hernias. Historically it was thought best to repair all such hernias because of the risk of incarceration. The annual probability of developing acute symptoms requiring emergency surgery with a watch and wait approach is around 1.1%. As a consequence, it has increasingly been recognized that adopting a watch-and-wait approach for asymptomatic and minimally symptomatic hernias is reasonable. Current practice favours a laparoscopic approach for symptomatic hernias where complete sac excision, primary crural repair with or without the use of mesh, and routine fundoplication is the standard of care in appropriate cases.

Stylopoulos N et al. Paraesophageal hernias: operation or observation? *Annals of Surgery* 2002; 236(4):492–501.

Lebenthal A et al. Treatment and controversies in paraesophageal hernia repair. *Frontiers in Surgery* 2015; 2:13.

23. d) Oesophageal manometry

The most likely diagnosis is oesophageal dysmotility and the patulous oesophagus suggests achalasia. Manometry would best discriminate the aetiology. Achalasia is an uncommon primary oesophageal motor disorder of unknown aetiology which is characterized manometrically by an inappropriate failure of relaxation of the lower oesophageal sphincter (LOS) combined with loss of oesophageal peristalsis. Endoscopically, typical findings are of a dilated oesophagus with retained saliva and food debris in the absence of any mucosal stricturing or tumour. However, on occasion endoscopy may not show an overt abnormality. Radiologically there is an absence of peristalsis during a barium swallow in association with oesophageal dilatation and a failure of relaxation of the LOS, giving rise to a 'bird-beak' appearance. Patients typically complain of dysphagia to solids and liquids in association with regurgitation, refractory reflux symptoms, chest pain ± weight loss. Manometry should be performed if achalasia is suspected. Based on manometry, achalasia can be divided into three subtypes. *This is the gold-standard treatment management*

- Type I: absent peristalsis without abnormal pressure
- Type II: absent peristalsis with abnormal pan oesophageal high pressure patterns
- Type III: absent peristalsis with distal oesophageal spastic contractions

Disruption of the lower oesophageal sphincter either by pneumatic dilatation (70–90% effective) or laparoscopic myotomy (88–95% effective) forms the mainstay of management. Patients with Type I achalasia have an intermediate prognosis that is inversely associated with the degree of oesophageal dilatation. Type II patients have a very favourable outcome and Type III have the least favourable outcome after lower oesophageal sphincter disruption.

Pandolfino JE and Gawron AJ. Achalasia: a systematic review. *Journal of the American Medical Association.* 2015; 313(18):1841–52.

24. c) Jackhammer oesophagus *Vigorous oesophageal Contraction* *Pneumatic / jackhammer*

The distal contractile integral (DCI) is a measure of the vigour of distal oesophageal contraction. A DCI value of >5000mmHg-s-cm defines a nutcracker oesophagus but such values are seen in up to 5% of normal subjects which makes the diagnosis non-specific and the term is now used less frequently. Hypertensive oesophageal contractions may also occur in the context of other oesophageal abnormalities such as OGJ obstruction, GORD, and eosinophilic oesophagitis.

A small subgroup of patients with oesophageal dysmotility display hypertensive contractions termed a jackhammer oesophagus or hypercontractile oesophagus. This is a rare disorder, currently defined as the occurrence of ≥20% of swallows with a DCI >8000mmHg-s-cm (within the context of normal oesophagogastric junction relaxation). The condition is commonly associated with multi-peaked contractions which can result in DCI values in excess of 50,000mmHg-s-cm. Such values are never observed in controls and almost always associated with oesophageal symptoms of dysphagia, reflux, and chest pain. *Calcium antagonists.*

Roman S et al. The Chicago classification of motility disorders: an update. *Gastrointestinal Endoscopy Clinics of North America* 2014; 24(4):545–61.

25. c) Child–Pugh class C

Child's score was initially proposed more than 30 years ago as a means of predicting mortality in cirrhotic patients who underwent after surgery for portal hypertension. The original score (termed the Child–Turcotte score) was modified by Pugh in 1973. The newer Child–Pugh classification replaced nutritional status with prothrombin time (cut-off at 4–6 seconds). The INR or prothrombin ratio is now commonly used with roughly equivalent values of 1.7–2.0. The patient in

Table 6.1 Child—Pugh classification

Factor	1 point	2 points	3 points
Total bilirubin (µmol/L)	<34	34–50	>50
Serum albumin (g/L)	>35	28–35	<28
INR:/ PT ratio	<1.7	1.71–2.30	>2.30
Ascites	None	Mild	Moderate to Severe
Hepatic encephalopathy	None	Grade I–II (or suppressed with medication)	Grade III–IV (or refractory)

Reproduced from *British Journal of Surgery*, 60, 8, Pugh RNH, Murray-Lyon IM, Dawson JL, Pietroni MC, Williams R., Transection of the oesophagus for bleeding oesophageal varices, pp. 646–9. Copyright © 1973 British Journal of Surgery Society Ltd.

the current scenario has a Child–Pugh score of 10 and would be in Class C. Class A patients have a score of <7 and Class C patients are scored >9. There is no Class D.

Although the Child–Pugh classification (Table 6.1) is one of the more commonly used prognostic indicators in patients who present with an acute variceal bleed, a number of other poor prognostic factors have been identified which include a high MELD score (model for end-stage liver disease score) and the presence of shock, renal failure, infection, hepatocellular carcinoma, active bleeding at the time of endoscopy, portal vein thrombosis, and a hepatic venous pressure gradient (HVPG) >20 mmHg.

Durand F and Valla D. Assessment of prognosis in cirrhosis. *Seminars in Liver Disease* 2008; 28(1):1101–22.

26. d) Absence of nonadrenergic, noncholinergic inhibitory ganglion cells

Achalasia is a primary oesophageal motility disorder characterized by impaired relaxation of the lower oesophageal sphincter (LOS) in association with absent oesophageal peristalsis. In addition to failure of relaxation of the LOS, the sphincter may also be hypertensive in up to 50% of patients.

LOS pressure and relaxation is mediated by excitatory (acetylcholine and substance P) and inhibitory (nitric oxide and vasoactive intestinal peptide) neurotransmitters. Patients with achalasia lack non-adrenergic, non-acetylcholine, inhibitory ganglion cells leading to excessive excitatory stimulation with a failure of relaxation.

There is increasing evidence that the condition is an autoimmune disease and many patients have single nucleotide polymorphisms in the major histocompatibility complex region of chromosome 6. Similar polymorphisms are seen at the same site in autoimmune disorders such as multiple sclerosis, SLE, and type I diabetes.

Gyawali CP. Achalasia: new perspectives on an old disease. *Neurogastroenterology & Motility* 2016; 28(1):4–11.

Gockel I et al. Common variants in the HLA–DQ region confer susceptibility to idiopathic achalasia. *Nature Genetics* 2014; 46(8):901–4.

27. a) D0 lymphadenectomy

The level described in the scenario an incomplete N1 dissection, as the nodes along the short gastric, supra-pyloric, and intra-pyloric nodes were not removed. An incomplete N1 dissection is termed a D0 lymphadenectomy.

Table 6.2 Japanese Research Society for the Study of gastric cancer lymph node classification

Lymph node station	Site of nodes	Node level
1	Right cardia	N1
2	Left cardia	N1
3	Lesser curvature	N1 — *right gastric*
4	Greater curvature	N1
4sa	Short gastric vessels	N1 - *from splenic arty.*
4sb	Left gastroepiploic vessels	N1
4d	Right gastroepiploic vessels	N1
5	Suprapyloric	N1 — *gastroduodenal*
6	Infrapyloric	N1

An incomplete N1 dissection is labelled as a D0 lymphadenectomy. A complete N1 dissection is labelled as a D1 lymphadenectomy.

7	Left gastric artery	N2
8	Common hepatic artery	N2
9	Coeliac trunk	N2
10	Splenic hilum	N2
11	Splenic artery	N2

A complete N2 dissection is labelled as a D2 lymphadenectomy.

12	Hepatic duodenal ligament	
13	Posterior surface of the head of the pancreas	
14	Root of the mesentery	D3
14A	Superior mesenteric artery	D3
14V	Superior mesenteric vein	D3

12 — 14

D3 dissections include dissection of lymph nodes at stations 12 through 14, along the hepatoduodenal ligament and the root of the mesentery (N3 level).

15	Para-aortic	N4
16	Paracolic	N4

15 - 16 D4.

D4 resections include stations 15 and 16 in the para-aortic and the paracolic region

Source data from Gastric Cancer, 14, Japanese Gastric Cancer Association
Japanese classification of gastric carcinoma: 3rd English edition. 2011,
The International Gastric Cancer Association and tThe Japanese Gastric Cancer Association.

The Japanese Research Society for the Study of Gastric Cancer published a manual standardizing lymph node dissection in gastric cancer (see Table 6.2). This recognizes 16 different lymph node stations surrounding the stomach. These are grouped according to location extending away from the primary tumour (N1–N4) and the extent of lymphadenectomy is classified according to the level of the lymph node section (D1–D4). In D1 dissections, nodes close to the greater and lesser curvatures of the stomach only are removed (stations 1–6, N1 level). See Figure 6.3.

Kim HJ et al. Standardization of the extent of lymphadenectomy for gastric cancer: impact on survival. *Advances in Surgery* 2001; 35:203–23.

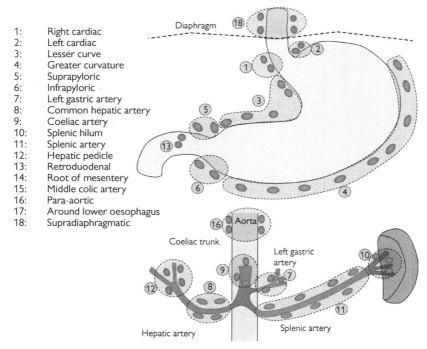

1: Right cardiac
2: Left cardiac
3: Lesser curve
4: Greater curvature
5: Suprapyloric
6: Infrapyloric
7: Left gastric artery
8: Common hepatic artery
9: Coeliac artery
10: Splenic hilum
11: Splenic artery
12: Hepatic pedicle
13: Retroduodenal
14: Root of mesentery
15: Middle colic artery
16: Para-aortic
17: Around lower oesophagus
18: Supradiaphragmatic

Fig. 6.3 Lymph node stations in gastric cancer

28. c) Age greater than 60 years

The Glasgow–Blatchford bleeding score (GBS) is a screening tool designed to assess the likelihood that a patient presenting with an upper GI bleed will need some form of medical intervention, such as an OGD or blood transfusion. It may also be used to help to identify patients that do not need to be admitted to hospital. The Rockall score may also be used to assess the severity of an upper GI bleed but is weighted towards assessing the risk of mortality. A score of six or more is associated with a greater than 50% risk of needing an intervention.

The Glasgow–Blatchford score is devised as follows in Table 6.3.

Blatchford O et al. A risk score to predict need for treatment for upper gastrointestinal haemorrhage. *Lancet* 2000; 356:1318–21.

29. c) Eosinophilic oesophagitis

This condition has gained increasing importance when evaluating patients who present with food impaction and dysphagia. The condition was first described in children but it is now increasingly recognized in adults. The underlying pathophysiology is not clear but it does seem that food allergy plays a role. It appears to have an autoimmune allergic component as it is associated with both asthma and coeliac disease. There may also be in association with reflux oesophagitis and heartburn.

Typically, patients present with difficulty with swallowing, food impaction, regurgitation, or vomiting. In children there may also be feeding difficulties and a failure to gain weight. The diagnosis is usually made on endoscopy (see Figure 6.4). Although endoscopy may be normal, histology shows

Table 6.3 Glasgow–Blatchford score

Admission risk marker	Score component value	
Blood urea (mmol/L)		
6.5–7.9	2	
8.0–9.9	3	
10.0–25.0	4	
>25.0	6	
Haemoglobin for men (g/L)		Haemoglobin for women (g/L)
120–129	1	100–119
100–119	3	
<100	6	<100
Systolic blood pressure (mmHg)		
100–109	1	
90–99	2	
<90	3	
Other markers		
Pulse >100bpm	1	
Presentation with malaena	1	
Presentation with syncope	2	
Hepatic disease	2	
Cardiac failure	2	

S – shock
M – haemoglobin
U – Urea.
C – comorbids.
P

Reprinted from *The Lancet*, 356, Blatchford, O., Murray W.R., Blatchford M., A risk score to predict need for treatment for uppergastrointestinal haemorrhage, pp. 1318–21. Copyright (2000) with permission from Elsevier.

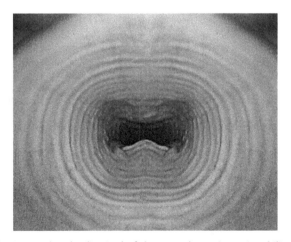

Fig. 6.4 Concentric rings or 'trachealization' of the oesophagus in eosinophilic oesophagitis

Autoimmune disease associated ō Schatzki rigs.

typical appearances of numerous eosinophils within the superficial epithelium. The eosinophilic _s_ inflammation may not be limited to the oesophagus alone and may extend throughout the gastrointestinal tract. On occasion micro abscesses and an expansion of the basal cell layer may be present. White plaques or exudates may be observed. Ridges, furrows, or rings may also be noted within the oesophageal wall. Concentric rings have been described which makes the oesophagus look like a trachea. The term 'corrugated oesophagus' is used. It may be that the syndrome of multiple Schatzki rings is in fact eosinophilic oesophagitis. *Pseudo - trachealion.*

Treatment is by dietary modification with an attempt to exclude any food allergens that are identified. Pump inhibitors are also used. Occasionally topical steroids are used. Mechanical dilatation of the oesophagus is rarely necessary.

Furuta GT and Katzka DA. Eosinophilic esophagitis. *New England Journal of Medicine* 2015; 373:1640–8.

30. e) Score cannot be calculated from these data

The Rockall risk scoring system is used to identify patients at risk of adverse outcome following an acute upper GI bleed (see Table 6.4). The scoring system is a combination of clinical data and endoscopic findings. A convenient mnemonic is ABCDE (i.e. Age, Blood pressure fall, Comorbidity, Diagnosis, and Evidence of bleeding). The system is helpful in predicting mortality although it requires both the results of an OGD and also the subjective assessment of major morbidity to calculate the score. A score of less than 3 carries a good prognosis and a total score of 8 or more carries a high risk of mortality. In the current scenario, the score cannot be calculated, as she has not had an upper GI endoscopy.

Rockall TA et al. Risk assessment after acute upper gastrointestinal haemorrhage. *Gut* 1996. 38(3):316–21.

Vreeburg EM et al. Validation of the Rockall risk scoring system in upper gastrointestinal bleeding. *Gut* 1999. 44(3):331–5. *This is definitely a post-OGD system*

Table 6.4 Rockall score

Variable	Score 0	Score 1	Score 2	Score 3
Age	<60	60—79	>80	
Shock	No shock	Pulse >100 BP >100 Systolic	SBP <100	
Co-morbidity	Nil major		CHF, IHD, major morbidity	Renal failure, liver failure, metastatic cancer
Diagnosis	Mallory—Weiss	All other diagnoses	GI malignancy	
Evidence of bleeding	None		Blood, adherent clot, spurting vessel	

Adapted from *Gut*, 38, 3, Rockall T.A., Logan, R.F., Devlin, H.B, and Northfield T.C, Risk assessment after acute upper gastrointestinal haemorrhage, pp. 316—21. Copyright © 1996, BMJ Publishing Group Ltd and the British Society of Gastroenterology

31. d) Associated with less late morbidity such as weight loss, dumping, and diarrhoea

Vagal-sparing oesophagectomy can be performed laparoscopically through cervical and gastric incisions. The oesophagus is stripped, preserving the vagal nerves. It can be used for intra-mucosal adenocarcinoma and high-grade dysplasia which do not require a lymphatic dissection. It should not be considered in cancers which have invaded into the submucosa or beyond because of the risk of nodal metastases.

The procedure offers the advantage of being easier to perform, does not require single lung ventilation or mediastinal dissection, avoids the need for a pyloroplasty, and is associated with reduced morbidity and a better functional outcome.

Both early and late complications are reduced including less perioperative morbidity and a shorter hospital stay compared to either a transhiatal or en bloc oesophagectomy. In addition, late morbidity including weight loss, dumping, and diarrhoea are less likely with a vagal-sparing approach.

DeMeester SR. Vagal-sparing esophagectomy: is it a useful addition? *Annals of Thoracic Surgery* 2010; 89(6):S2156–8.

Peyre CG et al. Vagal-sparing esophagectomy: the ideal operation for intramucosal adenocarcinoma and Barrett with high-grade dysplasia. *Annals of Surgery* 2007; 246(4):665–71.

32. b) T1a

T1 primary oesophageal squamous cell cancers are staged as Tis if there is evidence for high-grade dysplasia, T1a when the tumour invades the lamina propria or muscularis mucosa. T1b tumours invade the submucosa. Such lesions can be considered for endoscopic therapy including endoscopic mucosal resection, endoscopic submucosal dissection, or ablative procedures such as radiofrequency ablation.

Oyama T et al. Endoscopic submucosal dissection of early esophageal cancer. *Clinical Gastroenterology and Hepatology* 2005: 3;S67–S70.

Rice TW et al. 7th Edition of the AJCC Cancer Staging Manual: Esophagus and esophagogastric junction. *Annals of Surgery Oncology* 2010; 7:1721–4.

33. a) Female gender

Male gender, older age, and a history of reflux symptoms have consistently been shown to be predictors for increased risk of Barrett's oesophagus. There also appears to be an association with obesity, although some studies have failed to demonstrate a high BMI as a risk factor. A number of studies have also shown an association with cigarette smoking although this is not a consistent finding. Family clustering appears to occur in Barrett's oesophagus, which has been identified in up to 30% of relatives of patients with Barrett's high-grade dysplasia. Genetic factors may account for this familial association.

Fitzgerald RC et al. British Society of Gastroenterology guidelines on the diagnosis and management of Barrett's oesophagus. *Gut* 2014; 63(1):7–42.

34. c) 35–39.9

Obesity is generally classified using the WHO classification by body mass index (BMI) (see Table 6.5). This ranges from underweight (<18.5) to Obese Class III (>40).

Dixon JB et al. Bariatric surgery: an IDF statement for obese Type 2 diabetes. *Diabetic Medicine* 2011; 28:628–42.

35. b) BMI >35 and type 2 diabetes

Criteria for bariatric surgery are defined through the NICE and SIGN guidelines. In terms of their weight, patients should have a BMI of >40 or between 35 and 40 with a weight-loss-responsive disease although the SIGN guidelines suggest the threshold for surgery is a BMI >35 with at least one weight-loss-responsive disease.

Table 6.5 WHO classification of body mass index

WHO classification	BMI kg/m2
Underweight	< 18.5
Normal weight	18.5–24.9
Overweight	≥ 25.0
Preobese	25.0–29.9
Obese	≥ 30.0
Obese class I	30.0–34.9
Obese class II	35.0–39.9
Obese class III	≥ 40.0

Adapted from *WHO Technical Report Series*, 894, World Health Organization, Obesity: preventing and managing the global epidemic, 2000. Licence: Creative Commons BY 3.0 IGO (https://creativecommons.org/licenses/by/3.0/igo)

National Institute for Health and Care Excellence. Obesity, the prevention, identification, assessment and management of overweight and obesity in adults and children. NICE Guideline 43. 2006. <https://www.nice.org.uk/guidance/cg189/evidence/obesity-update-appendix-m-pdf-6960327447>.

Scottish Intercollegiate Guidelines Network. Management of Obesity. A national clinical guideline. 2010. <http://www.sign.ac.uk/assets/sign115.pdf>.

36. e) DVT/PE

The commonest cause of mortality following bariatric surgery is DVT/PE, accounting for approximately 50% of deaths. The overall risk of mortality following gastric banding is up to 0.1% and after gastric bypass is up to 0.2%

Podnos YD et al. Complications after laparoscopic gastric bypass a review of 3464 cases. *Archives of Surgery* 2003; 138:957–61.

37. e) Urgent decompression of the band using a Huber needle, contrast swallow, and laparoscopy

The clinical picture is consistent with an acute slippage of the gastric band and the key clinical finding is the severe abdominal pain which may be consistent with ischaemia/necrosis of the gastric pouch above the band. This is an urgent situation and the appropriate management involves decompression using a Huber needle, a contrast swallow, and laparoscopy to release the band.

ASMBS position statement on emergency care of patients with complications related to bariatric surgery. *Surgery for Obesity and Related Diseases* 2010; 6:115–7.

38. c) 3%

The risk of anastomotic leak following gastric bypass is approximately 3%. Anastomostic leak should be considered in the post-operative patient who develops tachycardia, complains of abdominal pain or just has a sense of impending doom. If anastomotic leak needs to be excluded, patients should have an urgent CT and/or immediate re-laparoscopy with either direct repair or T-tube placement. Other early complications of gastric bypass include bleeding from anastomoses and staple lines, closed loop obstructions from internal herniation or inaccurate Roux-limb reconstruction, and DVT/PE.

Lee S. Effect of location and speed of diagnosis on anastomotic leak outcomes in 3828 gastric bypass cases. *Journal of Gastrointestinal Surgery* 2007; 11:708–13.

Extended Matching Items

Therapeutic endoscopy

[handwritten: Caspofungin. Remembered]

1. F. Fully covered oesophageal stent

Clinically there is an oesophageal perforation. In a fasted patient, immediate placement of a fully covered stent should be considered, followed by broad-spectrum antibiotics and a proton pump inhibitor. *[handwritten: caspofungin also.]*

Oesophageal perforation carries a high morbidity and mortality if not appropriately and rapidly treated. Management depends on a number of factors including the location of the perforation, the mechanism of perforation, and the overall health of the patient. Cervical perforations are usually small and can often be treated conservatively as contamination is contained within the triangle of Killian in the neck. Thoracic perforations are more serious. Iatrogenic perforations secondary to sclerotherapy or balloon dilatation can usually be managed with endotherapy. Small tears may be clipped and larger perforations may be treated with a covered stent. However, in the absence of a stricture or cancer, such stents tend to migrate. Perforation of the intra-abdominal portion of the oesophagus is perhaps the most serious site and often results in the rapid development of severe abdominal pain, peritonitis, and sepsis and is more likely to require surgery. However, surgery should only be contemplated in patients who are fit for intervention.

Romero RV and Goh KL. Esophageal perforation: Continuing challenge to treatment. *Gastrointestinal Intervention* 2013; 2:1–6.

[handwritten: Iatrogenic perforation vs Boerhaave — much better to treat — less sicker as starved.]

2. D. Radiofrequency ablation

Comorbidities would preclude consideration of transhiatal or vagal-sparing oesophagectomy. Radiofrequency ablation would provide appropriate treatment for high-grade dysplasia in Barrett's. Barrett's oesophagus is a premalignant condition where the oesophageal squamous epithelium undergoes columnar change with metaplasia, which predisposes to the development of oesophageal adenocarcinoma. If there is no associated metaplasia, it is thought that the risk of developing cancer is low. Oesophageal adenocarcinoma is thought to develop following a stepwise progression from oesophagitis, metaplasia, dysplasia, and finally adenocarcinoma. Surveillance may be necessary in cases of indeterminate or low-grade dysplasia. Clinical follow-up and management of patients with high-grade dysplasia needs to be tailored to the individual patient. Resection may need to be considered in fit patients with high-grade dysplasia. Alternative ablative techniques such as radiofrequency ablation should be considered, particularly in unfit patients such as presented in this scenario. *[handwritten: ablative as not sorted by EMR-]*

Booth CL and Thompson KS. Barrett's esophagus: A review of diagnostic criteria, clinical surveillance practices and new developments. *Journal of Gastrointestinal Oncology* 2012; 3:232–42.

3. J. Pyloric balloon dilatation

[handwritten: Pyloromyomyotomy to reduce the idver of gas ... of pt ... oesophgets]

Delayed emptying of the gastric conduit following oesophagectomy is common and up to 20% of patients have evidence of frank gastric outlet obstruction. Endoscopic balloon dilatation of the pylorus following oesophagectomy has a success rate of up to 95%. Conservative management consists of prokinetic drugs, nasogastric drainage, and dietary alterations. Some surgeons routinely perform a pyloromyotomy at the time of oesophagectomy in order to improve gastric emptying. However, it is not clear if such an intervention actually reduces the incidence of gastric outlet obstruction following oesophagectomy.

Lanuti M et al. Management of delayed gastric emptying after esophagectomy with endoscopic balloon dilatation of the pylorus. *Annals of Thoracic Surgery* 2011; 91:11019–24.

4. C. Endoscopic mucosal resection

This nodular area requires further investigation. EMR will provide an adequate biopsy specimen for histological assessment and if there is no evidence of invasive disease, will also provide a flat mucosa for subsequent RFA.

5. A. Enteric stent

Stenting would be more appropriate than palliative laser in this setting, particularly in view of the burden of disease and frailty, by providing more immediate palliation of gastric outlet obstruction.

Treatment of upper gastrointestinal bleeding

6. I. Radiotherapy

In extensive gastric carcinoma laser is often unhelpful. Single-fraction palliative radiotherapy can help in reducing transfusion requirements.

7. G. ERCP

Presuming a post-sphincterotomy bleed, ERCP allows adrenaline injection therapy, tamponade with a balloon, endoscopic clip application, or insertion of a covered biliary stent. Failing this, interventional radiological embolization would be the next course of action.

8. E. Sengstaken–Blakemore tube

Endoscopic band ligation (EBL) is the treatment of choice for acute variceal haemorrhage and also for primary and secondary prophylaxis of oesophageal bleeding. Complications occur in 2–25% of patients and include oesophageal stricture formation, infection, and re-bleeding secondary to variceal haemorrhage or post-banding oesophageal ulceration (reported in 3–7% of patients). Post-banding ulcer haemorrhage occurs between 2 and 30 days. It can be managed with cyanoacrylate endoscopic injection, metallic stent, balloon tamponade, and trans-jugular intra-hepatic portosystemic shunt (TIPS).

In the current scenario, the patient is close to arrest and the only therapeutic option would be insertion of a Sengstaken–Blakemore tube. Assuming that this controlled the haemorrhage, the patient could be resuscitated with the view to undergoing upper GI endoscopy to assess and manage either repeat variceal bleeding or bleeding from oesophageal ulceration.

9. J. Cyanoacrylate endoscopic injection

Gastric varices are classified into either gastro-oesophageal varices or isolated gastric varices. They may be present in up to 20% of patients with cirrhosis. The majority (75%) are felt to be oesophageal varices that extend below the gastro-oesophageal junction along the lesser curve of the stomach. According to Sarin's classification, these are termed gastro-oesophageal varices 1 (GOV1). Around 20% are oesophageal varices that extend into the fundus of the stomach (GOV2). Isolated gastric varices (IGV) are much less common, affecting either the fundus of the stomach (IGV1) (2%) or ectopic varices elsewhere in the stomach (IGV2) (4%).

The one-year risk of bleeding from gastric varices is 10–15%. Some limited studies suggest that cyanoacrylate injection may be more effective than banding. In treatment failures, a trans-jugular intra-hepatic portosystemic shunt should be considered.

Garcia–Pagán JC et al. Management of gastric varices. *Clinical Gastroenterology and Hepatology* 2014; 12(6):919–28.

Upper GI functional disorders

10. B. Implantable gastric pacemaker

A number of publications have documented that gastric electrical stimulation (GES), via insertion of a gastric pacemaker, can lead to an improvement in quality of life and nutritional status for some patients. However, the quality of the data is poor and there is a lack of randomized controlled trials. Predictors of a good response to GES include diabetic-associated gastroparesis and patients where nausea and vomiting are the predominant symptoms. Unfortunately, it is not possible to predict with accuracy the likely individual response to GES. The mechanism of action of GES remains poorly understood. Despite this, GES may be of benefit in some patients with severe gastroparesis who fail to respond to medical therapy.

Soffer EE. Gastric electrical stimulation for gastroparesis. *Journal of Neurogastroenterology and Motility* 2012; 18(2):131–7.

11. F. Calcium channel antagonists

Manometry would suggest a hypercontractile oesophagus (Jackhammer oesophagus), which may respond to calcium channel antagonists, nitrates, and sildenafil.

12. H. Laparoscopic Heller's myotomy with partial fundoplication

The manometry results suggest achalasia. There is some argument regarding the efficacy of pneumatic dilatation versus laparoscopic Heller's myotomy (LHM) in the management of achalasia. Dilatation appears to be marginally better than LHM in treating Type II achalasia, although success rates of 90–100% are achieved with both interventions. Some authors have suggested that longer-term success rates may be possible with LHM. Success rates of around 80% with either pneumatic dilatation or LHM are possible in Type I achalasia. Type III patients may be best treated with LHM where success rates of around 85% are reported versus a success rate of 40% for dilatation.

Rohof WO et al. Outcomes of treatment for achalasia depend on manometric subtype. *Gastroenterology* 2013; 144:718–25.

Management of oesophageal cancer

13. L. Chemoradiotherapy

For those diagnosed with a localized squamous cell carcinoma of the oesophagus, definitive chemoradiotherapy is the management of choice, resulting in better outcomes in proximal and middle third tumours compared to surgical resection. No studies have shown an advantage by following definitive chemoradiotherapy with surgery.

Bedenne L et al. Chemoradiation followed by surgery compared with chemoradiation alone in squamous cancer of the oesophagus: FFCD 9102. *Journal of Clinical Oncology* 2007; 25:1160–8.

14. B. Neoadjuvant chemotherapy & Ivor–Lewis oesophagectomy

In a patient presenting with a resectable middle-third oesophageal adenocarcinoma, the two-phase Ivor–Lewis oesophagectomy (laparotomy and right thoracotomy) with two-field lymphadenectomy is the standard approach. For patients with resectable lower-third oesophageal adenocarcinomas the Ivor–Lewis, or alternatively the transhiatal approach (without thoracotomy), can be utilized. Nodal yield is less in the transhiatal approach, although there has been no statistically significant survival difference demonstrated between the two approaches. The decision often comes down to patient fitness in consideration of suitability for thoracotomy, as there is a lower morbidity particularly with regard to pulmonary complications with the transhiatal approach.

Some large studies have shown significantly better overall and disease free-survival with a carboplatin and paclitaxel-based neoadjuvant chemoradiotherapy regimen. This regimen was also associated with a 34% reduction in the risk of longer-term mortality compared to patients progressing straight to surgery. This regimen is also associated with a lower risk of developing high-grade toxicity. Although not currently standard practice in the United Kingdom, where ECF-based (epirubicin, cisplatin, and 5-fluorouracil) chemoradiotherapy regimens are used, it is likely to feature in future management algorithms.

Hulscher JB et al. Extended transthoracic resection compared with limited transhiatal resection for adenocarcinoma of the esophagus. *New England Journal of Medicine* 2002; 347(21):1662–9.

Cunningham D et al. Perioperative chemotherapy versus surgery alone for resectable gastroesophageal cancer. *New England Journal of Medicine* 2006; 355:11–20.

Van Hagen P et al. Preoperative chemoradiotherapy for esophageal or junctional cancer. *New England Journal of Medicine* 2012; 366:2074–84.

15. G. Transhiatal oesophagectomy

The transhiatal approach can also be used for resection in patients with Barrett's with high-grade dysplasia for whom endoscopic management is not an option, although the use of endoscopic therapies such as radiofrequency ablation and endoscopic mucosal resection should be considered first-line.

Management of gastric cancer

16. I. Neoadjuvant chemotherapy, distal gastrectomy, and adjuvant chemotherapy

The primary objective of gastric cancer surgery is the resection of the lesion with a clear longitudinal and circumferential margin. In patients with a resectable distal (middle or lower third) gastric adenocarcinoma, a distal gastrectomy would be the favoured approach. There is no survival benefit in total gastrectomy over distal gastrectomy assuming a minimal proximal resection margin of 3–5cm can be obtained. Perioperative chemotherapy should be considered in all patients being considered for resection, the only exception being early-stage gastric cancers.

Bozzetti F et al. Subtotal versus total gastrectomy for gastric cancer: five-year survival rates in a multicenter randomized Italian trial. Italian Gastrointestinal Tumour Study Group. *Annals of Surgery* 1999; 230:170–8.

Cunningham D et al. Perioperative chemotherapy versus surgery alone for resectable gastroesophageal cancer. *New England Journal of Medicine* 2006; 355:11–20.

17. F. Neoadjuvant chemotherapy, total gastrectomy, and adjuvant chemotherapy

In this scenario, the pathology is suggestive of a Lauren diffuse-type adenocarcinoma characterized by a linitus plastica growth pattern. A 5cm proximal resection margin will be required as an absolute minimum and sometimes more. As such, a total gastrectomy would be favoured over a distal gastrectomy. The standard of care for all patients (other than those with early-stage gastric adenocarcinomas) is the incorporation of perioperative chemotherapy into management.

Cunningham D et al. Perioperative chemotherapy versus surgery alone for resectable gastroesophageal cancer. *New England Journal of Medicine* 2006; 355:11–20.

18. B. Total gastrectomy

Patients with HDGC who have a germline mutation in the *CDH1* gene have a lifetime risk of gastric cancer of 83% in women and 67% in men. Those who have this condition and develop gastric adenocarcinoma have a much poorer prognosis than those without this mutation, with as few as

10% having potentially curable disease. In light of this it is recommended that patients with this condition undergo prophylactic total gastrectomy. The optimal extent of lymphadenopathy in these patients is controversial, as the majority of patients with this condition who undergo total gastrectomy will have a small foci of T1a cancer. These carry a risk of up to 6% for lymph node metastases and as such a D1 lymphadenectomy with resection of stations 1–7 would be acceptable.

Van der Post RS et al. Hereditary Diffuse Gastric Cancer: Updated clinical guidelines with an emphasis on germline CDH1 mutation carriers. *Journal of Medical Genetics* 2015; 52(6):361–74.

Investigations and staging of oesophageal cancer

[handwritten: Stage potentially resectable.]

19. G. PET–CT and EUS

[handwritten: OGD | CT Scan | PET + EUS.]

In patients with potentially resectable oesophageal adenocarcinoma, the use of both PET–CT and endoscopic ultrasound for staging has become routine. The main role of PET–CT is to ensure that there is no metastatic disease, especially in those with locoregional lymphadenopathy, given the higher potential for undetected metastases, including metastatic lymphadenopathy not seen on CT.

PET–CT is not a good investigation for the differentiation of nodal disease adjacent to the primary tumour and EUS provides a much better method of clarifying this. It is accepted that EUS and EUS–FNA are the most accurate methods for locoregional staging for oesophageal adenocarcinoma but their clinical impact is minimal. As such it is used selectively on a patient-by-patient basis to increase the accuracy of staging.

Puli SR et al. Staging accuracy of esophageal cancer by endoscopic ultrasound: a meta-analysis and systematic review. *World Journal of Gastroenterology* 2008; 14(10):1479–90.

20. D. Laparoscopy and peritoneal cytology

In patients with a junctional oesophageal adenocarcinoma the use of a staging laparoscopy with peritoneal cytology should be considered, as these have a significant potential for intra-abdominal metastatic disease resulting in their management being palliative.

DeGraaf GW et al. The role of staging laparoscopy in oesophagogastric cancers. *European Journal of Surgical Oncology* 2007; 33(8):988–92.

21. A. CT chest/abdomen

[handwritten: for re-staging – CT scan NOT to complete staging]

In patients who have undergone neoadjuvant chemotherapy, patients should be re-staged to determine response to chemotherapy and/or check for metastatic progression. It is noteworthy that the reduction in primary tumour volume following neoadjuvant chemotherapy must be in the region of 50% to accurately determine response.

22. C. Upper GI endoscopy

[handwritten: Even c palliative disease get primary tissue despite metastatic.]

Although the patient in this scenario clearly presents with metastatic disease, an OGD should be considered if an oesophagogastric cancer is suspected. This will allow for histopathological confirmation of the diagnosis and the potential for palliative chemotherapy. In patients with a new diagnosis of GIST, the use of CT scanning is the first-line investigation to assess the primary lesion and look for metastases. This may be complemented by the use of EUS–FNA.

23. A. CT chest/abdomen

Local increases in size, transperitoneal spread or metastatic spread to the liver are the most common methods of progression of GISTs. A contrast-enhanced CT of chest abdomen and pelvis is therefore appropriate for staging and follow-up. MRI or contrast-enhanced ultrasound may also be considered. Pelvic MRI is best for local staging of rectal GISTs. PET–CT can be used to assess early tumour response to molecular-targeted therapy.

Joensuu H et al. Management of malignant gastrointestinal stromal tumours. *Lancet Oncology* 2002; 3(11):655–64.

The ESMO/European Sarcoma Network Working Group. Gastrointestinal stromal tumors: ESMO Clinical Practice Guidelines for diagnosis, treatment and follow-up. *Annals of Oncology* 2012; 23 (suppl 7):vii49–vii55.

Staging of oesophagogastric cancer

24. E. T2 N1 M0 R0

Staging of oesophagogastric cancer is carried out using the TNM 7 classification which came into effect in January 2010. Junctional cancers are now staged within the oesophageal staging system. The patient in this scenario demonstrates disease through the muscularis propria but not adventitia making it T2, with nodal disease in one to two regional lymph nodes making it N1 disease.

Rice TW et al. Esophagus and esophagogastric junction. In: Amin MB et al. (eds). *AJCC Cancer Staging Manual*, 8th edn. New York, NY: Springer, 2017, pp. 185–202.

Sobin LH et al (eds). *TNM Classification of Malignant Tumours*, 7th edn. Oxford: Wiley-Blackwell, 2009.

25. H. T3 N2 M0 R0

This patient has disease invading through the subserosa, but not through to the visceral peritoneum or adjacent structures, making it a T3 cancer. Three to six positive regional lymph nodes classify this as an N2 tumour.

26. A. T4 N3 M1

This patient has advanced disease with tumour evident on the surface of the stomach suggesting T4 disease, with 7–15 nodes involved making it N3 disease. The presence of positive peritoneal cytology makes this case M1 and as such, a curative resectional procedure would be contraindicated.

Palliative management of oesophagogastric cancer

27. H. Insertion of oesophageal stent

Up to two-thirds of patients who present with oesophagogastric cancer are found to have disease that is not amenable to cure. There is a relative paucity of evidence for a survival benefit for palliative chemotherapy or radiotherapy in metastatic oesophageal adenocarcinoma and few patients survive for longer than one year. The management of symptoms is therefore critical in improving quality of life. One of the most distressing symptoms patients present with is dysphagia and the use of self-expanding metal stents is an effective method in palliating dysphagia. These can be inserted endoscopically or radiologically.

Sreedharan A et al. Interventions for dysphagia in oesophageal cancer. *Cochrane Database of Systematic Reviews* 2009; (4):CD005048.

28. G. Laparoscopic gastrojejunostomy

Gastric outlet obstruction is a common occurrence in patients with advanced distal gastric cancers. Options for palliation include the formation of a gastrojejunostomy to bypass the lesion, which may be performed laparoscopically. Alternatively, the use of a duodenal stent may also achieve the same effect. There is some evidence that duodenal stent placement may be a better option in patients with a very poor prognosis and a relatively short life expectancy, while laparoscopic

[handwritten: Young + fit → lap gastrojej | old + infirm → stent duodenum]

gastrojejunostomy may be a better option in fitter patients with a better prognosis as suggested in this scenario.

Ly J et al. A systematic review of methods to palliate malignant gastric outlet obstruction. *Surgical Endoscopy* 2010; 24(2): 290–7.

29. D. Combination chemotherapy and trastuzamab

Combination chemotherapy is the main treatment option for patients with inoperable gastric tumours, given that it has been shown to improve quality of life and prolong survival when compared to best supportive care. Patients who have tumours that strongly express HER-2 should also be offered trastuzumab (Herceptin®).

Trastuzumab is a monoclonal antibody that binds to the HER2/neu receptor. The HER receptor proteins are embedded in the cell membrane and communicate molecular signals from outside the cell (epidermal growth factors) to inside the cell, thereby turning genes on and off. The HER protein (human epidermal growth factor receptor), binds to human epidermal growth factor, which stimulates cell proliferation. In some cancers, notably certain types of breast cancer, colon, and gastro-oesophageal cancers, HER2 is over-expressed and causes cancer cells to reproduce uncontrollably.

Bang YJ et al. Trastuzumab in combination with chemotherapy versus chemotherapy alone for treatment of HER2-positive advanced gastric or gastro-oesophageal junction cancer (ToGA): a phase 3, open-label, randomized controlled trial. *Lancet* 2010; 376(9742): 687–97.

Causes of upper GI haemorrhage

30. I. Dieulafoy's lesion — *[handwritten: missed frequently.]*

Dieulafoy's lesion is a large tortuous arteriole within the submucosa of the stomach or other area of the gastrointestinal tract. It erodes through the mucosa to intermittently bleed. It is uncommon and accounts for less than 5% of all gastrointestinal bleeds in adults. Around 75% of documented lesions occur in the upper stomach within 6 cm of the gastro-oesophageal junction, most commonly on the lesser curvature. Lesions are twice as common in men and patients typically have multiple comorbidities including hypertension, cardiovascular disease, chronic renal disease, and diabetes.

Typically, they give rise to intermittent bleeding. Bleeding occurs through a minute defect in the mucosa which is almost impossible to see unless they are actively bleeding. Patients therefore often undergo several OGDs before they are diagnosed. Alternatively, angiography may be helpful but again, it is usually only diagnostic if performed when the patient is actively bleeding. The lesion can usually be treated endoscopically with injection, diathermy, heater probe, banding, or clipping.

Baxter, M and Aly EH. Dieulafoy's lesion: current trends in diagnosis and management. *Annals of The Royal College of Surgeons of England.* 2010; 92(7): 548–54.

31. J. Duodenal ulcer

Non-variceal upper GI bleeding accounts for at least 30—40% of upper GI bleeds in cirrhotic patients. Peptic ulcer disease accounts for at least 60% of such cases. Other causes include gastritis, hypertensive gastropathy, and oesophageal ulceration. Increasing age, male sex, diabetes, chronic renal disease, a history of gastro-oesophageal variceal bleeding, and the use of non-steroidal anti-inflammatory drugs have been shown to be risk factors for peptic ulcer bleeding in cirrhotic patients. It is therefore very important to confirm or exclude variceal bleeding as the cause for upper GI haemorrhage in patients with cirrhosis and to initiate appropriate treatment based on the site of the haemorrhage.

[handwritten: varices — 60% will be variceal — peptic ulcer as most common cause.]

Luo JC et al. Cirrhotic patients at increased risk of peptic ulcer bleeding. A nationwide population-based cohort study. *Alimentary Pharmacology & Therapeutics* 2012; 36(6): 542–50.

32. L. Haemobilia

Haemobilia is a rare cause of upper GI bleeding. At least two- thirds of cases follow on from medical interventions such as liver biopsy, transhepatic cholangiography, angiography, or endoscopic interventions such as ERC and insertion of biliary stents. However, blunt or penetrating trauma to the liver can also cause haemobilia. Other causes include inflammatory and neoplastic conditions in and around the liver, gallbladder, and biliary tree. On rare occasions, congenital or acquired vascular aneurysms, pancreatitis, and hepatitis may cause haemobilia. The classic presentation is that of acute biliary-type upper abdominal pain in association with jaundice and haematemesis or melaena. However, Quincke's classic triad of upper abdominal pain, upper gastrointestinal haemorrhage, and jaundice only occurs in about 20% of patients.

CT or MRI scanning is not always helpful in diagnosing the cause of bleeding although clot-like debris may be seen distending the bile ducts. Endoscopy or ERC may diagnose clot coming from the duodenal papilla. If it follows local intervention such as sphincterotomy, direct application of clips or injection with adrenalin may be possible. If bleeding is secondary to blunt or penetrating injury to the liver, angiography with embolization may control bleeding.

Chin MW and, Enns R. Hemobilia. *Current Gastroenterology Reports* 2010; 12: 121–9.

Merrell SW and, Schneider PD. Hemobilia—evolution of current diagnosis and treatment. *Western Journal of Medicine* 1991; 155: 621–5.

Causes of dysphagia

33. F. Pharyngeal pouch

This is a condition of elderly patients and rarely occurs before the age of 40 years. Symptoms are initially fairly minimal and patients frequently do not seek medical advice. The condition is more common in males. Typical symptoms include dysphagia, which is consistently present, regurgitation of undigested food in association with a choking sensation when eating. Patients may also complain of noise or borborygmi in the cervical region and symptoms of aspiration including chronic cough, halitosis, and weight loss. Hoarseness may also occur. As the pouch enlarges symptoms may become more severe and lead to malnutrition. There may be no specific findings on examination. However, weight loss and occasionally the identification of a swelling in the neck which gurgles on palpation (Boyce's sign) can occur. There may also be signs of infection—consolidation due to aspiration.

Siddiq MA et al. Pharyngeal pouch (Zenker's diverticulum). *Postgraduate Medical Journal* 2001; 77: 506–11.

34. A. Achalasia

Achalasia is characterized by difficulty in swallowing with regurgitation and sometimes chest pain. Endoscopy may show food debris within the oesophagus but it may also be normal. The diagnosis is established with a combination of oesophageal manometry and a barium swallow. The condition is characterized by incomplete or absent relaxation of the lower oesophageal sphincter (<75% relaxation upon wet swallow), increased lower oesophageal sphincter tone (>100mmHg, normal is <26mmHg), and a lack of peristalsis within the oesophagus. Biopsy is not necessary to establish the diagnosis but if performed may show hypertrophy of the musculature and an absence of ganglion cells within the myenteric plexus. See Figure. 6.5.

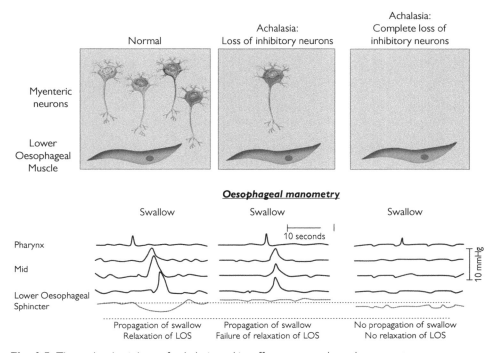

Fig. 6.5 The pathophysiology of achalasia and its effect on oesophageal manometry

35. C. Systemic sclerosis

Systemic sclerosis is an autoimmune disorder resulting in generalized connective tissue disease affecting the skin and the various internal organs. Gastrointestinal tract involvement is seen in more than 90% of patients. The oesophagus is the most frequently affected organ. Oesophageal motility is affected, which results in a reduction in lower oesophageal pressure with a loss of distal oesophageal body peristalsis leading to severe reflux. Patients may develop erosive oesophagitis and Barrett's oesophagus and ultimately oesophageal adenocarcinoma. Morphea, which is also known as localized cutaneous scleroderma, is characterised by predominant skin involvement and sparing of internal organs. However, the oesophagus can be involved in 5 to –10% of cases.

Arif T et al. Assessment of esophageal involvement in systemic sclerosis and morphea (localized scleroderma) by clinical, endoscopic, manometric and pH metric features: a prospective comparative hospital based study. BMC *Gastroenterology* 2015; 15: 24.

Single Best Answers

1. **A 54 year old woman attends the breast clinic. She has a lump in the left breast that has been present for several weeks. After clinical examination and mammography, what is the next investigation that should be considered?**
    a) Core biopsy of the lump
    b) Cytology smear from left nipple
    c) Fine needle aspiration of the lump
    d) MRI of both breasts
    e) Ultrasound of left breast

2. **A 46 year old woman has a 3-month history of blood-stained discharge from a single duct on the right nipple. Clinical examination and mammography are normal. Nipple smear from the single duct discharge is reported as showing epithelial cells and occasional red blood cells.**
    What is the next step?
    a) List for total duct excision
    b) List for microdochectomy
    c) Perform core biopsy under the nipple
    d) Reassure and discharge
    e) Repeat nipple smear in three months

3. **Which statement regarding the UK Breast Screening Programme is correct?**
    a) Breast cancer is detected in 5% of women screened
    b) Median uptake is 90%
    c) Two-view mammography is performed
    d) Women are screened every two years
    e) Women between the ages of 40 and 70 are invited

4. **Which of the following is true regarding breast-conserving surgery for breast cancer?**
    a) It is contraindicated in tumours greater than 5cm diameter
    b) It is contraindicated where there is bulky axillary nodal involvement
    c) Radiotherapy can be safely omitted following breast-conserving surgery
    d) Intraoperative radiotherapy has equivalent recurrence rates to external beam radiotherapy
    e) It has equivalent recurrence rates to mastectomy when combined with external beam radiotherapy

5. **Which of the following results with regard to the tumour margins would result in re-excision being recommended?**
    a) A margin of <1mm from the edge of the specimen
    b) A margin of <2mm from the edge of the specimen
    c) A margin of <5mm from the edge of the specimen
    d) A measurement does not matter as long as there is no tumour at the inked margin
    e) Clear margins are not required if radiotherapy is planned

6. **A patient with a previous history of left breast cancer attends for follow-up five years after having breast-conserving surgery and sentinel node biopsy followed by adjuvant radiotherapy. Her follow-up mammogram shows a new 1cm area of microcalcification in the left breast. Axillary ultrasound is normal. Stereotactic biopsy of the area of microcalcification reveals ductal carcinoma *in situ*.**

    What is the most appropriate treatment?
    a) Mastectomy
    b) Mastectomy and axillary node clearance
    c) Wide local excision
    d) Wide local excision and sentinel node biopsy
    e) Wide local excision and radiotherapy

7. **A 43 year old woman attends the breast clinic with a single, palpable, firm, enlarged lymph node in the left axilla. Clinical breast examination and mammography are otherwise normal. What is the most appropriate next step in this patient's management?**
    a) Axillary clearance
    b) Ultrasound of the axilla
    c) Excision biopsy of node
    d) Review in clinic in two months
    e) Sentinel lymph node biopsy

8. **What is the accepted best method to localize a sentinel node?**
   a) Axillary ultrasound
   b) Methylene blue plus technetium-labelled albumin
   c) One-step nucleic acid amplification
   d) Patent blue plus technetium-labelled albumin
   e) Technetium-labelled albumin

9. **Which of the following statements about patent blue dye is incorrect?**
   a) It can cause a widespread urticarial rash
   b) It can cause an artefactual drop in observed venous oxygen saturation
   c) It is contraindicated in pregnancy
   d) It is licensed for use in breast surgery
   e) There is a 0.1% chance of anaphylaxis

10. **Which of the following is true regarding management of the axilla in a patient with breast cancer and a positive sentinel node biopsy?**
    a) Axillary clearance is associated with higher rates of axillary recurrence than axillary radiotherapy
    b) Axillary radiotherapy is associated with a higher rate of lymphoedema than axillary clearance
    c) Radiotherapy is used after axillary clearance
    d) No further treatment is needed as the positive sentinel node has been removed
    e) There is no difference in survival between axillary clearance and axillary radiotherapy

11. **A 44 year old woman has latissimus dorsi breast reconstruction following mastectomy for breast cancer. Where is the pedicle of her latissimus dorsi flap most likely to be found?**
    a) Axilla
    b) Midline
    c) Parasternal
    d) Subareolar
    e) Subclavicular

12. **Which of the following is a contraindication to DIEP (deep inferior epigastric artery perforator) breast reconstruction following mastectomy for breast cancer?**
    a) Age over 65 years
    b) More than four axillary nodes involved by tumour
    c) Previous abdominoplasty
    d) Previous caesarean section
    e) Previous open cholecystectomy

13. **Therapeutic mammoplasty can be described as which of the following?**
    a) Breast-conserving surgery
    b) Free flap reconstruction
    c) Pedicled flap reconstruction
    d) Simple mastectomy
    e) Subcutaneous mastectomy

14. **A 31 year old woman has 3 first-degree relatives with breast cancer and 2 with ovarian cancer. She has declined *BRCA* testing at this time.**

    Which management strategy is most appropriate?
    a) Annual breast ultrasound
    b) Annual breast MRI
    c) Annual mammography
    d) Bilateral risk-reducing mastectomy
    e) Random core biopsies

15. **A 45 year old woman has been assessed by a geneticist as being at a high risk of breast cancer due to her family history. Which of the following would be most appropriate for her to take to reduce her risk of developing breast cancer?**
    a) Denosumab
    b) Goserelin
    c) Letrozole
    d) Progesterone
    e) Tamoxifen

16. **Which of the following confers an increased risk of breast cancer in women?**
    a) Birth of first child at age <20 years
    b) Excess alcohol consumption
    c) Lucent breast parenchyma on mammogram
    d) Premenopausal obesity
    e) Regular exercise

17. **Which of the following is true of Paget's disease of the breast?**
    a) It can be treated with topical steroids
    b) It is often bilateral
    c) Surgical management is with mastectomy
    d) The underlying breast cancer will be visible on mammogram
    e) The areola is affected after the nipple

18. **Which of the following statements is most accurate when considering a 2.5cm Phyllodes tumour?**
    a) It is a good prognosis breast cancer
    b) It is an aggressive form of breast cancer
    c) It is treated by wide local excision
    d) It is treated by wide local excision and sentinel node biopsy
    e) It is best treated with endocrine therapy

19. **An 80 year old man is undergoing an elective inguinal hernia repair. He had started Finasteride for prostate cancer six months previously. While the patient is under anaesthesia, the operating surgeon notices a hard lump beneath the patient's left nipple along with firm nodes in the left axilla.**

    What is the most appropriate management?
    a) Freehand core biopsy of lump later that day
    b) Intra-operative core biopsy of lump in breast
    c) Intra-operative core biopsy of lump in breast and axilla
    d) Stop finasteride straight away
    e) Ultrasound guided biopsy of breast and axilla the next week

20. **A 50 year old man has a mastectomy and sentinel node biopsy for an 18mm, grade 2, node-negative, ductal breast cancer. The tumour is ER8, PR8, HER2 negative.**

    Which is the most appropriate adjuvant treatment?
    a) Chemotherapy
    b) Herceptin
    c) No adjuvant treatment
    d) Radiotherapy
    e) Tamoxifen

21. **A 50 year old woman is recalled to breast screening after her mammogram is reported as showing a 1cm area of polymorphic microcalcification. Clinical examination is normal.**

    What is the most likely diagnosis?
    a) Artefact
    b) Benign microcalcification
    c) Ductal carcinoma *in situ*
    d) Invasive ductal breast cancer
    e) Mondor's disease

22. A 52 year old woman is about to commence adjuvant treatment for locally advanced breast cancer. Which of the following agents is most likely to cause hair loss?

a) Lapatinib
b) Tamoxifen
c) Docetaxel
d) Trastuzumab
e) Letrozole

23. A 39 year old premenopausal woman is diagnosed with a 2.5cm, node-negative, oestrogen receptor-positive breast cancer. Which hormone medication would be most appropriate as part of her adjuvant treatment?

a) Anastrozole
b) Exemestane
c) Letrozole
d) Raloxifene
e) Tamoxifen

24. Which of the following is true regarding neo-adjuvant chemotherapy for breast cancer?

a) After complete pathological response, surgery can safely be omitted
b) Complete pathological response is most likely in oestrogen receptor-positive, HER2-negative breast cancer
c) Overall survival is superior when compared with adjuvant chemotherapy
d) Lobular breast cancer responds well
e) The usual regimen is three cycles of fluorouracil/epirubicin/cyclophosphamide + three cycles of a taxane

25. In which of the following patients with HER2-positive breast cancer would it be appropriate to give Herceptin as part of treatment?

a) A 55 year old woman with a tumour measuring 9mm
b) A 50 year old woman who is unfit to receive cytotoxic chemotherapy
c) A 60 year old woman with congestive cardiac failure
d) A 65 year old woman with metastatic spread to the lungs
e) A 90 year old woman who is otherwise well

26. **A 55 year old patient has undergone a mastectomy and axillary clearance. She has a 40mm, grade 3, ductal cancer, with 3 of 18 nodes involved. The tumour is ER 8, PR 8, HER2 negative. There is LVI present and the deep resection margin is 1mm. What would be the most appropriate adjuvant treatment for this patient?**
    a) Adjuvant chemotherapy, chest-wall radiotherapy, and letrozole
    b) Chest wall radiotherapy but no adjuvant systemic therapy
    c) Adjuvant chemotherapy and letrozole
    d) After mastectomy radiotherapy is not needed as the whole breast has been removed
    e) After mastectomy systemic therapy is not needed as the whole breast has been removed

27. **Bisphosphonate treatment for bone metastases in breast cancer is contraindicated in which of the following situations?**
    a) Hyperparathyroidism
    b) Hypocalcaemia
    c) Hypomagnesemia
    d) Hyponatremia
    e) Recent malignant fracture

28. **Which of the following statements is correct regarding breast fibroadenomas?**
    a) Cytology is required to distinguish fibroadenoma from phyllodes tumour
    b) They most commonly present in childhood
    c) They are a precursor to lobular neoplasia
    d) They are of monoclonal origin
    e) They most commonly present in women less than 30 years of age

29. **Which of the following statements is correct in relation to duct ectasia?**
    a) It is a precursor to ductal carcinoma *in situ*
    b) It is a neoplastic condition
    c) It is characterized by a greenish-brown discharge from multiple ducts
    d) It occurs less commonly in smokers
    e) It is usually treated with surgery

30. **A 29 year old woman attends A&E with a tender, swollen left breast. Her temperature is 37.5°C. She is two weeks post-partum and is breastfeeding. Ultrasound shows a collection in the left breast.**

    What is the most appropriate next step in management?
    a) Advise to stop breastfeeding
    b) Arrange mammograms of both breasts
    c) Needle aspiration of the collection
    d) Book theatre for incision and drainage
    e) Start bromocriptine

31. **An anxious 45 year old woman presents with severe constant bilateral breast pain. She denies excess caffeine and wears a supportive sports bra day and night. On examination she is focally tender over her anterior chest wall.**

What is the most likely diagnosis?
a) Benign cyclical mastalgia
b) Breast cysts
c) Costochondritis (Tietze's syndrome)
d) Granulomatous mastitis
e) Inflammatory breast cancer

32. **A 19 year old man has pain and tenderness beneath the right nipple which has stopped him playing football. He is fit and well and on no prescribed medications. On examination there is a tender swelling beneath the right nipple.**

What is the most likely diagnosis?
a) Body dysmorphism
b) Male breast cancer
c) Male fibroadenoma
d) Gynaecomastia
e) Lipoma

Extended Matching Items

Breast lump

A. Breast abscess
B. Breast cancer
C. Breast cyst
D. Ductal carcinoma *in situ* (DCIS)
E. Fat necrosis
F. Fibroadenoma
G. Fibrocystic mastopathy
H. Gynaecomastia
I. Lipoma
J. Phyllodes tumour

Choose the most appropriate diagnosis for each of the following scenarios:

1. A 63 year old woman with a 3cm hard non-tender ill-defined breast lump
2. A 71 year old woman with a 3cm hard non-tender ill-defined breast lump. She gives a vague history of a fall with an injury to the breast about two weeks ago.

Diagnosis

A. Atypical lobular hyperplasia
B. Breast cyst
C. Duct ectasia
D. Fibroadenoma
E. Galactocoele
F. Inflammatory breast cancer
G. Lobular breast cancer
H. Mondor's disease
I. Paget's disease
J. Phyllodes tumour
K. Pregnancy-associated breast cancer
L. Tubular breast cancer

Choose the most appropriate diagnosis for each of the following scenarios:

3. A 79 year old woman attends for pathology results following wide local excision and sentinel node biopsy for breast cancer. She is told her pathology shows a good prognosis cancer.

4. A 36 year old woman who is breastfeeding her first child attends with a smooth mobile painless lump in the outer quadrant of the right breast. Core biopsy is attempted and a white opaque fluid is expressed.

Oncoplastic surgery

A. Abdominal advancement flap
B. Deep inferior epigastric artery perforator (DIEP) flap
C. Latissimus dorsi (LD) flap
D. Superior gluteal artery perforator (SGAP) flap
E. Lateral intercostal artery perforator (LICAP) flap
F. Thoracodorsal artery perforator (TDAP) flap
G. Transverse upper gracilis (TUG) flap

For each of the following scenarios, choose the most likely procedure from the list.

5. Which breast reconstruction procedure will typically leave a horizontal or oblique scar on the upper back?

6. Which procedure leaves a scar on the upper inner thigh?

7. Which procedure is combined with abdominoplasty?

Breast cancer and genetics

A. *BRCA1* mutation
B. *BRCA2* mutation
C. Cowden syndrome (*PTEN* mutation)
D. Gardner syndrome
E. Li–Fraumeni syndrome (*p53* mutation)
F. Lynch syndrome
G. Multiple endocrine neoplasia
H. Peutz–Jeghers syndrome
I. Von Hippel–Lindau syndrome

Choose the most appropriate diagnosis for each of the following scenarios:

8. In which condition in women is the lifetime breast cancer incidence 45% and ovarian cancer incidence 15%?

9. In which condition are carriers predisposed to breast cancer, sarcomas, adrenal cancer, and leukaemias?

10. Which condition is associated with an increased risk of benign and malignant breast tumours, follicular thyroid cancer, renal and endometrial cancers?

Endocrine therapy

A. Letrozole
B. Letrozole + tamoxifen
C. Goserelin + letrozole
D. Goserelin + tamoxifen
E. No endocrine therapy
F. Tamoxifen

For each of the following patients, choose the most appropriate adjuvant treatment from the options.

11. An 82 year old woman with a 15 mm grade 1, ER4, PR0, HER2-negative breast cancer. The sentinel node was negative.

12. A 34 year old woman who had a mastectomy and immediate breast reconstruction for a 4cm inflammatory breast cancer She has 11/12 positive nodes and is ER8, PR8, HER2 negative. She has finished her other adjuvant treatment.

13. A 68 year old woman who had a wide local excision for a grade 3 tumour. She has 0/2 nodes and is ER6, PR4, HER2 negative.

14. A 38 year old woman who had a WLE for a 16mm grade 2 tumour. The sentinel node was negative and her receptor status is ER8, PR8, HER2 negative. The patient is keen to start a family within the next few years.

Breast development

A. Amazia
B. Athelia
C. Gynaecomastia
D. Neonatal breast enlargement
E. Poland syndrome
F. Polymastia
G. Polythelia
H. Tuberous breast

Choose the most appropriate diagnosis for each of the following scenarios:

15. Presence of an accessory breast with or without an accessory nipple

16. This condition may include absence of pectoralis major

17. There is a small circular breast base and anterior projection of the nipple–areola complex

Gynaecomastia

A. Finasteride
B. Lansoprazole
C. Marijuana
D. Omeprazole
E. Ranitidine
F. Steroids
G. Tamoxifen

Choose the most appropriate drug from the list.

18. Which drug does not cause gynaecomastia?

Single Best Answers

1. e) Ultrasound of left breast

Patients with a discrete lump should have both mammography and ultrasound carried out. Imaging is carried out before core biopsy as haematoma may alter the images. Sensitivity of mammography to detect breast cancer is up to 95% in lucent breasts, but as low as 40% in dense breasts. Targeted ultrasound at a focal site of concern has up to 95% sensitivity and 90% specificity, though it is less accurate as a screening tool. MRI has a high sensitivity but low specificity for detection of breast cancer. It tends to overestimate lesion size and has been shown to increase mastectomy rate without reducing re-excision or local recurrence rate. MRI is indicated in the following situations: if there is discrepancy regarding the extent of the disease from clinical examination, mammography, and ultrasound assessment; if breast density precludes accurate mammographic assessment; to assess tumour size and multifocality if breast conserving surgery is being considered for invasive lobular cancer. MRI can be useful in imaging for suspected local recurrence; for diagnosis in patients with breast implants; to monitor response to neoadjuvant chemotherapy; and in screening of women at high risk of breast cancer.

Killelea BK et al. Trends and clinical implications of preoperative breast MRI in Medicare beneficiaries with breast cancer. *Breast Cancer Research Treatment* 2013; 141(1): 155–63.

Houssami N et al. An individual person data meta-analysis of preoperative magnetic resonance imaging and breast cancer recurrence. *Journal of Clinical Oncology* 2014; 32(5):392–401.

National Institute for Health and Care Excellence. Early and locally advanced breast cancer: diagnosis and treatment. NICE Guidelines [CG 80] February 2009. <https://www.nice.org.uk/guidance/cg80>.

2. b) List for microdochectomy

The most likely diagnosis is an intraductal papilloma. This is diagnosed by excising the affected duct. The operation is carried out to obtain a diagnosis. Any nipple smear with epithelial cells is abnormal. Intraductal papilloma can cause blood-stained or clear duct discharge which can be copious, usually from a single point on the nipple. Imaging is often normal. Ultrasound will sometimes diagnose the papilloma. The pathology of intraductal papilloma is usually benign but can be associated with atypia—atypical ductal hyperplasia or DCIS. The rate of finding DCIS or even invasive cancer is 22–75% where atypia is present and much lower when the papilloma is benign.

Warrick JI and Allred DC (eds). Pathology of papilloma with atypia or ductal carcinoma *in situ*. <https://emedicine.medscape.com/article/2069668-overview>. Updated November 2015.

Breast screening most effective @ screening for Cancer than bowel screening.

3. c) Two-view mammography is performed

The UK Breast Screening Programme invites women aged 50–70 years for two-view digital mammography every 3 years. Patients between the ages of 47–73 years are being screened in some centres as part of the UK Age Extension Trial. Women can continue to attend after 70 years on request. One-third of breast cancer in the United Kingdom presents via the screening programme. Breast cancer or ductal carcinoma *in situ* (DCIS) is detected in approximately 0.8% of women screened. Median uptake annually is around 72%. *Good Screening.*

%

An independent panel chaired by Professor Sir Michael Marmot reviewed the evidence of benefit and harm in relation to the UK Breast Screening Programme in 2012. It found that breast screening prevents 1300 deaths in the United Kingdom per year. For every 10,000 women screened for 20 years, 681 cancers/DCIS are diagnosed, of which 129 are 'over-diagnosed' (excess diagnoses compared to non-screened population), and 43 breast cancer deaths are prevented. Thus 1 death is prevented per 233 women screened for 20 years. Three women are 'over-diagnosed' (and therefore 'over-treated') to prevent one death.

4. e) It has equivalent recurrence rates to mastectomy when combined with external beam radiotherapy

Meta-analysis of studies comparing mastectomy to conservation surgery with external beam post-operative radiotherapy show no difference in overall or disease-free survival. In four of the six studies, breast conservation was associated with a significantly increased risk of loco-regional recurrence, but this did not impact on survival. Four centimetres is often given as an arbitrary cut-off for tumour size requiring mastectomy but this can vary with the size of the affected breast and the patient's suitability for oncoplastic resection.

The TARGIT-A and ELIOT trials compared intra-operative radiotherapy with post-surgery external beam radiotherapy. The TARGIT-A trial showed no difference in recurrence between the groups but has been criticized for reporting too early. The ELIOT trial showed a significantly higher rate of local recurrence with intra-operative radiotherapy (though no survival difference was shown).

In order to reduce early and late morbidity associated with radiotherapy, trials have attempted to identify subgroups of excellent prognosis groups where radiotherapy is not necessary. BASO 2 showed a 2% annual risk of recurrence in patients with tumours <2cm, grade 1 and node negative, without adjuvant treatment, reduced to 0.2% with adjuvant tamoxifen and radiotherapy. PRIME 2 looked at low-risk disease in patients over 65 years. The authors concluded that without radiotherapy, of 100 patients, 5 would have a local recurrence, of which 1 would have had a local recurrence with radiotherapy. Therefore, 96% had unnecessary treatment. *errors*

A rare late complication of breast radiotherapy is angiosarcoma, with a median latency of 10 years. CREST syndrome, lupus, morphoea, and scleroderma are relative contraindications to radiotherapy, as sufferers can have a severe adverse reaction with skin tightening and erythema.

Jatoi I and Proschan MA. Randomized trials of breast-conserving therapy versus mastectomy for primary breast cancer: a pooled analysis of updated results. *American Journal of Clinical Oncology* 2005; 28(3):289–94.

Vaidya JS et al. Risk-adapted targeted intraoperative radiotherapy versus whole breast radiotherapy for breast cancer: 5-year results for local control and overall survival for the TARGIT—A randomized trial. *Lancet* 2014; 383:603–13.

Veronesi U et al. Intraoperative radiotherapy versus external radiotherapy for early breast cancer (ELIOT): a randomized controlled equivalence trial. *Lancet Oncology* 2013; 14(13):1269–77.

Complications radiotherapy - erythema.
                            - contracture.

- angiosarcoma.
- pneumonitis

Kunkler IH et al. Breast-conserving surgery with or without irradiation in women aged 65 years or older with early breast cancer (PRIME II): a randomised controlled trial. *Lancet Oncology* 2015; 16(3):266–73.

Blamey RW et al. Radiotherapy or Tamoxifen after conserving surgery for breast cancers of excellent prognosis: BASO II trial. *European Journal of Cancer* 2013; 49(10):2294–302.

5. a) A margin of <1mm from the edge of the specimen

Same for RO as HPB/CMC etc.

The UK Association of Breast Surgeons 2009 guidelines were updated at a consensus meeting in January 2016. At this meeting a resection margin of 1mm was recommended for both invasive cancer and DCIS. These are the current UK guidelines on resection margins for breast-conserving surgery. Clear margins according to local guidelines are required before commencing radiotherapy.

The American Association of Breast Surgeons guidelines published in 2014 after review of 33 studies concluded that, as long as no tumour is present at the inked margin, recurrence rates (median 5.2% at 6.6 years) were not improved by taking a wider margin and that further excision was unnecessary, regardless of tumour biology or patient age.

6. a) Mastectomy

The patient needs a mastectomy as they cannot have radiotherapy a second time and radiotherapy is needed after breast-conserving surgery for DCIS. If the patient did not receive radiotherapy the first time then wide local excision and radiotherapy would be treatment of choice the second time, as the area is small.

Stereotactic biopsy is the technique used to carry out a radiological-guided biopsy where the abnormal area is not visible on ultrasound scanning. The technique involves using the mammogram X-ray machine to locate the area of interest and guide a needle to the correct lesion. This technique is usually required to biopsy an area of microcalcification.

Even though radiotherapy is fractionated to reduce morbidity to healthy tissues and skin, the skin cannot tolerate further radiotherapy treatment and would break down.

As this is a small area of DCIS, sentinel node biopsy would not be needed.

7. b) Ultrasound of the axilla

Imaging tests are always done before biopsy, whether in the breast or axilla. In this patient's case it is likely that a core biopsy would be required but only after the ultrasound scan. For some conditions, such as lymphoma, it may not be possible to achieve a diagnosis with core biopsy and excision biopsy may be needed to get more tissue. Ultrasound features of an involved axillary node include: increased cortical thickness (>3mm); round shape (loss of ovoid shape); absence of well-defined margin; loss of hyperechoic fatty hilum.

8. d) Patent blue plus technetium-labelled albumin

With the combined technique of patent blue dye and radioisotope, the detection rate of sentinel node biopsy is 97%. Using one or other technique the detection rate decreases by 3%.

Goyal A, Newcombe RG, Chhabra A, Mansel RE. ALMANAC Trialists Group. Factors affecting failed localisation and false-negative rates of sentinel node biopsy in breast cancer—results of the ALMANAC validation phase. *Breast Cancer Research and Treatment* 2006; 99(2):203–208.

9. d) It is licensed for use in breast surgery

Patent blue dye is not licensed for use in breast surgery. Serious allergic reactions to blue dye occurred in 0.1% of cases in the UK ALMANAC trial and the Government UK safety update

(10 February 2012) uses the same figure. Milder reactions can also occur such as urticarial rash. Patent blue dye should not be used in pregnancy.

Mansel RE et al. Randomized mulitcenter trial of sentinel node biopsy versus standard axillary in operable breast cancer: the ALMANAC trial. *Journal of the National Cancer Institute* 2006; 98:599–609.

10. e) There is no difference in survival between axillary clearance and axillary radiotherapy

Axillary clearance has been considered the standard treatment for node-positive patients until recently. The EORTC AMAROS trial randomized patients with a positive sentinel node to axillary clearance or axillary radiotherapy and showed that axillary recurrence rates were similar between both treatments, but that lymphoedema rates were lower after axillary radiotherapy. The recurrence rates were in fact lower after axillary clearance but both had very low recurrence rates, albeit with short follow-up of about five years. Patients with node positive axillas on core biopsy and bulkier axillary disease may still benefit more from axillary clearance.

Zhang J and Wang C. Axillary radiotherapy: an alternative treatment option for adjuvant axillary management of breast cancer. *Scientific Reports* 2016; 6(26304). doi:10.1038/srep26304.

11. a) Axilla

In breast reconstruction, the latissimus dorsi (LD) flap is brought through the axilla as a pedicled flap. In plastic surgery, the LD flap can also be transposed to another location as a free flap. A pedicled flap remains attached to its original blood supply. A free flap is detached from its original blood supply and re-anastomosed elsewhere.

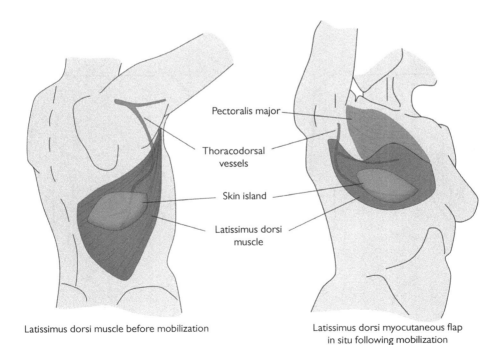

Pectoralis major

Thoracodorsal vessels

Skin island

Latissimus dorsi muscle

Latissimus dorsi muscle before mobilization

Latissimus dorsi myocutaneous flap in situ following mobilization

Fig. 7.1 Latissimus dorsi myocutaneous pedicle flap

The latissimus dorsi muscle is a fan-shaped muscle of wide origin (see Figure 7.1):

- Origin: Spinous processes of T7–T12 vertebrae, thoracolumbar fascia, iliac crest, inferior angle of scapula.
- Insertion: Narrows to a tendon that inserts into the floor of intertubercular groove of the humerus.
- Blood supply: Thoracodorsal artery (branch of subscapular artery); thoracodorsal vein.
- Innervation Thoracodorsal nerve (branch of posterior cord of brachial plexus: C5–C9).
- Action Extension, adduction, and medial rotation of the shoulder (think of a butler with hand behind back and the dorsum of hand flat against the lower back).

Functional difficulties reported by patients following LD reconstruction include lifting down heavier items from a high shelf or pushing up onto the side of a swimming pool. However, most patients regain baseline DASH (disability of the arm, shoulder, and hand) scores for shoulder function by 6–12 months.

The inferior edge of the LD muscle forms the posterior margin of Petit's triangle, and lumbar herniae have occasionally been reported as a complication of LD harvest.

Hudak PL et al. Development of an upper extremity outcome measure: The DASH (Disabilities of the Arm, Shoulder and Head). *American Journal of Industrial Medicine* 1996; 29: 602–8.

Button J et al. Shoulder function following ALD breast reconstruction. *Journal of Plastic, Reconstructive & Aesthetic Surgery* 2010; 63:1505–12.

12. c) Previous abdominoplasty

Abdominoplasty removes the tissue that is used in DIEP reconstruction (see Figure 7.2). Age is not a contraindication provided the patient is otherwise fit and well. Extensive nodal involvement is not a contraindication to a DIEP flap but patients should be staged and counselled prior to undergoing

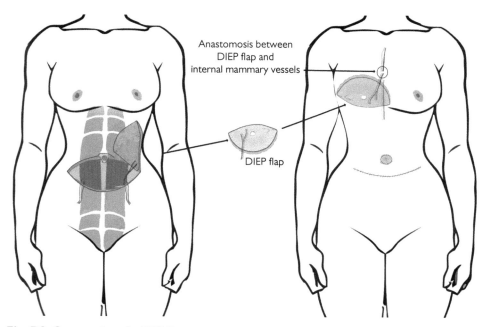

Anastomosis between DIEP flap and internal mammary vessels

DIEP flap

Fig. 7.2 Construction of a DIEP flap

any such major operation if they have a high risk of developing recurrent disease. It is unusual for caesarean section or open cholecystectomy scars to disrupt the deep inferior epigastric vessels. In many centres, patients undergoing a DIEP flap will have pre-op MR angiography to assess the presence and suitability of abdominal vessels. DIEP breast reconstruction is a free flap technique utilizing a horizontal ellipse of skin and fat from the lower abdomen. The surgeon dissects the rectus abdominis to retrieve sufficient vessel length but doesn't detach the muscle (as in a TRAM flap). This minimizes, but doesn't exclude, later muscle weakness or hernia. Each DIEP flap operation yields two half-ellipse-shaped free flaps, each on its perforator. DIEP flaps can be bilateral but only if both sides are reconstructed at the same time. The DIEP flap is re-anastomosed onto the internal mammary artery and vein by removing a section of third or fourth rib cartilage just lateral to the sternum (or alternatively onto the thoracodorsal vessels in the axilla).

13. a) Breast-conserving surgery

A therapeutic mammoplasty is a wide local excision using breast reduction and mastopexy (uplift) techniques. Adjuvant radiotherapy is still given as with wide local excision.

Oncoplastic breast surgery with therapeutic mammoplasty is classified as follows:

> Level 1: <20% of breast volume excised and no skin resection required.
> Level 2: up to 50% of breast volume excised plus skin resection.

Clough KB et al. Improving breast cancer surgery: a classification and quadrant per quadrant atlas for oncoplastic surgery. *Annals of Surgical Oncology* 2010; 17:1375–91.

14. b) Annual breast MRI

NICE gives surveillance recommendations for women in different risk categories. Women with >30% probability of being a *BRCA* carrier should be offered annual breast MRI from age 30–49, with annual mammography to start by age 40.

$1/4$ 3 – any age
$1/3$ 2 – 2 <50
$1/6$ 1 – 1 <40

Table 7.1 Population risk of breast cancer in UK women

Decade of age	Risk
30	1 in 2000
40	1 in 200
50	1 in 50
60	1 in 22
70	1 in 13
80	1 in 8

The lifetime risk of breast cancer for women in the UK is 11%. See Table 7.1.

Patients who should be referred to a breast unit for family history assessment include:

- One first-degree relative under 40 $1/2$ 15%
- Two first-degree relatives under 50 $1/3$ ↓ 30%..
- Two first-degree relatives with ovarian or breast cancer at any age
- Three second-degree relatives at any age $1/4$.
- One male first-degree relative with breast cancer at any age

Table 7.2 Risk of breast cancer in patients with a family history

	Risk at age 40–50	Lifetime risk
Population risk ('Low' risk)	<3%	<17%
Moderate risk	3–8%	17–30%
High risk (non-gene carrier)	>8%	>30%

In secondary care, risk can be assessed using Manchester, BOADICEA, or Tyrer Cuzick scores. Patients should be referred for genetic testing if they have >10% probability of being a gene carrier, or if they are of Ashkenazi Jewish descent. Patients not found to be gene carriers are stratified into high- and moderate-risk groups based on their calculated percentage risk. See Table 7.2.

Bilateral mastectomy has been shown to improve survival in patients with proven *BRCA* gene mutation including those diagnosed with breast cancer. There is no evidence that it improves survival in high/moderate risk non-*BRCA* patients or in patients with contralateral breast cancer.

National Institute for Health and Care Excellence. Familial breast cancer. NICE Guidelines [CG 164] June 2013. <https://www.nice.org.uk/guidance/cg164>.

Evans DG et al. A new scoring system for the chances of identifying a *BRCA1/2* mutation outperforms existing models. *Journal of Medical Genetics* 2004; 41:474–80.

Antoniou AC et al. The BOADICEA model of genetic susceptibility to breast and ovarian cancer. *British Journal of Cancer* 2004; 91:1580–90.

Tyrer J et al. A breast cancer prediction model incorporating familial and personal risk factors. *Statistics in Medicine* 2004; 23:1111–30.

Rebbeck TR et al. Bilateral prophylactic mastectomy reduces breast cancer risk in *BRCA1* and *BRCA2* mutation carriers: the PROSE study group. *Journal of Clinical Oncology* 2004; 22(6):1055–62.

Metcalfe K et al. Contralateral mastectomy and survival after breast cancer in carriers of *BRCA1* and *BRCA2* mutations: retrospective analysis. *British Medical Journal* 2014; 348:g226.

Fayanju OM et al. Contralateral prophylactic mastectomy after unilateral breast cancer: a systematic review and meta-analysis. *Annals of Surgery* 2014; 260(6):1000–10.

15. e) Tamoxifen

Chemoprevention with 5 years of tamoxifen or raloxifene reduces breast cancer incidence by about 50%. The results of the IBIS I trial showed that 22 patients needed to be treated with 5 years of tamoxifen to prevent 1 breast cancer over 20 years. There was no difference in overall survival. The incidence of uterine cancer was higher in the tamoxifen group (0.8% vs 0.6%) but low overall with no difference in survival. NICE guidelines state that premenopausal women at high risk of breast cancer should be offered five years of tamoxifen (raloxifene has not been tested in premenopausal women). Post-menopausal women should be offered five years of tamoxifen or raloxifene. Women at moderate risk should be offered chemoprevention and can use the Manchester Decision Aid as a guide. Of 1000 women who take tamoxifen for 5 years, 5 will suffer DVT and 60 will require investigation for uterine bleeding. The IBIS II study evaluated the effect of anastrozole on breast cancer incidence and mortality in high-risk post-menopausal women. Although incidence of breast cancer was reduced by 50%, there was no increase in overall survival. Bilateral prophylactic salpingo-oophorectomy has been shown to reduce the risk of breast cancer by approximately 50% in women at high risk.

Fisher B et al. Tamoxifen for the prevention of breast cancer: Current status of the NSABP P-1 Study. *Journal of the National Cancer Institute* 2005; 97(22):1652–62.

Vogel VG et al. NSABP P-2 Study of Tamoxifen and Raloxifene (STAR). *Journal of the American Medical Association* 2006; 295:2727–41.

Cuzick J et al. Tamoxifen for prevention of breast cancer: extended long-term follow-up of the IBIS I breast cancer prevention trial. *Lancet Oncology* 2015; 16:67–75.

Making Choices (2014). Nightingale and Genesis Breast Cancer Prevention Centre, University Hospital of South Manchester. <http://www.uhsm.nhs.uk>.

Cuzick J et al. Anastrozole for prevention of breast cancer in high-risk postmenopausal women (IBIS-II). *Lancet* 2014; 383:1041–8.

Guillem JG et al. ASCO/SSO review of current role of risk-reducing surgery in common hereditary cancer syndromes. *Journal of Clinical Oncology* 2006; 24(28):4642–60.

16. b) **Excess alcohol consumption**

A first full-term pregnancy at a young age reduces breast cancer risk.

Alcohol intake increases breast cancer risk in a dose-related fashion. Even moderate alcohol usage increases risk.

Increased breast density is an independent risk factor for breast cancer. In the past, Woolfe patterns were used, now BI-RADS (Breast Imaging and Reporting Data System) density grades are used to classify density from A (fatty) to D (dense).

Post-menopausal obesity increases breast cancer risk but premenopausal obesity has no effect on risk. This is because after the menopause obese women produce more oestrogen in peripheral fat.

Exercise reduces the risk of developing breast cancer and most other cancers. Moderate exercise is enough to produce this effect.

Allen NE et al. Moderate alcohol intake and cancer incidence in women. *Journal of the National Cancer Institute* 2009; 101:296–305.

Dam MK et al. Five year change in alcohol intake and risk of breast cancer and coronary heart disease among postmenopausal women: prospective cohort study. *British Medical Journal* 2016; 353:i2314.

17. e) **The areola is affected after the nipple**

Paget's disease affects the nipple before the areola, unlike nipple eczema which affects the areola before the nipple. Nipple eczema is often bilateral whereas Paget's is unilateral. In both cases a red scaly rash appears. Paget's cells are similar to DCIS. Often there are no abnormalities on a mammogram (15–65% normal mammograms). Treatment may involve removing the nipple and subareolar tissue followed by radiotherapy, or mastectomy.

18. c) **It is treated by wide local excision**

Phyllodes tumours are clinically similar to fibradenomas but occur in older patients. The history is often of a rapidly enlarging lump. They are either benign (85–90%), borderline or malignant (10–15%) and are treated by local excision with a margin. They arise from breast stroma cells and are therefore not breast cancers but part of the sarcoma spectrum. Sentinel node biopsy or axillary clearance is not part of the treatment. Malignant phyllodes tumours spread like sarcomas with haematogenous spread to the lungs, bones, heart, and liver.

19. e) Ultrasound guided biopsy of breast and axilla the next week

Male breast cancer is uncommon, accounting for approximately 0.5–1% of breast cancers. Incidence is commonest between the ages of 60–70 and is associated with hyper-oestrogenism (Klinefelter's, obesity, gynaecomastia, cirrhosis) and with lifetime radiation exposure. Patients presenting with asymmetric gynaecomastia or a discrete breast mass should therefore undergo core biopsy +/− imaging with ultrasound or mammography. It can be linked to *BRCA2* gene mutation, and families with a history of male breast cancer at any age, as well as female relatives fitting the moderate risk criteria, should be referred for genetic screening.

The patient should be informed of the finding once he has recovered from anaesthesia and core biopsy performed with his informed consent. As in female breast cancer, image-guided core biopsy is the gold standard, although in many units freehand core biopsy of the lump is performed. Ultrasound of the axilla should be performed with core biopsy of any suspicious nodes.

20. e) Tamoxifen

Treatment of male breast cancer usually takes the form of mastectomy and sentinel node biopsy with the need for further axillary treatment and adjuvant therapy determined by pathological findings. Tamoxifen is the usual agent in ER+ve disease. Data on aromatase inhibition in men is limited and concerns exist regarding its efficacy due to testicular oestrogen production. Pathology, natural history, and prognosis is similar to stage-matched disease in women.

Giordano SH et al. Breast carcinoma in men: a population-based study. *Cancer* 2004; 101(1):51–7.

National Institute for Health and Care Excellence. Familial breast cancer: classification, care and managing breast cancer and related risks in people with a family history of breast cancer. NICE Guidelines [CG164] June 2013. <https://www.nice.org.uk/guidance/cg164>.

21. c) Ductal carcinoma *in situ*

Microcalcifications on mammography are suspicious for DCIS and can be associated with invasive cancer. Benign calcification is more commonly coarse or large (described as 'tea-cupping') related to skin or vascular calcification, or smooth, round areas.

Ductal carcinoma *in situ* is primarily a radiological and histological diagnosis describing cells with the cytological features of malignancy which have not yet crossed the basement membrane. It cannot be differentiated from invasive cancer on FNA (fine needle aspiration) due to the absence of tissue architecture. Prior to the introduction of the breast screening programme it was rarely diagnosed, as it is usually impalpable. Untreated DCIS confers a very high risk of subsequent breast cancer, though not all DCIS will progress to invasive malignancy. By contrast lobular carcinoma *in situ* (LCIS) is not a clearly pre-malignant condition and is best considered a marker of increased risk of breast cancer of 1–2% per year, with a lifetime risk of 30–40%.

Patients with technically conservable DCIS are usually offered conservation surgery. Sentinel node biopsy is only performed if histology reveals a focus of invasive cancer in the surgical specimen. Adjuvant radiotherapy to the breast is offered in high-grade disease in most centres, though use of radiotherapy in grade 1 or 2 DCIS (low or intermediate grade) varies widely throughout the United Kingdom. Widespread or multifocal DCIS, or a large area where conservation would lead to a poor cosmetic outcome is usually treated with mastectomy and synchronous sentinel node biopsy, with or without reconstruction. There is some evidence that tamoxifen reduces the rate of local recurrence in DCIS but this does not form part of the current NICE recommendations.

Fisher B et al. Lumpectomy and radiation for the treatment of intraduct breast cancer: findings from the National Surgical Adjuvant Breast and Bowel Project B-17. *Journal of Clinical Oncology* 1998: 16;441–52.

Association of Breast Surgery at BASO 2009. Surgical guidelines for the management of breast cancer. *European Journal of Surgery Oncology* 2009; 35 suppl 1:1–22.

Simpson PT et al. The diagnosis and management of pre-invasive breast disease: pathology of atypical lobular hyperplasia and lobular carcinoma *in situ. Breast Cancer Research* 2003; 5(5):258–62.

22. c) Docetaxel

Taxotere is commonly used in breast cancer and is the most likely of the drugs listed to cause hair loss. Lapatinib is used in metastatic HER-2+ve disease and does not cause hair loss. Tamoxifen and letrozole can cause hair thinning, but this is usually mild. Herceptin does not cause hair loss.

Most chemotherapy drugs cause hair loss. Epirubicin, given as part of the FEC (fluorouracil, epirubicin, cyclophosphamide) regimen for breast cancer, causes total scalp and body hair loss in most patients. Use of a cooling cap to cause scalp vasoconstriction prior to, during, and after drug administration allows some patients to avoid total hair loss. It is, however, uncomfortable and difficult to tolerate. Patients who wish to try to keep their hair should be advised to wash it as seldom as possible, to minimize brushing, and to avoid straighteners and hairdryers.

23. e) Tamoxifen

This woman is likely to be premenopausal given her age, and therefore is not suitable for an aromatase inhibitor such as a), b), or c) alone. Raloxifene is used for chemoprevention in post-menopausal women at high risk of breast cancer, although it is inferior to tamoxifen in terms of disease prevention and is not currently used in the adjuvant setting.

Tamoxifen is a mixed oestrogen agonist/antagonist with antagonistic effects in the breast. Aromatase inhibitors act by preventing the conversion of androgens into oestrogen by peripheral fat. They have no effect on ovarian production of oestrogen (possibly even up-regulating it) and therefore are not suitable for premenopausal women.

The SOFT trial compared: tamoxifen alone; tamoxifen and ovarian suppression; and exemestane and ovarian suppression in a group of premenopausal women. There was no benefit to ovarian suppression in the study population overall, but in patients under 35, most of whom remained premenopausal after chemotherapy, there was statistical evidence of survival benefit with exemestane and ovarian suppression.

Francis PA et al. Adjuvant ovarian suppression in premenopausal breast cancer. *New England Journal of Medicine* 2015; 372:436–46.

24. e) The usual regimen is three cycles of fluorouracil/epirubicin/cyclophosphamide + three cycles of a taxane

Neo-adjuvant chemotherapy (NAC) has been demonstrated to be equivalent in terms of disease-free and overall survival compared to conventional adjuvant chemotherapy. Polychemotherapy regimens involving taxanes can achieve clinical response in 60–90%, and pathological complete responses of 10–30%, particularly in ER–ve, Her2+ve disease. Lobular cancer does not respond well to NAC (complete pathological response rates 6% vs 18% for non-lobular breast cancer).

The current SIGN guidelines state that NAC should be considered for patients with inoperable cancer and for patients whose disease is not presently conservable but might become so after chemotherapy. The NSABP B-18 trial showed that the NAC group were more likely to undergo conservation vs mastectomy (67.8% vs 56.8%) with similar rates of local recurrence. Additional prognostic information is gained by assessing the extent of pathological response in the resected specimen. Patients with a pathological complete response (pCR) show an improved disease free survival of 85.7% compared to 76.9% in those without a pCR. The Cochrane Review suggests that omitting surgery is not demonstrably safe but may in future be a possibility for patients who achieve a pCR.

Scottish Intercollegiate Guidelines Network. Treatment of Primary Breast Cancer. SIGN Guideline 134. September 2013. <http://www.sign.ac.uk/sign-134-treatment-of-primary-breast-cancer.html>.

National Institute for Health and Care Excellence. Early and locally advanced breast cancer: diagnosis and treatment. NICE Guidelines [CG80] February 2009. <https://www.nice.org.uk/guidance/cg80>.

Fisher B et al. Effect of preoperative chemotherapy on the outcome of women with operable breast cancer. *Journal of Clinical Oncology* 1998; 16:2672–85.

Mieog JS et al. Preoperative chemotherapy for women with operable breast cancer. *Cochrane Database of Systematic Reviews* 2007; 2:CD005002.

25. d) A 65 year old woman with metastatic spread to the lungs

The HER-2 receptor is overexpressed in about 15% of breast cancers and is associated with poor prognosis compared to matched HER-2 negative disease. Herceptin is a monoclonal antibody targeting the HER-2 receptor demonstrated to improve disease-free survival, first in the HERA trial and subsequently in the NSABP-B31 and NCCTG-N9831 trials. In early breast cancer, it is usually given at three-weekly intervals for one year. It is also given in the metastatic setting. Although age alone is not a direct contraindication to Herceptin, risk of cardiotoxicity increases with age and it would not form part of routine treatment of early breast cancer in very elderly patients.

Cardiac toxicity is the main side effect. 5% develop a significant drop in LV ejection fraction (1% of controls). 2% develop congestive cardiac failure. (0% of controls). Cardiac functional assessments should be repeated every 3 months during trastuzumab treatment, with treatment suspended if LVEF (left ventricular ejection fraction) drops by ≥10 percentage (ejection) points from baseline and to below 50%.

The N9831 study showed a trend towards better disease-free survival with concurrent administration of Herceptin and chemotherapy. NICE guidance suggests Herceptin should be given with chemotherapy, and not in low-risk cancers smaller than 1cm. In these cases, where chemotherapy would not be offered, the disadvantages of Herceptin are likely to outweigh the benefits.

Piccart-Gebhart MJ et al. Trastuzumab after adjuvant chemotherapy in HER2-positive breast cancer. *New England Journal of Medicine* 2005; 353:1659–72.

National Institute for Health and Care Excellence. Trastuzumab for the adjuvant treatment of early-stage HER2-positive breast cancer. NICE technology appraisal guidance [TA107] August 2006. <https://www.nice.org.uk/guidance/ta107>.

26. a) Adjuvant chemotherapy, chest-wall radiotherapy, and letrozole

The patient would require both systemic adjuvant therapy and chest-wall radiotherapy. Many consensus statements and guidelines recommend chest-wall radiotherapy for patients with four or more nodes involved following the publication of the Danish Radiotherapy trials in 2007 (Overggard et al.). A sub-study of the Danish trials also showed a benefit for chest-wall radiotherapy in women with one to three nodes involved, both in terms of local recurrence and overall survival. The Oxford overview of 2014 looking at the effects of radiotherapy after mastectomy and axillary surgery showed that radiotherapy had no benefit for node-negative women, but that for women with 1–3 nodes involved the risk of local recurrence was 0.68 and overall survival 0.8. These benefits are similar to women with four or more nodes involved. The SUPREMO trial, which stopped recruiting in 2013, randomized women with one to three involved nodes to RT or no RT (radiotherapy), and the results are awaited.

EBCTCG (Early Breast Cancer Trialists' Collaborative Group). Effect of radiotherapy after mastectomy and axillary surgery on 10-year recurrence and 20-year breast cancer mortality: meta-analysis of individual patient data for 8135 women in 22 randomised trials. *Lancet* 2014; 383 (9935):2127–35.

27. b) Hypocalcaemia

[handwritten: Make more calcium available + Suppress the PTn secretion by ↑ vitamin D]

Bone-modifying agents (BMAs) used in breast cancer include bisphosphonates and denosumab. Bisphosphonates cause apoptosis of osteoclasts. They increase bony uptake of serum calcium and are contraindicated in hypocalcaemia. Calcium and vitamin D supplements should be given prior to bisphosphonates in this case. The main side effects of bisphosphonates are oesophago-gastric irritation (oral preparations only) and more rarely, osteonecrosis of the jaw. Caution is also required in renal impairment due to nephrotoxicity. Denosumab is a human monoclonal antibody that blocks osteoclast formation. It can also cause hypocalcaemia and osteonecrosis of the jaw. Bisphosphonates can be given orally or IV. Denosumab is given subcutaneously every four weeks.

In early (non-metastatic) breast cancer, oral bisphosphonates are given for aromatase-inhibitor-induced osteoporosis. The AZURE trial and an EBCTCG meta-analysis investigated the addition of bisphosphonates as part of adjuvant treatment and have shown some improvement in bone recurrence and overall survival in post-menopausal women.

In women with radiological evidence of bone metastases, BMAs reduce pain and skeletal-related events: fracture; requirement of radiotherapy or surgery to bone; and spinal cord compression. Bisphosphonates are given IV for bone metastases due to greater bioavailability. Denosumab is given subcutaneously and less frequently than bisphosphonates and avoids hospital attendance for IV infusion. In long-bone metastases, the Mirels score can be used to identify patients at high risk of fracture in whom fixation may be indicated prior to radiotherapy.

Reid DM et al. Guidance for the management of breast cancer treatment-induced bone loss: a consensus position statement from a UK expert group. *Cancer Treatment Reviews* 2008; 34:S1–18.

Coleman RE et al. Breast-cancer adjuvant therapy with zoledronic acid. *New England Journal of Medicine* 2011; 365:1396–405.

EBCTCG. Adjuvant bisphosphonate treatment in early breast cancer. *Lancet* 2015; 386:1353–61.

Van Poznak C et al. ASCO clinical practice guideline update of the role of bone-modifying agents in metastatic breast cancer. *Journal of Clinical Oncology* 2011; 29(9):1221–7.

Mirels H. Metastatic disease in long bones: a proposed scoring system for diagnosing impending pathologic fractures. *Clinical Orthopaedics and Related Research* 2003; 415:S4–13.

28. e) They most commonly present in women less than 30 years of age

Fibroadenomas are most common in women in their late teens and 20s. They are composed of mixed glandular and connective tissue. Giant fibroadenoma are fibroadenomas greater than 5cm in diameter. Fibroadenoma and phyllodes tumour are two distinct pathological entities with very similar clinical, radiological, and cytological features. Fibroadenoma and giant fibroadenoma are of polyclonal origin, while phyllodes tumours are monoclonal in origin.

Phyllodes tumours are fibroepithelial tumours with a histological continuum from benign to malignant. They can behave similarly to sarcoma and recur locally or, more rarely, metastasize to distant sites including lung or bone.

Juvenile fibroadenoma present in children or adolescents, and can grow rapidly. When planning excision of juvenile fibroadenoma, it is important to refer to a specialist breast team. Excision is usually via submammary incision to avoid cutting into the breast bud, which can cause later breast deformity and/or hypoplasia.

Noguchi S et al. Demonstration of polyclonal origin of giant fibroadenoma of the breast. *Virchow's Archiv* 1995; 427(3);343–7.

29. c) It is characterized by a greenish-brown discharge from multiple ducts

Duct ectasia is a smoking-related disorder characterized by multiple duct discharge on both sides, which can be yellow, green, or brown in colour. Duct ectasia predisposes to periductal mastitis. If the discharge of duct ectasia is brown it can be difficult to know if it is blood stained. Nipple smear is the best test to identify red blood cells if present. If blood or epithelial cells are present on the nipple smear then microdochectomy may be indicated, but the majority of patients will never need surgery.

30. c) Needle aspiration of the collection

A patient with a lactational abscess should be encouraged to continue breastfeeding. Mammograms would not be appropriate for a 29 year old. Antibiotics would be given but needle aspiration should be carried out without delay. Theatre for incision and drainage would not be recommended and would be reserved for cases that had failed with aspiration under the care of the specialist breast team.

Bromocriptine is no longer recommended. The commonest organism in breast abscess formation is Staphylococcus aureus. The best initial antibiotic to use would be flucloxacillin. A patient who is systemically unwell or septic may need hospital admission.

31. c) Costochondiritis (Tietze's syndrome)

Breast pain is the commonest reason for referral to the Breast Clinic and is usually benign. The guidelines of the Association of Breast Surgery UK suggest non-urgent referral from primary care in patients with persisting breast pain and no palpable abnormality.

A clinical history can be useful in differentiating between the classically benign premenstrual cyclical breast pain, and non-cyclical breast pain, which is often constant. Bilateral clinical examination should be performed to exclude any associate abnormality of breast, skin, axillae, and the underlying chest wall.

Treatment for cyclical breast pain usually involves reassurance, advice to wear a well-fitting and supportive bra, and prescription of simple analgesia or NSAIDS. There is no evidence that reduction in caffeine intake is beneficial. RCTs suggest that danazol, tamoxifen, gestrinone, goserelin, and toremifene improve cyclical breast pain. However, they are associated with unpleasant and potentially severe side effects and are usually reserved for the most severe and persistent cases. Treatment for non-cyclical breast pain depends on the underlying cause. Mammography is usually offered in cases of unilateral post-menopausal breast pain, although most abnormalities detected are unrelated to the pain.

Tietze's syndrome is inflammation of the costochondral joints characterized by tenderness in the affected area and usually responds well to NSAIDs.

Willett AM et al. Best practice diagnostic guidelines for patients presenting with breast symptoms. Association of Breast Surgery UK (2010). <https://associationofbreastsurgery.org.uk/media/1416/best-practice-diagnostic-guidelines-for-patients-presenting-with-breast-symptoms.pdf>.

Scurr J et al. The prevalence, severity, and impact of breast pain in the general population. *The Breast Journal* 2014; 20(5):508–13.

National Institute for Health and Care Excellence. Breast pain—cyclical. NICE Clinical Knowledge Summaries, September 2012. <https://cks.nice.org.uk/breast-pain-cyclical>.

32. d) Gynaecomastia

When taking a history in a patient with gynaecomastia, ask about medication from the GP, recreational drugs, the use of anabolic steroids for body-building, alcohol use, and changes in sexual functioning. Investigation of gynaecomastia may include the following blood tests: FBC, U&E, LFT, TFT, oestradiol, testosterone, prolactin, FSH, LH, hCG, aFP, SHBG, and LDH. Core biopsy gives a definitive diagnosis.

Extended Matching Items

Breast lump

1. B. Breast cancer

A new firm breast lump should raise suspicion of breast cancer until proven otherwise, particularly in post-menopausal women.

DCIS can present as a discrete mass but is more usually ill-defined or impalpable.

Fibrocystic mastopathy, breast cysts, and fibroadenomata can present with a discrete firm lump, but all are uncommon in post-menopausal women.

2. B. Breast cancer

A new firm breast lump should raise suspicion of breast cancer until proven otherwise, particularly in post-menopausal women. It is not uncommon for a minor injury to the breast to 'trigger' a woman to notice a breast lump for the first time.

Fat necrosis can mimic breast cancer on clinical examination. It results from saponification of damaged fat with oil cysts and eventual fibrosis. It may occur after a minor injury not recalled by the patient, or after a more significant injury with resorbing haematoma. It can also occur after breast surgery or radiotherapy.

Diagnosis

3. L. Tubular breast cancer

Numerous subtypes of breast cancer exist and can be differentiated on histology. Ductal cancer accounts for 80–90% of all breast cancers, also known as no special type (NST).

Lobular cancer makes up 10%, and are more commonly multifocal. 20% of lobular cancers are bilateral at presentation. Histologically they look more favourable but outcomes are similar to ductal cancers as they may be chemo-resistant, larger at presentation, and hard to feel. Lobular cancers stain negative for E-cadherin (unlike ductal cancer).

Medullary breast cancer is a rare subtype characterized by large cells with a clear histological boundary and white cells. It can be associated with the BRCA1 gene.

Tubular cancer accounts for just 1% of all breast cancers. It has an excellent prognosis with characteristic tubular appearance of cells on histology. Mucinous breast cancer (2%) also has a good prognosis.

4. E. Galactocoele

A galactocoele is a cyst containing milk or milky fluid. It is caused by a protein plug blocking a breast duct. It is usually seen in young lactating women or women who have recently stopped breastfeeding.

Pregnancy associated breast cancer describes breast cancer diagnosed during pregnancy or within a year of delivery. Although traditionally believed to be associated with poor outcomes, when matched stage for stage with non-pregnancy associated cancer in age-matched controls, results are comparable. However, diagnosis may be delayed due to the physiological changes of the breast in pregnancy.

Inflammatory breast cancer presents with a hot, inflamed breast, either with a palpable underlying mass or sometimes a diffusely swollen breast with no focal lesion. It is inoperable at presentation and standard practice is to downstage with neoadjuvant chemotherapy prior to surgery (usually mastectomy). It can be misdiagnosed as mastitis and therefore mastitis in the older woman should be investigated with a high degree of suspicion.

Phyllodes tumour is a stromal tumour of the breast, named after the 'leaf-like' pattern of tumour growth. Commonest in women in their 40s and 50s, >50% are benign. The remainder are borderline or malignant. Risk of recurrence is around 10% with clear margins at initial excision.

Atypical lobular hyperplasia is the term used to describe proliferation with cellular atypia causing distortion of lobular units. It is not usually palpable and can present as an incidental finding. It confers a three to fivefold relative risk of developing cancer in either breast.

Oncoplastic surgery

5. C. Latissimus dorsi flap

A latissimus dorsi (LD) flap leaves an oblique or horizontal scar on the upper back. This is one of the most common and robust flaps used for breast reconstruction.

The lateral intercostal artery perforator (LICAP) flap utilizes the fold of skin and fat just beneath the axilla. The thoracodorsal artery perforator (TDAP) flap uses some of the skin and fat overlying the LD flap (therefore any future LD more difficult and of reduced volume). Both LICAP and TDAP are usually too small for complete breast reconstruction but can be used to fill defects resulting from larger wide local excision.

6. I. Transverse upper gracilis flap

The transverse upper gracillis (TUG) flap is taken from the upper inner thigh; while the superior gluteal artery perforator (SGAP) flap leaves a scar across the upper buttock. Thigh/lower back flaps are less common in most units and are generally used as 'second-line' techniques.

7. C. Deep inferior epigastric perforator (DIEP) flap

Transverse rectus abdominus myocutaneous (TRAM), Superficial inferior epigastric artery (SIEA), and deep inferior epigastric artery perforator (DIEP) flaps leave a horizontal scar along the lower abdomen and a circular scar around the umbilicus. An SIEA flap is only possible in patients who have a large enough superficial epigastric artery (about 15% of population) to avoid dissecting into the rectus muscle to retrieve the deep artery.

In an abdominal advancement flap procedure, the skin of the abdomen down to umbilicus is mobilized to 'advance' over a mastectomy defect. This is a skin coverage technique (for example in extensive skin involvement or local cancer recurrence in a mastectomy flap) rather than a breast reconstruction.

Breast cancer and genetics

8. B. *BRCA2* mutation

BRCA is a tumour suppressor gene involved in repairing double-strand DNA breaks. Mutation in the autosomal dominant *BRCA1* tumour suppressor gene (*c17*) gives a lifetime risk of breast cancer (60–80%) and ovarian cancer (40–65%) in women. In men the lifetime risk of breast cancer is 2%. Carriers are also at increased risk of pancreatic and prostate cancer.

Mutation in the autosomal dominant *BRCA2* tumour suppressor gene (*c13*) causes a lifetime risk of breast cancer of 50–75%. The risk of ovarian cancer (15–40% is less when compared to *BRCA1*. Male *BRCA2* carriers are at greater risk of breast and prostate cancer than for *BRCA1*. The lifetime risk of male breast cancer in *BRCA2* is 6%. Carriers are also at increased risk of pancreatic and colon cancer, melanoma, and leukaemias.

BRCA1-associated cancers are mostly triple negative, while *BRCA2*-associated cancers have a similar subtype distribution to sporadic breast cancers. *BRCA*-associated ovarian cancer tends to be high grade serous or endometrioid.

PARP (poly-ADP ribose polymerase) inhibitors (e.g. Olaparib) are an emerging treatment for *BRCA*-associated breast cancer that exploits the *BRCA* mutation. Broadly, PARP is critical in single-strand DNA repair and if it is inhibited single-strand breaks become double-strand breaks, which cannot be repaired by the *BRCA*-deficient cell, leading to cell death.

The ongoing Olympia trials are investigating Olaparib as a neoadjuvant, adjuvant, and second-line treatment in *BRCA*-associated early and metastatic breast cancer. See Figure 7.3.

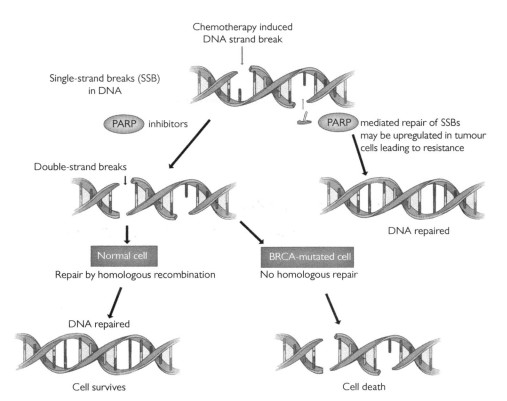

Fig. 7.3 Mechanism of action of PARP inhibitors in BRCA mutated cancers

Chen S et al. Meta-analysis of *BRCA1* and *BRCA2* penetrance. *Journal of Clinical Oncology* 2007; 25(11):1329–33.

Evans DG et al. Penetrance estimates for *BRCA1* and *BRCA2* based on genetic testing in a clinical cancer genetics service setting. *BMC Cancer* 2008; 8:155.

Tutt A et al. OlympiA, Neo-Olympia and OlympiAD: Randomised phase III trials of olaparib in patients with breast cancer and a germline *BRCA1/2* mutation. *Annals of Oncology* 2014; 25(s4):iv85–iv109.

9. E. Li–Fraumeni syndrome (*p53* mutation)

Li–Fraumeni syndrome is caused by mutation in the autosomal dominant *TP53* and/or *CHEK2* tumour suppressor gene. It is also known as 'SBLA' syndrome (sarcoma breast leukaemia adrenal). Patients are radiation-sensitive and should not have mammograms. NICE recommends surveillance with annual breast MRI between ages 20–50.

10. C. Cowden syndrome (*PTEN* mutation)

Cowden syndrome is linked to mutation in the autosomal dominant *PTEN* tumour suppressor gene. This results in multiple hamartomas (skin, mucous membranes) and macrocephaly. There is an increased risk of breast, follicular thyroid, endometrial, renal, colorectal cancer, and melanoma.

Multiple endocrine neoplasia (MEN) type 1 (Wermer syndrome) is caused by mutation in the autosomal dominant *MEN1* gene. It is associated with parathyroid, pancreatic islet cell and pituitary tumours. In women it carries a threefold increased risk of breast cancer.

Peutz–Jeghers syndrome is associated with mutation in the autosomal dominant *STKII* tumour suppressor gene. The condition causes hyperpigmented patches on the hands, feet, oral, and perianal mucosa. Benign gastrointestinal (GI) hamartomatous polyps predispose to obstruction and intussusception. There is an increased risk of many cancers by middle age, including pancreatic, breast, ovarian, and GI tract.

Gardner syndrome, Lynch syndrome, and Von Hippel–Lindau syndrome are not known to be associated with a higher risk of breast cancer than that of the general population.

Endocrine therapy

11. F. Tamoxifen

This elderly lady has a low-grade, node-negative cancer associated with good prognosis. Even with weakly ER+ve disease she is likely to get benefit from tamoxifen, though her overall risk of recurrence is low.

12. C. goserelin and exemestane

This patient is premenopausal with very high-risk disease. The SOFT trial showed a significant advantage with ovarian suppression and an aromatase inhibitor compared to tamoxifen in the high-risk subgroup.

13. A. Letrozole

The BIG 1-98 trial compared letrozole to tamoxifen in the post-menopausal population and showed superiority in disease-free survival and time to distant recurrence in the letrozole arm, especially in the higher risk subgroup. NICE guidelines suggest offering an aromatase inhibitor (AI) to all post-menopausal patients not in the low-risk group. Low risk is defined as excellent or good NPI group, or 10-year predictive survival of >93%. In practice this means all patients with grade 2 or 3 disease, or node positivity, or adverse pathological features such as LVI are offered an AI.

14. F. Tamoxifen

This young woman should be offered tamoxifen for ten years and unlike the patient in Q44 is unlikely to obtain benefit from ovarian suppression + AI. She should be counselled against becoming pregnant while on tamoxifen due to potential teratogenicity.

Discontinuing tamoxifen in order to start a family involves balancing the increased risk of recurrence against the patient's desire for a family and is often a difficult decision. Many clinicians would advise waiting three years after diagnosis before trying to conceive, after which time the rate of recurrence diminishes. She can be reassured that there is no evidence that pregnancy is associated with recurrence or adverse outcome. Some oncologists may offer three years of goserelin plus exemestane as an alternative to tamoxifen in patients who wish to try to conceive, as this may be superior to tamoxifen over a shorter time frame, though this has not been proven.

Breast development

15. F. Polymastia

Polymastia is the presence of an accessory or supernumerary breast(s)

16. E. Poland syndrome

Poland syndrome includes congenital unilateral underdevelopment of the breast and pectoralis major muscle. This is usually right-sided and may have associated ipsilateral webbing of the fingers.

17. H. Tuberous breast

Tuberous breast describes congenital breast hypoplasia with a constricted breast base, constricted skin envelope, and central pseudoherniation of parenchyma and the nipple-areolar complex.

Amazia is absence of the breast (the nipple and areola are present). Athelia is absence of the nipple (rare).

Gynaecomastia is enlargement of the male breast.

Polythelia is the presence of an accessory nipple(s), which may occur with or without polymastia. They arise along the mammalian milk line from the axilla to the pubis and are present in about 2% of the population.

Neonatal breast enlargement is a normal consequence of maternal oestrogen and progesterone. It occurs independent of the sex of the baby and subsides within weeks to months.

Gynaecomastia

18. G. Tamoxifen

When assessing a patient with gynaecomastia, a careful drug history is important, both prescription and illicit drugs, including steroids commonly used in body-building. If the patient has recently started on medication it is more likely to be the cause than a long-standing treatment. Tamoxifen can be used to treat gynaecomastia although it not licensed for this use. It may be important for the patient to stay on the causative medication and all that is required is reassurance. If in doubt look up the agent or seek advice from a pharmacist.

Single Best Answers

1. **A 27 year old euthyroid female presents with a 2-year history of a thyroid swelling. An ultrasound demonstrates a 2cm solid mass in the left lobe of the thyroid with mixed vascularity. Fine needle aspiration cytology (FNAC) is reported as showing 'a scanty specimen that is heavily blood stained and is inadequate for cytological interpretation THY 1'. What is the most appropriate next step?**
   a) A diagnostic hemithyroidectomy
   b) An urgent repeat FNAC
   c) A core biopsy
   d) A hemithyroidectomy with on-table frozen section
   e) A repeat FNAC after three months

2. **A 32 year old female presents with a 3-week history of a right-sided neck mass that moves with swallowing. An ultrasound confirms a 5cm thin-walled cyst in the right lobe of the thyroid. This is aspirated to dryness and the specimen is sent to cytology. Cytology is reported as 'an acellular specimen THY 1'. What is the next most appropriate step in managing this?**
   a) Hemithyroidectomy
   b) Urgent repeat FNAC
   c) Open biopsy
   d) Clinical review after three to six months
   e) Repeat FNAC after three months

3. **Which of the following statements is true in relation to imaging of the neck?**
   a) Contrast CT is the best imaging for the thyroid gland
   b) Ultrasound of the neck is indicated in patients with a possible parapharyngeal abscess
   c) PET–CT is the primary investigation of differentiated thyroid carcinoma
   d) Incidental thyroid nodules are the most common incidental findings in imaging of the neck
   e) Ultrasound guided FNAC is required for assessment of simple thyroid goitre

4. **What is the commonest complication after total thyroidectomy for Grave's disease?**
    a) Seroma formation
    b) Hypocalcaemia
    c) Permanent vocal cord palsy
    d) Post-operative haemorrhage requiring re-operation
    e) Keloid scar formation

5. **A 54 year old male with a long-standing thyroid mass has recently noticed a change in his voice. Laryngoscopy shows a right vocal cord palsy. An ultrasound of his neck reveals a multinodular goitre with a 3cm U3 (indeterminate lesion) on the right side. An ultrasound guided FNAC is performed and shows follicular cells consistent with a follicular lesion (THY3F/Bethesda 3). What is the next most appropriate step in management?**
    a) Diagnostic hemithyroidectomy
    b) Total thyroidectomy
    c) Core biopsy
    d) Hemithyroidectomy with on-table frozen section
    e) Repeat FNAC after three months

6. **A 34 year old female is hoping to become pregnant. She has been thyrotoxic for the past two years. Previously she developed agranulocytosis on carbimazole. Her TSH is 0.2U/mL (normal range 1–4U/mL) and T4 is 30µg/dL (normal Range 9–21µg/dL). She has been treated with propranolol and propylthiouracil for the last six months. An ultrasound shows a diffuse symmetrical goitre. What is the best treatment option in this situation?**
    a) Bilateral subtotal thyroidectomy
    b) Total thyroidectomy
    c) Radioactive iodine treatment
    d) Lugol's iodine treatment for three months
    e) Continue with current medical treatment

7. **A 54 year old male has undergone a total thyroidectomy and left neck dissection (level 2a, 3, 4, 5b, and central compartment) for a FNAC proven papillary thyroid cancer (THY5) 2 days previously. He was previously well with no cardiac history. He is due for discharge with planned radioiodine remnant ablation (RRA) in four weeks. His adjusted calcium is 2.34mmol/L (normal range 2.2–2.5mmol/L). His drugs on discharge should include:**
    a) Calcium 1000mg TDS for 8 weeks
    b) Levothyroxine (T4) 100mcg TDS with adjustment depending on TFTs at 3 months
    c) Levothyroxine 150mcg TDS for 2 weeks then liothyronine (T3) for 2 weeks
    d) Thyrogen (rhTSH) for 6 weeks
    e) Liothyronine (T3) 20mcg TDS for 2 weeks

8. **A 35 year old lady with a history of papillary thyroid cancer diagnosed 12 years before presents with a 2cm neck mass on the left, level 5a. An ultrasound-guided core biopsy confirms metastatic papillary thyroid cancer. Which of the following descriptions best describes the anatomical boundaries of the posterior triangle of the neck (level 5):**
    a) Posterior border of sternomastoid muscle, anterior border of trapezius, and the clavicle
    b) Anterior border of trapezius, the nuchal line posteriorly, and upper border of the scapula
    c) Anterior border of sternomastoid muscle, anterior border of trapezius, and the clavicle
    d) Omohyoid muscle inferomedialy, digastric muscle superiorly, and trapezius posteriorly
    e) Posterior border of sternomastoid muscle, the nucal line posteriorly, and the clavicle

9. **A 57 year old male with a history of a previous CABG presents with a 2-month history of an enlarging right-sided thyroid lump. He is noted to be hoarse, although he states that his voice has not changed in years. What is the likely cause of his hoarseness?**
    a) Right recurrent laryngeal nerve palsy
    b) Laryngeal malignancy
    c) Left recurrent laryngeal nerve palsy
    d) Lung cancer
    e) Acute laryngitis

10. **A 54 year old female undergoes a CT of neck, chest, and abdomen following a haemoptysis. An incidental thyroid mass is seen. She also has nodal disease in her neck and mediastinum but there is no pulmonary involvement and no other disease found. Her calcitonin is 1206. An ultrasound-guided FNAC confirms medullary thyroid cancer. A total thyroidectomy, bilateral neck dissection, and mediastinal clearance via a sternotomy is planned. What other investigations should be performed before surgery?**
    a) 24-hour urinary catecholamine
    b) Oesophagogastroscopy
    c) Genetic testing
    d) Abdominal USS
    e) PTH level

11. **A 23 year old patient with primary hyperparathyroidism is noted to also have a history of severe gastroesophageal reflux and peptic ulceration. He is also noted to have numerous telangiectasia around his nasolabial folds. There is no significant family history of note. What is the most likely underlying condition?**
    a) Hereditary haemorrhagic telangiectasia
    b) Multiple endocrine neoplasia type 2
    c) Parathyroid adenoma
    d) Multiple endocrine neoplasia type 1
    e) Overuse of NSAIDs for bone pain

12. **A 65 year old lady is diagnosed with Cushing's syndrome which is thought to be ACTH-independent. What is the single best investigation to confirm the diagnosis?**
    a) MRI pituitary
    b) CT scan abdomen/pelvis
    c) High-dose dexamethasone suppression test
    d) Inferior petrosal sinus catheterization
    e) 24-hour urinary cortisol

13. **A 60 year old male with a long-standing right parotid mass presents with difficulty drinking fluids, difficulty raising his lip on the right side, and an inability to hold an air seal around the lip on the right side of his mouth. An ultrasound-guided FNAC suggests this is an acinic cell carcinoma. What is the likely cause of weakness of his lips?**
    a) Complete paralysis of the maxillary division of the trigeminal nerve
    b) Direct invasion of the buccal nerve
    c) Upper motor neuron lesion of facial nerve
    d) Partial weakness of the mandibular division of trigeminal nerve
    e) Paralysis of the buccal branch of the facial nerve

14. **A 54 year old male smoker presents with a mass in the tail of his left parotid that has been present for the last 6 weeks. Ultrasound of the neck is performed that shows this is a 5cm cystic mass adjacent to the tail of his left parotid gland. There is no obvious solid component. FNAC is performed that shows scanty necrotic sheets of squamous cells consistent with a branchial cyst. What is the most appropriate next step in his management?**
    a) Excision of the cyst
    b) Aspiration of the cyst and clinical review after three months
    c) Core biopsy
    d) FDG PET scan
    e) Repeat FNAC after three months

15. **A 54 year old female patient has an acute abscess secondary to a submandibular duct stone. The abscess involves the floor of the mouth and extends around the mylohyoid muscle into the neck. She is to be taken to theatre for an incision and drainage through the neck. What structures are potentially at risk through this approach?**
    a) Marginal mandibular nerve, accessory nerve, greater auricular nerve
    b) Deep cervical nerve, marginal mandibular nerve, inferior alveolar nerve
    c) Lingual nerve, hypoglossal nerve, submental nerve
    d) Lingual nerve, marginal mandibular nerve, hypoglossal nerve
    e) Accessory nerve, greater auricular nerve, deep cervical nerve

16. **A 42 year old lady presents with a painful lump in the left submandibular gland. FNAC is inconclusive so she undergoes an US and core biopsy. Histology reveals the most common submandibular gland malignancy. The pathologist also comments on a 'Swiss cheese' pattern. Which assessment is particularly relevant in terms of prognosis?**
    a) Neck examination
    b) Intra-oral bimanual palpation of the submandibular glands
    c) Flexible nasendoscopy of the larynx
    d) Unstimulated saliva test
    e) Cranial nerve examination

17. **An 87 year old Muslim lady presents with a 3-hour history of acute abdominal pain. She has previously been fit and well but has been diagnosed with osteoporosis after a fractured neck of femur six months previously. Blood tests are as follows:**

    Chloride 105mmol/L, potassium 5mmol/L, urea 6.7mmol/L, creatinine 123μmol/L, amylase 1000U/L, albumin 34g/L, calcium 2.40mmoll/L, adjusted calcium 2.69mmol/L (normal range 2.05–2.60mmol/L), PTH 40nmol/L (normal range 1.3–6.8nmol/L)

    She improves slowly over a 72-hour period. An abdominal CT shows diffuse enlargement of the pancreas and retroperitoneal oedema. There is no evidence of gallstones. What is the most appropriate next step in her management?
    a) Laparoscopic cholecystectomy after six weeks
    b) Open cholecystectomy
    c) Sestamibi scan
    d) Oesophagogastroduodenoscopy
    e) Abdominal MRI after six weeks

18. **A 37 year old lady who has a history of left hemithyroidectomy for a THY 3 lesion and known permanent left recurrent laryngeal nerve (RLN) paralysis now requires excision of a right-sided parathyroid adenoma. What important issue should be discussed during consent?**
    a) Surgery may be unsuccessful and repeat exploration may be required
    b) Careful monitoring of serum calcium will be required post-operatively
    c) The same anterior neck incision can be used for this surgery
    d) There is a 1% risk of right RLN paralysis with consequent potential need for tracheostomy
    e) The surgery may be more difficult than usual because she has had previous thyroid surgery

19. **Regarding parathyroid anatomy, which of the following statements is correct?**
    a) The inferior parathyroid glands arise from the fourth branchial pouch
    b) Approximately 60% of the population have 4 parathyroid glands
    c) A parathyroid gland typically weighs 50–60mg
    d) The superior parathyroids are typically superior and lateral to the recurrent laryngeal nerve and the inferior parathyroids lie inferior and medial to the nerve
    e) The inferior parathyroids have a more consistent location in the neck

20. **A 45 year old man with primary hyperparathyroidism has pre-operative imaging including a Technetium 99mTc Sestamibi scan which has suggested a right inferior parathyroid adenoma. At operation an obvious right inferior parathyroid adenoma is excised. However, his intra-operative parathyroid hormone level fails to fall following removal of the suspect gland. What is the most likely problem?**
    a) Parathyroid cancer
    b) MEN 2b
    c) Double adenoma
    d) Paget's disease
    e) Renal failure

Extended Matching Items

Neck swellings

    A. Hashimoto's thyroiditis
    B. Graves' disease
    C. Toxic nodule
    D. Multinodular goitre
    E. Thyroid lymphoma
    F. Fourth branchial arch cyst
    G. Bleed into a thyroid cyst
    H. Follicular adenoma
    I. Papillary thyroid cancer

For each of the following scenarios, select the most likely diagnosis from the preceding list. Each answer can be used once, more than once, or not at all.

1. A 27 year old female presents with a 3-month history of excessive sweating and palpitations. She has a diffuse swelling of the root of her neck. The thyroid peroxidize (TPO) level is normal.

2. A 14 year old male presents with a recurrent erythematous swelling of the left lower neck. He has had two previous thyroid abscesses drained. He is pyrexial at 38.2° and has an indurated swelling overlying the left lobe of the thyroid gland associated with a poorly healed scar.

3. A 34 year old Ukrainian lady presents with a 5-month history of a swelling in the root of the neck. She also complains of choking on liquids. Examination confirms a right-sided

neck mass that moves on swallowing but not when protruding her tongue. Laryngoscopy confirms a right vocal cord palsy.

4. A 67 year old lady with a 7-day history of a 'cold' presents with acute noisy breathing. Her saturations are 99% on 28% oxygen and her respiratory rate is 22. Her pulse is 102bpm and irregular. Her GP recently diagnosed atrial fibrillation and she was started on digoxin and apixaban three months ago. She has a firm swelling on the right side of the root of her neck that she reports developed over the last six hours. Laryngoscopy shows left-sided deviation but normal vocal cord movement.

Head and neck swellings

A. Warthin's tumour
B. Pleomorphic salivary adenoma
C. Sjögren's syndrome
D. Mucoepidermoid cancer
E. Masseteric hypertrophy
F. Dental abscess
G. Submandibular sialolithiasis
H. Mumps
I. Reactive lymph nodes
J. Preauricular sinus

For each of the following scenarios, select the most likely diagnosis from the preceding list. Each answer can be used once, more than once, or not at all.

5. A 62 year old female smoker with a BMI of 44 presents with a 3-month history of discrete bilateral pre-auricular masses, larger on the left side than the right. The masses are non-tender and facial nerve function is preserved.

6. A 67 year old lady with primary hyperparathyroidism presents with right-sided neck pain and swelling that comes on when eating and resolves after about 30 minutes. There is nothing to feel on examination of the neck and intra-oral examination is normal.

7. A 55 year old lady with a history of dry eyes and mouth is concerned that she has developed bilateral, tender, swelling of her face. It does not vary with eating. Examination confirms bilateral, diffuse, parotid swelling.

8. A 25 year old male has been referred with a pre-auricular sebaceous cyst. Clinical examination reveals a 1cm hard mass with no obvious punctum. An ultrasound reveals a well-circumscribed rounded mass in the superficial lobe of the right parotid gland.

Endocrine tumours

A. Addison's disease
B. MEN 1
C. MEN 2a
D. MEN 3
E. Conn's syndrome
F. Adrenal adenoma
G. Cushing's syndrome
H. Phaeochromocytoma
I. Adrenocortical carcinoma

For each of the following scenarios, select the most likely diagnosis from the preceding list. Each answer can be used once, more than once, or not at all.

9. A 41 year old man presents to his GP with poor vision, headaches, and muscle weakness, and is found to have a BP of 165/95 and potassium of 3.0mmol/L. What is the most likely diagnosis?

10. A 45 year old woman is admitted to A&E following a fall at work. She has minor injuries but is found to be hypertensive and routine bloods show evidence of mild hypercalcaemia. During further questioning she explains that her sister has recently undergone thyroid surgery for a medullary thyroid cancer. What is her underlying condition most likely due to?

11. A 30 year old male presents to his GP with headaches. His blood pressure is 170/95. He is known to suffer from Von Hippel–Lindau (VHL) syndrome.

12. A 65 year old woman presents with post-menopausal bleeding and a 5cm mass in her left adrenal gland. This mass has increased in size by 3cm over the last year and has marked enhancement on CT scan. What is the most likely diagnosis?

Investigation of endocrine tumours

A. Tc scincitigraphy
B. T3 serology
C. Fine needle aspiration cytology (FNAC)
D. Excision biopsy
E. CT scan neck and chest
F. Serum alkaline phosphatase
G. Iodine uptake scan
H. Thyroglobulin and thyroglobulin antibody serology
I.   TPO antibody levels
J.   MRI scan neck
K. Serum creatinine kinase

For each of the following scenarios, select the most likely diagnosis from the preceding list. Each answer can be used once, more than once, or not at all.

13. A 27 year old female is on long-term follow-up for T3N1 papillary thyroid cancer. She underwent a total thyroidectomy and selective neck dissection four years previously. This was followed by successful radioiodine ablation therapy. She remains well. What surveillance investigation should be done to look for recurrent disease?

14. A 45 year old man is on the waiting list for a thyroidectomy for thyrotoxicosis. A routine ultrasound has shown a 1.5cm benign nodule in the right lobe of his thyroid. What is the most appropriate investigation to define the extent of surgery?

15. A 35 year old lady presents with mild hypothyroidism and a moderate goitre. An ultrasound scan confirms diffuse thyroid enlargement and multiple reactive-looking nodes. What investigation should be done to further investigate this?

16. A 64 year old male smoker presents with a 3-month history of weight loss, epigastric pain, and mild dysphagia. On examination he is cachectic. He is noted to have a right-sided mass at the root of the neck. It lies behind the sternocleidomastoid muscle and does not appear to move on swallowing. The rest of his neck examination is normal. His bloods, including TFTs, are normal. What is the most appropriate investigation to diagnose the problem?

17. A 16 year old girl with thyrotoxicosis is concerned about the risk of post-operative hypocalcaemia. What preoperative test may indicate that she is at increased risk of developing this post-operatively?

Surgical management of patients with endocrine disorders

A. Open adrenalectomy
B. Laparoscopic adrenalectomy
C. CT-guided biopsy
D. MRI scan adrenals
E. Discharge
F. Observe and repeat CT scan in six months
G. Endocrine assessment
H. Bleeding
I. Has not received IV hydrocortisone
J. Sepsis
K. Effects of post-operative analgesia
L. Alpha and beta blockade

For each of the following scenarios, select the most likely diagnosis from the preceding list. Each answer can be used once, more than once, or not at all.

18. A 68 year old lady with weight loss undergoes a CT scan of her chest, abdomen, and pelvis. This shows a 5cm right-sided adrenal lesion which predominately contains fat. Endocrine tests show this to be a non-functioning lesion. What is the most appropriate next step in her management?

19. A 55 year old man has just undergone an uncomplicated laparoscopic right-sided adrenalectomy for a phaeochromocytoma. He is noticed to be hypotensive six hours post-operatively. What is the most likely cause for this gentleman's low BP?

20. A 71 year old woman undergoes a routine CT scan of chest abdomen and pelvis as follow-up for a previous colon cancer. This shows a 4cm left-sided adrenal lesion. What is the most appropriate management in this case?

Single Best Answers

1. e) A repeat FNAC after three months

This is an indeterminate lesion on ultrasound. The THY1 result should be repeated, given the size and ultrasound findings, to ensure it is benign. If this is repeated too soon, the residual inflammation from the previous biopsy may change the cytological features of the specimen, potentially giving a false positive result. Therefore, a delay of at least three months is usually recommended before re-sampling. This can be modified if there are any features of concern, such as a rapid increase in size, vocal cord palsy, or evidence of local invasion on ultrasound. The THY system is the most commonly used system of categorizing thyroid cytology specimens (see Table 8.1), whereas in the

Table 8.1 The THY classification

Thy1: Non-diagnostic. Poor samples due to aspiration of a cyst or poor operator or preparation technique, such as insufficient epithelial cells or only poorly preserved cells.

Thy2: Non-neoplastic. Samples with adequate cellularity which suggests a non-neoplastic lesion such as normal thyroid tissue, a colloid nodule, or thyroiditis.

Thy3: Neoplasm possible. Subdivided into:

Thy3a: Atypical features present but not enough to place into another category.

Thy3f: Follicular neoplasm is suspected. The histological possibilities include a hyperplastic nodule, follicular adenoma, or follicular carcinoma. These cannot be distinguished on cytology alone.

Thy4: Suspicious of malignancy but definite diagnosis of malignancy is not possible.

Thy5: Diagnostic of malignancy (unequivocal features of papillary, medullary, or anaplastic carcinoma, or of lymphoma or metastatic tumour).

Source data from *Guidance on the Reporting of Thyroid Cytology Specimens,* Cross P, Chandra A, Giles T. 2016, The Royal College of Pathologists.

United States, the Bethesda system is commonly used.

The Royal College of Pathologists (2016) Guidance on the Reporting of Thyroid Cytology Specimens. London. <http://ukeps.com/docs/thyroidfna.pdf>.

Ali SZ and Cibas ES (eds). *The Bethesda System for Reporting (2010) Thyroid Cytopathology: Definitions, Criteria and Explanatory Notes.* New York, NY: Springer, 2010.

2. d) Clinical review after three to six months

A simple thyroid cyst will not contain cellular contents and unless suitably labelled as a 'Thyroid Cyst' on the request, the cytology will be reported as being a THY1 (inadequate) specimen. If it is completely aspirated, a period of observation for a few months to allow any recurrence to declare itself is reasonable management. If the cyst does not recur, no further management is required. However, if the cyst recurs, symptomatic treatment with a hemithyroidectomy is appropriate. As there is no solid component to sample, there is no benefit in repeating the FNAC and an open biopsy is not going to help the diagnosis.

3. d) Incidental thyroid nodules are the most common incidental findings in imaging of the neck

Unlike superficial neck abscesses, deep neck space abscesses are best assessed with contrast CT. The best modality for assessing the thyroid gland is ultrasound. However, it is not always necessary to combine this with FNAC, which is only indicated in certain situations: FNAC may be indicated when ultrasound identifies microcalcifications; hypo-echogenicity; irregular margins; intranodular flow; and the absence of a halo (referred to as a U classification). ← halo. = Cyst

Incidental thyroid nodules are common and may result in additional and potentially unnecessary investigations, procedures and health care costs. The management of incidental thyroid nodules (incidentalomas) varies and has led to calls that such patients should be investigated using defined protocols such as in Figure 8.1, which has been suggested by the American College of Radiology. In practice, most patients will have an ultrasound of the thyroid, which involves no risk to the patient.

Hoang JK et al. Managing incidental thyroid nodules detected on imaging: white paper of the ACR Incidental Thyroid Findings Committee. *Journal of the American College of Radiology* 2015; 12:143–50.

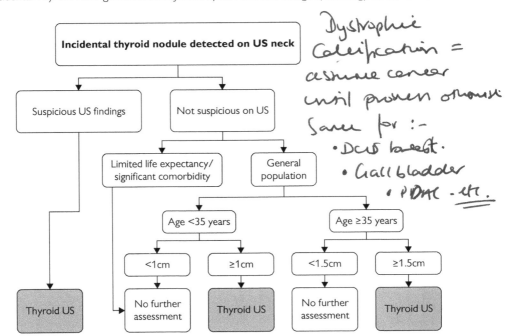

Dystrophic Calcification = assume cancer until proven otherwise

Same for :-
• DCIS breast.
• Gall bladder
• PDAC - etc.

Fig. 8.1 Proposed protocol to investigate incidental thyroid nodules

4. b) Hypocalcaemia

Whilst the best-known complication of thyroid surgery is vocal cord palsy, this is a relatively rare problem occurring in 1–2% of operations. Ideally, all patients undergoing thyroid surgery should have both pre- and post-operative vocal cord checks, looking specifically for nerve palsy. However, this is not universally performed at present and in some centres the vocal cords are only assessed if there is a change in voice post-operatively. Such an approach is likely to miss compensated vocal cord palsy.

Post-operative haemorrhage has always been feared in thyroid surgery due to the risk of acute airway compromise. Post-operative patients should be closely observed for signs of neck swelling that might herald such an event. It is occasionally necessary to open the wound on the ward to decompress the trachea in the event of sudden airway compromise. The incidence after total thyroidectomy is 1%.

The incidence of seroma formation after thyroid surgery ranges from 1–7%.

Hypocalcaemia is reported in 25% of patients undergoing thyroid surgery in the British Association of Endocrine and Thyroid Surgeons (BAETS) audit (adjusted calcium <2.10mmol/L within 24 hours of surgery) but 12% require long-term calcium supplementation at follow-up.

Keloid scar formation varies in incidence depending upon the racial origin of the patient (4.5–16%). It is commoner in people of Mediterranean or African origin but can occur in all races. Asking about previous scar problems in at-risk patients can assess susceptibility. Triamcinolone injection into the fresh site of scar may be considered. Silicone scar treatments may also reduce the severity of scarring and keloid.

Marneros AG et al. Clinical Genetics of Familial Keloids. *Archives of Dermatology* 2001; 137(11):1429–34.

BAETS Audit 2012. <http://www.baets.org.uk/wp-content/uploads/2013/05/4th-National-Audit.pdf>.

5. b) Total thyroidectomy

The finding of a follicular lesion on the FNAC can represent either a benign follicular adenoma or a follicular carcinoma. The two pathologies are differentiated by capsular or vascular invasion of the lesion as shown by histology of the whole specimen. The ultrasound findings are consistent with this. The U Classification gives a range from 1–5 of the risk of a lesion being malignant based on the ultrasound findings and defines the need for a biopsy.

The ipsilateral vocal cord palsy is very concerning in this context and so there is a high likelihood that this is a malignant follicular carcinoma. In this clinical context, the management should be a total thyroidectomy. Other situations including clinical or radiological evidence of local invasion to either the adjacent vascular structures or the upper airway, or known distant metastasis, would also be an indication for total thyroidectomy.

A hemithyroidectomy would confirm the diagnosis but is not suitable management for this likely malignant lesion and repeat biopsies are unlikely to clarify the situation, as the original sample was a satisfactory specimen.

On-table frozen section is unlikely to be helpful as the finding of local invasion requires careful histological evaluation of the whole specimen, which is not possible in this time interval.

Guidelines for the management of thyroid cancer, 3rd edn. British Thyroid Association 2014. <http://www.british-thyroid-association.org/Guidelines/Docs/BTA_DTC_guidlines.pdf>.

6. b) Total thyroidectomy

This patient is not controlled with medical treatment and she has had a reaction to carbimazole so continuing with medical treatment is not suitable. Her wish to start a family is a relative contraindication to receiving radioactive iodine treatment within 12 months of becoming pregnant. This also presents a problem if there are young children at home as they should avoid close contact for a few weeks post-treatment. *Lugol ↓ T3/T4 secretion + ↓ vascularity.*

Lugol's iodine can be used for preoperative treatment of thyrotoxic patients to help render them euthyroid. It works by blocking the release of thyroid hormones, diminishing biosynthesis, and preventing peripheral conversion of T4 to T3 before surgery. Once Lugol's has been started, surgery should take place within 14 days because of the risk of a rebound 'thyroid storm'. Thyroid storm is a potentially fatal complication of thyrotoxicosis where massive sympathetic stimulation causes pyrexia, tachycardia, cardiac arrhythmias, vomiting, and diarrhoea.

Subtotal thyroidectomy is no longer recommended as a treatment for thyrotoxicosis. The aim was to reduce the size of the thyroid whilst leaving a variable amount of tissue behind to give both residual thyroid hormone replacement and potentially preserve vascularity of the parathyroid glands. With the advent of reliable hormone replacement and good assays for assessing thyroid function the residual tissue is no longer necessary. Residual thyroid tissue can also cause problems with replacement regimens and patients can develop future problems with both thyroid enlargement and hyperthyroidism requiring further surgery. Revision surgery in this instance can be very complex.

Wolff J and Chaikiff IL. The temporary nature of the inhibitory action of excess iodine on organic iodine synthesis in the normal thyroid. *Endocrinology* 1949; 45:504.

7. e) Liothyronine (T3) 20 micrograms TDS for 2 weeks

This patent has a thyroid cancer with locoregional disease (hence the need for a neck dissection). He has normal adjusted calcium levels so calcium supplementation is unnecessary. In order for RRA to be effective, it is important that any residual thyroid cells are stimulated/producing thyroid hormone at the time of the treatment. This can be achieved indirectly by withholding hormone replacement, thereby stimulating natural TSH production or directly by giving recombinant TSH (rhTSH).

Levothyroxine needs to be withheld for at least four weeks prior to RRA. This causes patients to become symptomatically hypothyroid (which they don't enjoy). However, patients treated with liothyronine only need to stop treatment for two weeks prior to RRA. During the two weeks prior to treatment they should be off all treatment and go on a low-iodine diet.

Levothyroxine is given once a day and liothyronine is given three times a day. Rather than multiple changes in hormone types, some centres simply put patients on liothyronine post-operatively rather than change over.

The other option is continuing on levothyroxine but administer rhTSH at 48 and 24 hours before RRA treatment. This has the advantage of avoiding hormone changes but is a more expensive option.

Perros P et al. Guidelines for the management of thyroid cancer. *Clinical Endocrinology* 2014; 81:1–122.

8. a) Posterior border of sternomastoid muscle, anterior border of trapezius and the clavicle

The anterior neck has been traditionally divided into the anterior and posterior triangles. These do not include the trapezius and para-spinal muscles. Historically, other subdivisions were used including areas such as the submandibular triangle. However, these have been superseded by the levels of the neck. The levels of the neck were originally developed in the Memorial Sloan–Kettering Cancer Center as an easy and reproducible means of describing regional nodal involvement in cancer of the head and neck. It has now been universally accepted. See Table 8.2 and Figure 8.2.

Table 8.2 Levels of the neck

Level	Medial boundary	Lateral boundary	Superior boundary	Inferior boundary	Likely location of head and neck primary lesion
IA	Midline	Anterior belly of digastric			Floor of mouth, anterior oral tongue, lower lip, anterior mandibular alveolar ridge
IB	Anterior belly of digastric	Posterior belly of digastric	Body of mandible	Stylohyoid muscle	Oral cavity, anterior nasal cavity, soft tissue structures of the midface, and the submandibular gland
IIA	Lateral border of sternohyoid	Spinal accessory nerve	Skull base		Oral cavity, nasal cavity, nasopharynx, oropharynx, hypopharynx, larynx, and parotid gland
IIB	Spinal accessory nerve	Posterior border of sternocleidomastoid muscle		Inferior border of hyoid bone	Oral cavity, nasal cavity, nasopharynx, oropharynx, hypopharynx, larynx and parotid gland
III	Lateral border of sternohyoid	Posterior border of sternocleidomastoid	Inferior border of hyoid bone	Inferior border of cricoid cartilage	oral cavity, nasopharynx, hypopharynx, and larynx
IV	Lateral border of sternohyoid	Posterior border of sternocleidomastoid	Inferior border of cricoid cartilage	Clavicle	Hypopharynx, cervical oesophagus, and larynx
VA	Posterior border of the sternocleidomastoid muscle	Anterior border of the trapezius muscle	Apex formed by a convergence of the sternocleidomastoid and the trapezius muscles	Horizontal plane marking the inferior border of the arch of the cricoid cartilage	Nasopharynx and oropharynx
VB	Posterior border of the sternocleidomastoid muscle	Anterior border of the trapezius muscle	Horizontal plane marking the inferior border of the arch of the cricoid cartilage	Clavicle	Thyroid gland
VI	Midline	Common carotid artery	Hyoid bone	Suprasternal notch	Thyroid gland, glottic and subglottic larynx, apex of the pyriform sinus, and cervical oesophagus

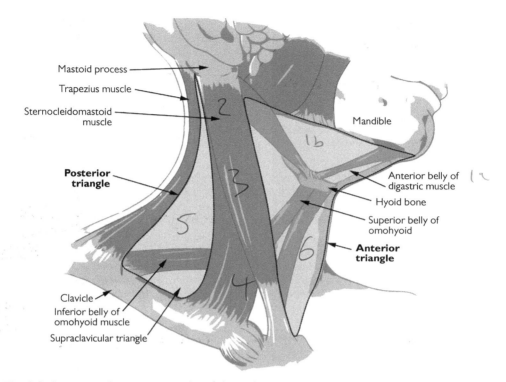

Mastoid process

Trapezius muscle

Sternocleidomastoid muscle

Mandible

Posterior triangle

Anterior belly of digastric muscle

Hyoid bone

Superior belly of omohyoid

Anterior triangle

Clavicle

Inferior belly of omohyoid muscle

Supraclavicular triangle

Fig. 8.2 Anterior and posterior triangles of the neck

Deschler DG et al (eds). *Quick Reference Guide to TNM Staging of Head and Neck Cancer and Neck Dissection Classification*, 4th edn. Alexandria, VA: American Academy of Otolaryngology–Head and Neck Surgery Foundation, 2014. Available for download at: <http://www.entnet.org/sites/default/files/ChapterThreeFINAL.pdf>.

9. c) Left recurrent laryngeal nerve palsy

Given the gentleman's voice has been hoarse for years and the thyroid lump has only been present for two months, it is likely he has a long-standing left vocal cord palsy from previous cardiothoracic surgery. The recurrent laryngeal nerve (RLN) hooks under the aortic arch on the left and is at risk in cardiothoracic surgery. On the right it can be non-recurrent or hook under the subclavian artery (see Figure 1.4).

In clinic, a fibreoptic laryngoscopy should be performed to determine the vocal cord mobility. This is an important part of the patient's management, especially for the consent process should a malignancy be proven and surgery required. The patient will have to be warned of the possibility of tracheostomy.

Dankbaar JW and Pameijer FA. Vocal cord paralysis: anatomy, imaging and pathology. *Insight Imaging* 2014; 5:743–51.

10. a) 24-hour urinary catecholamines

Medullary thyroid cancer is a rare disease that accounts for 3–5% of all thyroid cancers. It originates from the parafollicular (C cells), which produce the hormone calcitonin. Most commonly it is sporadic but a quarter of cases are familial. It can occur in association with multiple endocrine neoplasia (MEN) type 2A, which is also associated with phaeochromocytoma (33–50% of cases) and primary hyperparathyroidism. Medullary thyroid cancer also occurs in MEN type 3 (formerly 2B), which is also associated with phaeochromocytoma (50% of cases) and digestive neurofibromatosis. + Morton's.

All cases should undergo a thorough investigative work-up including genetic testing looking for RET mutation analysis (even in the absence of a family history). However, the only essential investigation that should be performed prior to neck surgery is 24-hour urinary catecholamines, given the potential for anaesthetic complications if one operated on a patient with an unsuspected phaeochromocytoma.

Wells SA et al. Multiple Endocrine Neoplasia Type 2 and familial medullary thyroid carcinoma: an update. *The Journal of Clinical Endocrinology & Metabolism* 2013; 98(8):3149–64.

11. d) Multiple endocrine neoplasia type 1

MEN type 1 (also called Wermer syndrome) is usually autosomal dominant but can occur spontaneously with sporadic mutation of the tumour suppressor gene MEN1, situated on chromosome band 11q13. Hyperparathyroidism is one of the most common presentations and is present in >90% of affected individuals. It is due to parathyroid hyperplasia (important surgically as at least 3½ glands will need to be excised to control the hyperparathyroidism). MEN1 is also associated with gastrinomas, insulinomas, glucagonomas, pancreatic polypeptidomas, carcinoid tumours, pituitary tumours, and cutaneous tumours such as angiofibromas. The life expectancy is poor with 50% probability of death by 50 years.

Norman J. Multiple Endocrine Neoplasia Type 1. Disorders of the Parathyroid, Pituitary, and Pancreas. Review on EndocrineWeb. <http://www.endocrineweb.com/conditions/pituitary-disorders/multiple-endocrine-neoplasia-type-1>.

Williams L. Wermer Syndrome (MEN Type 1). Review on Medscape website. <http://emedicine.medscape.com/article/126438-overview>.

12. b) CT scan abdomen/pelvis

If Cushing's syndrome is ACTH-independent then it is due to adrenal pathology, that is an adrenal adenoma, carcinoma, or hyperplasia. A CT scan of her abdomen will confirm any of these pathologies. If she had ACTH-dependent Cushing's syndrome then the cause is either from excess ACTH production from the pituitary, excess ACTH administration, or excess production in an ectopic ACTH-producing tumour.

Aspinall S et al. The adrenal glands. In: Lennard TWJ (ed.). *Endocrine Surgery*, 4th edn. Philadelphia, PA: Elsevier Saunders, 2009, pp. 73–99.

13. e) Paralysis of the buccal branch of the facial nerve

The combination of facial nerve weakness and a parotid mass is highly suggestive of a malignant process. A lower motor neurone weakness is differentiated from an upper motor neurone weakness which spares forehead movement as there is bilateral innervation of the facial motor nucleus for the forehead. The muscles of facial expression are all innervated by the facial nerve. The muscles of mastication are innervated by the mandibular division of the trigeminal nerve. The inability to hold an air seal of the lips is caused by paralysis of the buccal branch of the facial nerve (not the buccal nerve, which is from the trigeminal nerve and is a sensory nerve). Facial nerve weakness can be graded according to the House–Brackmann Facial Nerve Grading System that has been in routine clinical use for many years (see Box 8.1).

Box 8.1 House–Brackmann Facial Nerve Grading System

Grade I—Normal

Normal facial function in all areas.

Grade II—Slight dysfunction

Gross: slight weakness noticeable on close inspection; may have very slight synkinesis.

At rest: normal symmetry and tone.

Motion: forehead—moderate to good function; eye—complete closure with minimum effort; mouth—slight asymmetry.

Grade III—Moderate dysfunction

Gross: obvious but not disfiguring difference between two sides; noticeable but not severe synkinesis, contracture, and/or hemi-facial spasm.

At rest: normal symmetry and tone.

Motion: forehead—slight to moderate movement; eye—complete closure with effort; mouth—slightly weak with maximum effort.

Grade IV—Moderate severe dysfunction

Gross: obvious weakness and/or disfiguring asymmetry.

At rest: normal symmetry and tone.

Motion: forehead—none; eye—incomplete closure; mouth—asymmetric with maximum effort.

Grade V—Severe dysfunction

Gross: only barely perceptible motion.

At rest: asymmetry.

Motion: forehead – none; eye—incomplete closure; mouth—slight movement.

Grade VI—Total paralysis

No movement.

Reproduced from *Otolaryngology—Head and Neck Surgery*, 93, House JW, Brackmann DE., Facial nerve grading system, pp. 146–7. Copyright © 1985, © SAGE Publications.

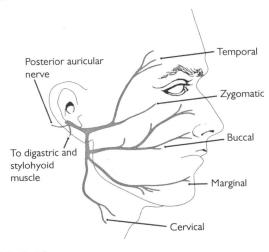

Fig 8.3 Branches of the facial nerve

House JW and Brackmann DE. Facial nerve grading system. *Journal of Otolaryngology—Head & Neck Surgery* 1985; 93:146–7.

Head and neck and spine. In: Sinnatamby CS (ed.). *Last's Anatomy Regional and Applied*, 12th edn. London: Churchill Livingstone Elsevier, 2011, pp. 329–83.

14. e) FDG PET scan

The presence of a squamous lined cyst in a patient over the age of 35 years is concerning for metastatic squamous cell carcinoma (SCC). A thorough examination for a primary cancer should be undertaken including the nasopharynx, oropharynx, tongue base, larynx, and hypopharynx. If no obvious primary is found on clinical examination, cross-sectional imaging including CT, MRI, or PET scan should be undertaken before surgical excision is considered.

Simple excision of the cyst is contraindicated until a complete assessment has been made as there is a high risk of incomplete excision and seeding of malignant cells in the surgical field, if the diagnosis is that of a metastatic SCC.

If an excision is performed (after all other evaluations have come back as negative) then a selective neck dissection removing all the lymph nodes at that level of the neck should be performed. A core biopsy would only be of value if there were a solid component to be sampled. As this is not seen on USS (ultrasound scan) this would not be helpful. A repeat FNAC after three months is not going to change the situation even if repeat cytology is benign (given concerns regarding the possibility of a sampling error).

15. d) *Lingual nerve, marginal mandibular nerve, hypoglossal nerve*

In the traditional approach to the deep lobe of the submandibular gland, the nerves at risk are:

Cn VII

- **The marginal mandibular nerve** (from the facial nerve) that lies deep to platysma and can descend up to 2cm below the mandible into the neck. Damage to this nerve can result in weakness of the depressor anguli oris, labii inferioris muscles, and mentalis muscle, which gives rise to an inability to lower the lip on the affected side.

Cn XII • **The hypoglossal nerve** that lies deep to the digastric muscle, ascends to supply the intrinsic muscles of the tongue. Damage leads to weakness of the tongue muscles and is tested by observing wasting and deviation of the tongue to the affected side.

Cn V • **The lingual nerve** (mandibular division of trigeminal nerve) provides sensory innervation to the tongue and also carries fibres of the Chorda tympani (facial nerve) that provide special sense taste to the anterior two-thirds of the tongue. See Figure 8.4.

V + VII sensation anterior tongue

16. e) **Cranial nerve examination**

The most common malignancy of the submandibular gland is an adenoid cystic carcinoma. Although this tumour accounts for only 10% of all salivary gland neoplasms, adenoid cystic carcinoma is the most common tumour type in the minor salivary glands. It has equal gender prevalence and often presents as an otherwise asymptomatic lump. However, given its predilection to perineural spread, it can cause pain and nerve palsies. Cranial nerve examination is therefore essential.

Although not always evident on examination, perineural involvement occurs in up to 80% of cases. Nerve resection and or adjuvant radiotherapy targeted to the nerve course may be considered. Long-term follow-up is required due to the insidious nature and preponderance for late local recurrence or distant metastasis (possible >20yrs).

Yuan Shin Butt F et al. Salivary glands. In: Lalwani AK (ed.). *Current Diagnosis and Treatment. Otolaryngology Head and Neck Surgery*, 3rd edn. New York, NY: McGraw Hill Lange, 2012, pp. 317–45.

Adenoid cystic carcinoma → comes from Warthin's.

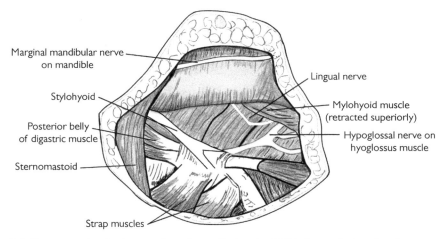

Marginal mandibular nerve on mandible

Stylohyoid

Posterior belly of digastric muscle

Sternomastoid

Lingual nerve

Mylohyoid muscle (retracted superiorly)

Hypoglossal nerve on hyoglossus muscle

Strap muscles

Fig. 8.4 Structures that lie deep to the submandibular gland. This figure displays the deep structures within the bed of the right submandibular gland after excision.

17. c) Sestamibi scan

This lady has acute pancreatitis. She also has primary hyperparathyroidism given the elevated calcium, PTH (parathyroid hormone), and normal renal function. This is likely to account for the acute pancreatitis. In this situation, cholecystectomy is not going to be of help in management.

A sestamibi scan is a nuclear medicine scan using Tc99m sestamibi. This is concentrated in the mitochondria of parathyroid and thyroid cells but the washout rate from abnormal parathyroid tissue is much slower than normal thyroid tissue. An early initial image is obtained 10–15 minutes after injection. This is followed by delayed imaging at 1.5–3 hours. Single-photon emission CT imaging can also be performed for improved anatomic localization (SPECT). Sestamibi scans have a reported sensitivity of 80–90%. Most endocrine surgeons advocate dual imaging by both ultrasound and sestamibi scanning to identify the site of disease definitively before proceeding with surgery.

18. d) There is a 1% risk of right RLN paralysis with consequent potential need for tracheostomy

All of the answers except e) are true (as the previous surgery was the contralateral side). However, the best answer is d), because this patient has a known contralateral palsy and although the risk is rare, the potential outcome has serious health and lifestyle implications. Thus, the patient should be fully informed of the possibility of tracheostomy and its implications, including the fact that it may be permanent.

Perros P et al. Guidelines for the management of thyroid cancer. *Clinical Endocrinology* 2014; 81:1–122.

19. d) The superior parathyroids are typically superior and lateral to the recurrent laryngeal nerve and the inferior parathyroids lie inferior and medial to the nerve

The parathyroid glands are derived from the third (inferior parathyroids) and fourth (superior parathyroids) brachial pouches around five to six weeks gestation. The majority of the population (85–90%) have 4 glands. The inferior parathyroids descend caudally with the thymus. They can have a much more variable location as they travel a greater distance, whereas the superior parathyroids descend with the thyroid gland itself. The average normal parathyroid will weigh between 20–40mg. See Figure 8.5.

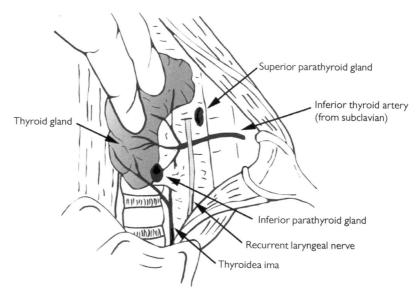

Fig. 8.5 Location of parathyroid glands in relation to the recurrent laryngeal nerve

Head and neck and spine. In: Sinnatamby CS (ed.). *Last's Anatomy Regional and Applied*, 12th edn. London: Churchill Livingstone, Elsevier, 2011, pp. 329–83.

20. c) Double adenoma

Primary hyperparathyroidism is most commonly caused by a single adenoma (87–90%). Less common causes include double or multiple adenomas, parathyroid hyperplasia, and carcinoma (1%).

Sestamibi scanning has a sensitivity of around 80% and a specificity of around 90%. The sensitivity falls to 30% in cases of double or multiple adenomas or hyperplasia. In the present scenario, a persistent elevation in the PTH level despite removal of an obvious adenoma suggests a second adenoma which was missed on preoperative imaging.

Parathyroid disease. In: Lennard TWJ (ed.). *Endocrine Surgery*, 4th edn. Philadelphia, PA: Elsevier Saunders, 2009, pp. 1–39.

Extended Matching Items

Neck swellings

1. B. Grave's disease

This patient has thyrotoxicosis with a diffuse goitre, ruling out a toxic nodule. This could be the early manifestation of Hashimoto's thyroiditis except that the TPO level is normal (this would normally be elevated with Hashimoto's thyroiditis). The diagnosis could be confirmed by checking for thyroid receptor antibodies (TRAb).

Lee JC et al. The thyroid gland. In: Lennard TWJ (ed.). *Endocrine Surgery*, 5th edn. Philadelphia, PA: Elsevier Saunders, 2014, pp. 41–70.

2. F. Fourth branchial arch cyst

Fourth branchial arch abnormalities are rare congenital problems caused by failure of the pharyngobranchial duct to degenerate in the seventh week of gestation. They present either with recurrent lateral neck abscesses or acute suppurative thyroiditis. They are more common on the left hand side. Typically, a sinus tract extends from the apex of the piriform sinus into the soft tissue of the neck. The diagnosis is confirmed by the presence of a tract in the piriform fossa either by direct examination, barium swallow (after acute infection has settled), or CT scan. Surgery is aimed at removal of any tract and closing the opening into the piriform sinus.

3. I. Papillary thyroid cancer

The presence of a neck mass that moves with swallowing but not tongue protrusion suggests either thyroid or laryngeal origin. Coming from Eastern Europe there would have been a potential for radiation exposure from the nuclear accident in Chernobyl that increases the risk of developing thyroid cancer. The finding of a vocal cord palsy is highly suspicious for malignant invasion of the recurrent laryngeal nerve. This is rarely caused by lymphoma but is seen in thyroid cancers.

4. G. Bleed into a thyroid cyst

Bleeding into a thyroid cyst may occur following a mild upper respiratory tract infection and excessive coughing. This acute event can give rise to significant airway obstruction. The risk of bleeding is higher in anticoagulated patients (in this case the diagnosis of AF and treatment with apixaban) but can occur with no such history. Initial management is to improve the airway problem. As there is usually an inflammatory component, nebulized adrenaline 2ml of 1 in 1000 can be helpful. Coagulation should be normalized and an ultrasound-guided aspiration of the cyst (or if necessary, freehand) should be performed. Patients should be observed for 24 hours following aspiration to ensure it does not re-accumulate.

Head and neck swellings

5. A. Warthin's tumour

Warthin's tumour (also known as papillary cystadenoma lymphomatosum) primarily affects older individuals. It is associated with cigarette smoking. The tumour is slow-growing and painless. In approximately 10% of cases, the tumour is bilateral and/or can be multifocal. They can spontaneously involute. It is very unlikely to become malignant. Investigation is by ultrasound and FNAC, but it has been reported that this can initiate an aggressive local inflammation (possibly related to leakage of cyst contents). This may lead to a sudden increase in size and pain in the area, which can mimic malignant transformation. Sjögren's syndrome may also present with generalized parotid enlargement but this is a diffuse process without discrete lesions on examination.

6. G. Submandibular sialolithiasis

The history of primary hyperparathyroidism raises the possibility of submandibular gland stones. These can cause intermittent pain and swelling of the affected partially obstructed gland. If intra-oral examination confirms a stone in the submandibular duct, direct removal can be performed under local anaesthetic. In the absence of a palpable stone, an ultrasound can identify a stone in the hilum of the gland or intra-glandular duct dilatation. Sialography is no longer commonly performed as more modern imaging techniques that are less invasive give similar information. A tumour would be unlikely as they do not usually present with intermittent swelling and infections do not resolve after just 30 minutes.

Bradley P et al. The salivary glands. In: Lennard TWJ (ed.). *Endocrine Surgery*, 5th edn. Philadelphia, PA: Elsevier Saunders, 2014, pp. 191–210.

7. C. Sjögren's syndrome

Sjögren's syndrome is an autoimmune condition that presents with dry eyes and mouth. Patients may also develop enlargement of the parotid glands. It can occur independently of other health problems (primary Sjögren's syndrome) or in association with other connective tissue disorders (secondary Sjögren's syndrome). Blood tests looking for other autoimmune conditions (ANA (antinuclear antibody), Rh factor, and others) should be performed. The diagnosis can be confirmed by sub-labial biopsy of the minor salivary glands of the lip. Biopsy of the major salivary glands is rarely necessary.

8. B. Pleomorphic salivary adenoma

Pleomorphic adenomas account for 80% of parotid gland tumours. Although the majority are benign, malignant transformation within a pre-existing adenoma has been reported to occur at a rate of 10% at 20 years. They present as isolated nodules but have small outgrowths from the main nodule that if left behind will lead to recurrence. For this reason, surgery is aimed at an extra-capsular dissection with a cuff of normal tissue where feasible. Frequently these are closely related to the facial nerve and so careful consideration of the operative approach is needed and specialist referral is advised.

Endocrine tumours

9. E. Conn's syndrome   — low renin aldosterone

Conn's syndrome or primary hyperaldosteronism occurs secondary to excess production of aldosterone by the adrenal cortex (zona glomerulosa). This results in low renin levels. The most common cause of primary hyperaldosteronism is an adrenal adenoma (Conn's syndrome). Other less common causes include adrenal cancer and familial hyperaldosteronism. Primary hyperaldosteronism accounts for between 5–15% of people who are found to have hypertension. Peak onset is between 30 and 50 years and is more common in women. Patients are often asymptomatic; however, muscle spasms, muscle weakness, and a low serum potassium and calcium may be present.   — lethargy from hypocalaemia.

Schirpenbach C and Reincke R. Primary hyperaldosteronism: current knowledge and controversies in Conn's syndrome. *Nature Clinical Practice Endocrinology & Metabolism* 2007; 3(3):220–7.

10. C. MEN 2a   MPP — MTC / para / phaeo

MEN 2a is an autosomal dominant familial cancer syndrome characterized by medullary cancer of the thyroid, phaeochromocytoma, and primary hyperparathyroidism, and occasionally cutaneous lichen amyloidosis. Phaeochromocytoma can cause paroxysmal symptoms of catecholamine excess often triggered by stress. In this scenario the patient sustained a fall and on admission to hospital was found to be hypertensive. She also had hypercalcaemia (most likely primary hyperparathyroidism) and describes a sibling who has had a medullary thyroid cancer.

Moline J and Eng C. Multiple endocrine neoplasia type 2: an overview. *Genetic Medicine* 2011; 9(13):755–64.

11. H. Phaeochromocytoma

Phaeochromocytomas are neuroendocrine tumours originating in the medulla of the adrenal gland. They produce excessive catecholamines. Up to 25% are familial. Mutations of the *VHL* and *NF1* genes are known to cause familial phaeochromocytoma. In *VHL*, phaeochromocytoma has an earlier onset

VHL = phaeo

than in the sporadic forms and is usually benign. Phaeochromocytoma can occur in approximately 1% of patients with *NF1* and has a mean age of around 42 years. Tumours are bilateral in approximately 10%, which is similar to the incidence of bilateral tumours in the sporadic form.

Parenbti G et al. Updated and new perspectives on diagnosis, prognosis, and therapy of malignant pheochromocytoma/paraganglioma. *Journal of Oncology* 2012. doi:10.1155/2012/872713.

12. I. Adrenocortical carcinoma

Adrenocortical carcinoma is a rare tumour affecting one to two people per 1 million every year. It has a bimodal age distribution, affecting children under 5 years and adults between 30 and 40 years old. Adrenocortical cancer has often invaded or metastasized at the time of diagnosis and the survival at 5 years is only 20–35%.

Most tumours secrete excess amounts of one or more hormones and are usually rapidly growing. CT characteristics for malignancy include non-homogenous gland enlargement, marked enhancement after contrast, evidence of local invasion, and metastasis. In this patient's case the tumour is producing high levels of oestrogen which have resulted in post-menopausal bleeding. Although previously open adrenalectomy was advocated as the treatment of choice, recent evidence suggest that a laparoscopic approach can be just as successful.

Wooten MD et al. Adrenal Cortical Carcinoma. Epidemiology and treatment with mitotane and a review of the literature. *Cancer* 1993; 72:3145–55.

Investigation of endocrine tumours

13. H. Thyroglobulin and thyroglobulin antibody serology

Thyroglobulin (TG) is performed as a part of the routine follow-up of patients who have been treated for thyroid cancer. A rising level of this tumour marker may be an indicator for recurrent disease and will direct further investigation. It is standard practice to test for the TG antibody level also, as the presence of antibodies may give rise to a false low TG result. In this situation, the TG antibody trend can be used to predict disease recurrence. An iodine uptake scan is routinely performed at three to six months following radioiodine ablation therapy but is not done as a routine surveillance investigation unless recurrence is suspected by either a rising TG or TG Ab or clinically.

14. A. Tc scincitigraphy

Technetium scanning is now rarely used for assessment of the malignant potential of thyroid nodules (hot nodules are likely to be benign and cold nodules may be malignant) having been superseded by more sensitive investigations like ultrasound and FNAC. However, it is still of use when there is a need to identify if a toxic patient has a 'hot nodule', in which case a hemithyroidectomy will cure the thyrotoxicosis whilst preserving the uninvolved lobe. This reduces the risk of complications and will likely obviate the need for post-operative thyroxine. Radioactive iodine could be used but is more expensive, involves a higher radiation dose, and is now almost exclusively used for cases of proven thyroid cancer.

15. I. TPO antibody levels

The finding of diffuse thyroid enlargement, hypothyroidism, and reactive lymph nodes raises the possibility of Hashimoto's thyroiditis (chronic lymphocytic thyroiditis). It is an autoimmune condition in which the thyroid gland is attacked by both antibody and cell mediated processes. It is more common in women than men. It is diagnosed by the finding of antibodies against thyroid peroxidize (TPO). Patients with Hashimoto's thyroiditis have an increased risk of developing thyroid lymphoma (normally B-cell Non-Hodgkin lymphoma).

Lee JC et al. The thyroid gland. In: Lennard TWJ (ed.). *Endocrine Surgery*, 5th edn. Philadelphia, PA: Elsevier Saunders, 2014, pp. 41–70.

16. C. Fine needle aspiration cytology (FNAC)

The history of weight loss, smoking, and a neck mass in a man of this age raises the possibility of metastatic malignancy. A primary site in the head and neck is likely (larynx pharynx, oropharynx, or thyroid given the position). However, a metastasis from a distant site such as lung or genitourinary tract should also be considered. Gastrointestinal malignancy rarely presents with neck metastases.

The appropriate investigation is FNAC (ideally under ultrasound guidance). Excision biopsy of an isolated metastatic neck node is not recommended as it carries the risk of locally spreading the disease and worsening prognosis. If FNAC is suggestive of lymphoma, formal histology is needed for accurate tissue typing. In this circumstance, a core biopsy or excision biopsy is appropriate.

CT scanning of the neck and chest should also be performed but this is of secondary importance to obtaining a tissue diagnosis.

17. F. Serum alkaline phosphatase

Post-operative hypocalcaemia after thyroid surgery may be secondary to hypoparathyroidism as a result of inadvertent removal or devascularization of the parathyroid glands. However, it may also be caused by hungry bone syndrome (HBS). This is characterized by the early post-operative development of prolonged hypocalcaemia associated with hypophosphataemia and hypomagnesaemia. It is exacerbated by suppressed parathyroid hormone levels in patients with high preoperative bone turnover and is frequently seen in patients who have had a parathyroidectomy for hyperparathyroidism. It can also occur in patients undergoing total thyroidectomy for thyrotoxicosis due to the rapid reversal of thyrotoxic osteodystrophy. The most appropriate and cost-efficient investigation is the alkaline phosphatase level. One recent study reported that an alkaline phosphates level of <340U/L is unlikely to result in HBS.

A vitamin D level is also useful but may be normal in some patients still at risk. However, any vitamin D deficiency should be corrected preoperatively. Vitamin D supplementation may also be required in conjunction with post-operative calcium replacement to ensure adequate intestinal absorption.

Cheong Loke S et al. Pre-operative serum alkaline phosphatase as a predictor for hypocalcemia post-parathyroid adenectomy. *International Journal of Medical Sciences* 2012; 9(7):611–16.

Surgical management of patients with endocrine disorders

18. B. Laparoscopic adrenalectomy

The most appropriate next line in this patient's management, excluding any other reason for her weight loss is laparoscopic adrenalectomy. The risk for malignant adrenal tumours increases with tumour size. For adrenal masses from 4 to 6 cm, the risk of malignancy is 6% and over 6 cm the risk increases to 25%. The scan also suggests that it is not entirely made up of fat (potential benign myelolipoma). In either scenario, excision is recommended. She has completed an endocrine assessment which has shown a non-functioning lesion and so the surgery in the form of a laparoscopic approach can go ahead safely. There is controversy around the appropriateness of laparoscopic adrenalectomy for patients with potential adrenocortical carcinomas. Laparoscopic adrenalectomy is the gold standard for benign masses as it results in significantly less pain, less morbidity, shorter recovery times and hospital stays compared to open adrenalectomy. Adjuvant therapies for adrenal cancers are limited and so a complete resection at initial surgery is essential.

Alexandraki KI, Grossman AB. Adrenal Incidentalomas: 'The rule of four' *Clinical Medicine* 2008; 8:201–4.

19. L. Alpha and beta blockade

Any patient undergoing adrenalectomy for phaeochromocytoma will require pre-operative medical therapy combining alpha and beta blockade to ensure that the patient is stable for surgery and to prevent an intra-operative hypertensive crisis. Alpha blockade is particularly important to prevent a crisis. High levels of catecholamines stimulate alpha receptors on blood vessels and cause vasoconstriction. Unopposed alpha-adrenergic receptor stimulation can precipitate a hypertensive crisis and so beta blockers are not administered until adequate alpha blockade has been established. Alpha-blockade is usually started 10–14 days preoperatively with beta blockers introduced thereafter.

Post-operative hypotension occurs because of changes in vascular compliance after excision of a phaeochromocytoma and also because of the residual effects of alpha and beta blockers. It takes three half-lives (36 hours) to dissipate the effects of phenoxybenzamine, and therefore following removal of the catecholamine drive, a drop in BP can occur.

20. G. Endocrine assessment

With advances in CT and MRI, incidental adrenal lesions are found with increasing frequency. So-called incidentalomas are present in approximately 3–4% of CT scans in the general population. Most are benign (>80%). However, all patients require a thorough endocrine assessment to evaluate the adrenal lesion fully.

Surgical excision is recommended for all adrenal incidentalomas >6cm. Current literature now suggests that the threshold for excision should be lowered to 4cm because adrenal cortical carcinomas are usually >4cm in size. However, any recommendations for surgery must take into account patient age, comorbidities, clinical judgement, and hormonal activity of the lesion. Laparoscopic adrenalectomy should be the gold standard for the surgical removal of adrenal masses following endocrine assessment.

Nieman L et al. Approach to the patient with an adrenal incidentaloma. *Journal of Clinical Endocrinology & Metabolism* 2010; 95(9):4106–13.

TRANSPLANT SURGERY

QUESTIONS

Single Best Answers

1. **You are performing a liver donation after brainstem death retrieval of the liver and kidneys. While performing the hilar dissection in preparation for liver retrieval, you notice an anatomical variant of the blood supply. Which of the following is the most commonly encountered?**
   a) Common hepatic artery is a branch of the superior mesenteric artery
   b) Common hepatic artery arises from the aorta
   c) Replaced or accessory right hepatic artery arises from the superior mesenteric artery
   d) Replaced or accessory left hepatic artery arises from the superior mesenteric artery
   e) Both right and left hepatic arteries arise from the superior mesenteric and left gastric arteries respectively

2. **A Spanish transplant team presents a research paper on the outcomes of renal transplantation from donors who have donated after planned withdrawal of treatment in an intensive care unit, leading to circulatory arrest. To which Maastricht category do these donors belong?**
   a) Maastricht I
   b) Maastricht II
   c) Maastricht III
   d) Maastricht IV
   e) Maastricht V

3. **Which of the following is not part of the brainstem death criteria used in the United Kingdom?**
   a) Two sets of tests performed on separate occasions by two separate doctors, only one of whom needs to be a consultant
   b) Absent gag reflex on posterior pharyngeal wall stimulation
   c) No respiratory effort in conjunction with a $PaCO_2$ of 5.9kPa
   d) Two complete sets of tests performed only one hour apart
   e) No motor response to supraorbital stimulation

4. **A patient is undergoing organ donation after brainstem death. What time of death should be recorded on the death certificate?**
    a) When the retrieval team commence the procedure to retrieve organs
    b) When the retrieval team complete the procedure
    c) The moment ventilation is ceased
    d) The completion of the first set of brainstem death tests
    e) The completion of the second set of brainstem death tests

5. **A 48 year old male with end-stage renal failure due to advanced type I diabetes is being assessed for simultaneous pancreas and kidney (SPK) transplant. He is currently on dialysis and has a number of complications related to his diabetes. Which of the following would you advise him is least likely to improve through successful SPK transplantation?**
    a) The requirement for insulin to control his diabetes
    b) Five-year survival
    c) Reversal of peripheral neuropathy
    d) Unawareness of hypoglycaemia
    e) The requirement for ongoing dietary restriction

6. **A 67 year old male presents to the surgical outpatient clinic with a symptomatic inguinal hernia. He has a functioning renal transplant and is maintained on sirolimus, ciclosporin, and prednisolone immunosuppression. What potential complication are you most concerned about?**
    a) Acute kidney injury
    b) Haematoma
    c) Mesh infection
    d) Nerve injury
    e) Seroma

7. **A 32 year old male presents 10 weeks post-transplant with acute transplant dysfunction. An ultrasound demonstrated good global perfusion and no evidence of hydronephrosis. A renal transplant biopsy is reported as showing T-cell mediated rejection with significant interstitial inflammation and moderate tubulitis. C4d stain is negative. There is no evidence of arteritis or capillaritis. How would this report be described in the Banff classification system?**
    a) Banff 1A
    b) Banff 1B
    c) Banff 2A
    d) Banff 2B
    e) Banff 3

8. **A 24 year old female is 3 months following a live donor renal transplant. She has recently completed a course of clarithromycin for a chest infection. She attends the transplant clinic complaining of a tremor. Her serum creatinine has risen from a baseline of 110μmol/L to 140μmol/ L. What is the most likely explanation for the deterioration in graft function?**
   a) Antibody-mediated rejection
   b) BK nephropathy
   c) Cell-mediated rejection
   d) Tacrolimus toxicity
   e) Urinary tract infection

9. **A 55 year old female presents 3 months following a live donor renal transplant complaining of abdominal cramps and profuse diarrhoea. Routine blood tests demonstrate a white cell count of 1.5 × 10⁹/L. The patient is receiving an immunosuppressive regimen of tacrolimus, mycophenolate mofetil, and prednisolone, in addition to prophylaxis with valganciclovir and co-trimoxazole. Which drug is most likely to have caused the patients symptoms?**
   a) Co-trimoxazole
   b) Mycophenolate mofetil
   c) Prednisolone
   d) Tacrolimus
   e) Valganciclovir

10. **A 45 year old male received his second renal transplant from a cadaveric donor. He had induction immunosuppression with anti-thymocyte globulin, then maintenance therapy of tacrolimus, mycophenolate mofetil, and steroids along with valganciclovir prophylaxis. Eight months following his transplant he presents with fever, malaise, and aching joints. Routine blood tests reveal a white cell count of 1.2 × 10⁹/L. What is the most likely diagnosis?**
   a) Aspergillosis
   b) BK-nephropathy
   c) Cryptococcosis
   d) Cytomegalovirus
   e) Epstein–Barr virus

11. **A 62 year old male presents 6 months following a cadaveric renal transplant with deterioration in graft function. A transplant ultrasound is unremarkable. The transplant kidney is biopsied which reveals cytopathic changes with evidence of tubulitis. Staining for SV40 is positive. What is the first-line treatment?**
    a) High-dose leflunomide
    b) High-dose oral steroids
    c) Intravenous methylprednisolone
    d) Oral ciprofloxacin
    e) Reduction in immunosuppression

12. **A 55 year old female presents 4 weeks following a cadaveric renal transplant with general malaise and frank haematuria. Her creatinine has risen from a baseline of 110–160µmol/L. What is the most likely diagnosis?**
    a) Acute rejection
    b) Arterial thrombosis
    c) Perinephric haematoma
    d) Urinary tract infection
    e) Venous thrombosis

13. **A 65 year old gentleman received a deceased donor renal transplant. A ureteric stent was inserted intra-operatively. Six days post-operatively there is a serous discharge from the wound. Biochemical analysis confirms the creatinine in the fluid to be >2000µmol/L (serum creatinine 200µmol/L). What is the best first-line management?**
    a) Percutaneous drainage of collection
    b) Percutaneous nephrostomy
    c) Remove ureteric stent
    d) Reinsert urinary catheter
    e) Urgent re-exploration of transplant kidney

14. **Which of the following is an absolute contraindication to renal transplantation?**
    a) Body mass index (BMI) >35kg/m²
    b) HIV infection with CD4 count <200/µL
    c) IgA nephropathy as primary renal disease
    d) Malignant melanoma Breslow thickness 2mm excised 5 years ago
    e) Previous renal transplant lost to non-compliance

15. **A 42 year old male with end-stage renal disease secondary to IgA nephropathy receives a pre-emptive live donor renal transplant from his sister. The transplant renal artery and vein are anastomosed onto the recipient external iliac artery and vein. What term correctly describes the transplanted kidney?**
    a) Heterotopic allograft
    b) Heterotopic autograft
    c) Orthotopic allograft
    d) Orthotopic autograft
    e) Orthotopic isograft

16. **A 45 year old male with adult polycystic kidney disease on haemodialysis is called in for a potential DCD kidney transplant. He is blood group AB and the donor is blood group A. He is currently well, has had no recent blood transfusions, and has up-to-date HLA antibody monitoring results in the Histocompatibility and Immunology laboratory for the last year. His calculated reaction frequency (CRF) is 0% and it is a 1,0,0 mismatched offer. In order to proceed with this transplant which of the following tests is required?**
    a) Complement dependent cytotoxicity (CDC) crossmatch assay
    b) Flow cytometry crossmatch assay
    c) A virtual crossmatch after discussion with a consultant clinical scientist
    d) No crossmatch assessment
    e) Anti B antibody titres

17. **A 30 year old female (blood group O) attends for transplant assessment. She has had two pregnancies and has a CRF of 77%. Several of her friends and family have come forward as potential live donors and have had initial bloods tests including blood group and crossmatch. Which of the following potential donors is most appropriate to take forward for further investigation?**
    a) Mother 67 years, blood group O, positive CDC HLA crossmatch
    b) Male friend 45 years, blood group A (subtype A2), negative HLA crossmatch
    c) Step-sister 37 years, blood group A (subtype A1), negative HLA crossmatch
    d) Husband 33 years, blood group O, positive CDC crossmatch
    e) Father 65 years, blood group O negative crossmatch, diagnosed 2 days ago with prostate cancer

18. **Which of the features listed is least likely to be a contraindication to live kidney donation?**
    a) Poorly controlled hypertension
    b) Diabetes mellitus
    c) High suspicion of donor coercion
    d) High suspicion of illegal financial exchange
    e) Age over 65

19. **Which of the following conditions is an absolute contraindication to liver transplantation?**
    a) Portal vein thrombosis
    b) Extra-hepatic malignancy
    c) Hepatitis C positivity
    d) Hepatitis B DNA positivity
    e) Hepatocellular carcinoma (size 4cm)

20. **A 55 year old obese female with IgA nephropathy who had been on dialysis for 7 years undergoes a renal transplant. On the third post-operative day she discharges 250mls of fluid from her transplant wound. The donor was a 42 year old female who died after brainstem death with a traumatic brain injury. The cold ischaemic time was seven hours. She had induction therapy with basaliximab and the mismatch was 100. Her current creatinine is 700umol/L. What is the most appropriate first investigation?**
    a) Renal transplant ultrasound
    b) CT abdomen and pelvis with IV contrast
    c) MRI
    d) Renal transplant biopsy
    e) Check the wound fluid for urea and electrolytes

Extended Matching Items

Simultaneous pancreas/kidney transplant

A. Renal artery thrombosis
B. Renal vein thrombosis
C. Pancreatic venous thrombosis
D. Pancreatic arterial thrombosis
E. Acute renal rejection
F. Acute rejection of the pancreas
G. Graft pancreatitis
H. Acute haemorrhage
I. Anastomotic leak from enterically drained pancreas
J. Hyperacute rejection of transplant

Choose from the following list the most likely post-operative complication in each scenario following simultaneous pancreas and kidney transplantation.

1. A patient who undergoes an emergency laparotomy eight hours after returning to the ward.

2. A 48 year old male develops severe pain over his renal transplant on the second post-operative day with cessation of urine output. On examination the kidney is tender and appears swollen. His amylase is 101U/L.

3. A 30 year old with new-onset abdominal pain on post-operative day 2. The amylase is 390U/L. The kidney transplant is working well and has a pulsatility index (PI) of 1.1 on ultrasound.

Complications of renal transplantation

A. Post-transplant lymphoproliferative disease (PTLD)
B. Acute cell-mediated rejection
C. Acute antibody-mediated rejection
D. Acute myocardial infarction
E. Post-transplant diabetes mellitus
F. Transplant renal artery stenosis
G. Squamous cell carcinoma of the skin
H. Pulmonary thrombo-embolism
I. Post-transplant hypertension
J. BK nephropathy
K. Urinary tract infection

Choose from the options which is the most likely complication in each scenario following kidney transplantation.

4. A 54 year old male transplant recipient who received ATG (anti-thymocyte globulin) induction presents with transplant dysfunction and transplant biopsy is positive for SV40 stain.

5. A 65 year old obese Asian male with a history of IgA nephropathy develops urinary frequency and blurred vision in the 2–3 weeks following a successful kidney transplant.

6. A 45 year old female 3 months post-renal transplant has persistently elevated blood pressure of 170/100mmHg despite titration of 3 anti-hypertensives. She is admitted as an emergency with breathlessness.

7. A 32 year old female who has received two previous transplants presents with acute transplant dysfunction 3–4 weeks post-transplant. A transplant biopsy demonstrates peritubular capillaritis with positive C4d staining. She is also noted to have serum donor-specific antibodies.

Liver transplant

A. Hepatic artery thrombosis
B. Primary non-function
C. Disease recurrence
D. Ischaemic cholangiopathy
E. Bile leak
F. Bile duct anastomotic stricture
G. Acute rejection
H. Transmitted donor infection

For each of the following scenarios select the most likely complication after liver transplantation. Each option may be used once, more than once or not at all.

8. A 23 year old female who took a paracetamol overdose receives an orthotopic liver transplant. In the following 24 hours her liver enzymes deteriorate, her coagulopathy deteriorates, and she develops acute kidney injury. She requires continuous dextrose to treat hypoglycaemia. Doppler USS demonstrates a patent hepatic artery.

9. A 45 year old female with primary biliary cirrhosis received a DCD (donation after cardiac death) liver transplant from a donor in whom the agonal phase prior to asystole was 30 minutes. Her graft functioned well in the initial post-transplant period but she returns to the clinic with deranged LFTs. Her bilirubin is 120μmol/L and ALP 600IU/L. Doppler ultrasound confirms a patent hepatic artery. An MCRP demonstrates diffuse intra-hepatic strictures.

10. A 40 year old man presents with jaundice, rigors, and pyrexia 5 months after a liver transplant which was complicated by a bile leak. His radiological assessment demonstrates a patent hepatic artery, intrahepatic and extrahepatic dilatation with no evidence of hepatic abscess.

Organ donation

A. Live genetically related donor
B. Live emotionally related donor
C. Donor after circulatory death
D. Donor after brainstem death
E. Directed altruistic donor
F. Non-directed altruistic donor

For each of the following potential organ donors select the most likely description from the list. Each option may be used once, more than once, or not at all.

11. A 42 year old male was involved in an RTA and sustained a catastrophic intracranial haemorrhage. Life-sustaining treatment is being withdrawn in ICU.

12. A 60 year old male has come forward as a potential donor for a local man who had posted on Facebook that he needed a kidney transplant.

13. A 55 year old female has contacted the transplant coordinators as she wishes to donate her kidney.

Organ preservation

A. University of Wisconsin solution
B. Histidine tryptophan ketoglutarate solution
C. Hypothermic pulsatile perfusion
D. Normothermic regional perfusion
E. *Ex vivo* normothermic machine perfusion
F. Static cold storage
G. Collins solution
H. Ross–Marshall citrate solution

For each of the following methods of organ or tissue preservation select the most likely answer from the list. Each option may be used once, more than once, or not at all.

14. A 44 year old man is declared brainstem dead and consent/authorization for organ donation is obtained. He sustained a head injury and the intent is to retrieve all abdominal organs for transplant. What cold preservation method is most appropriate?

15. A kidney retrieved from a 65 year old DCD donor is cold-perfused *in situ* and then placed on a machine with a centrifugal pump system for transport to the recipient centre. What method of preservation is described?

16. A 55 year old man has treatment withdrawn in ICU. After declaration of death and a five-minute standoff period he is transferred to theatre where a donor-after-circulatory-death retrieval is performed. What technique might be used in this scenario to optimize organ recovery after a period of warm ischaemia that precedes this type of retrieval?

Immunosuppressive drug therapy

A. Calcineurin inhibitor
B. Monoclonal antibody to CD-52
C. Anti-CD20 antibody
D. Interleukin-2 (IL-2) receptor blocker
E. Inhibitor of inosine monophosphate dehydrogenase (IMPDH)
F. Rabbit derived polyclonal antibodies to human T-cells
G. Chimeric human-murine anti-human tumour necrosis factor (TNF) monoclonal antibody
H. Purine analogue

For each of the following drugs, select the most appropriate description from the preceding list. Each option may be used once, more than once, or not at all.

17. Basiliximab

18. Alemtuzumab

19. Rituximab

20. Mycophenolate mofetil

Single Best Answers

1. c) Replaced or accessory right hepatic artery arises from the superior mesenteric artery

In a review of 1000 patients undergoing retrieval of the liver for transplantation, Hiatt and colleagues classified the most common anatomical anomalies into 6 subgroups:

- Type I Common hepatic artery arises from the coeliac axis to form the gastroduodenal and proper hepatic arteries, and the proper hepatic dividing distally into right and left branches (frequency 75.7%)
- Type II A replaced or accessory left hepatic artery arising from the left gastric artery (frequency 9.7%)
- Type III A replaced or accessory right hepatic artery arising from the superior mesenteric artery (frequency 10.6%)
- Type IV Both right and left hepatic arteries arising from the superior mesenteric artery and left gastric artery respectively (frequency 2.3%)
- Type V Entire common hepatic artery arising as a branch of the superior mesenteric artery (frequency 1.5%)
- Type VI Common hepatic artery originating directly from aorta (frequency 0.2%)[1]

The commonest abnormality is a replaced or accessory right hepatic artery which arises from the superior mesenteric artery. See Figure 9.1.

Hiatt JR et al. Surgical anatomy of the hepatic arteries in 1000 cases. *Annals of Surgery* 1994; 220(1):50–2.

Watson CJE and Harper SJF. Anatomical variation and its management in transplantation. *American Journal of Translational Research* 2015; 15:1459–71.

2. c) Maastricht III

The Maastricht categories on organ donation relate to the criteria used to classify the mode of organ donation. In this case, the research paper is based on donation after circulatory arrest (DCD), which is an example of controlled donation. It differs from donation after brain death (DBD). DCD donation is classified as per the Maastricht criteria, which differentiates between controlled and uncontrolled methods of donation after circulatory death. The Maastricht categories are summarized as follows:

[1] Adapted from Annals of Surgery, 220, Hiatt J, Gabbay J, and Busuttil R, Surgical Anatomy of the Hepatic Arteries in 1000 Cases, pp. 50–2. Copyright © 1994, © Lippincott-Raven Publishers.

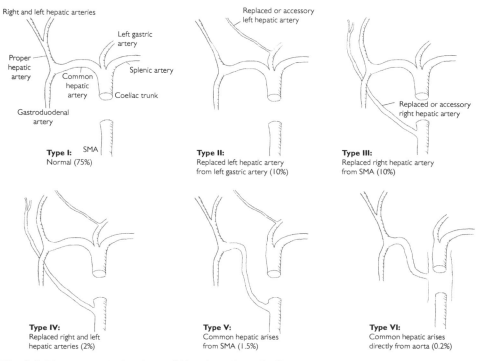

Fig. 9.1 Main anatomical variants of blood supply to the liver

Maastricht I—Brought in dead

Maastricht II—Unsuccessful resuscitation

Maastricht III—Awaiting cardiac arrest

Maastricht IV—Cardiac arrest after brainstem death

Maastricht V—Cardiac arrest in a hospital inpatient

[handwritten: already arrested.]

[handwritten: Planned withdraw].

[handwritten: dead in I Td.]

Koostra G et al. Categories of non-heart-beating donors. *Transplantation Proceedings* 1995; 27(5):2893–4.

3. c) No respiratory effort in conjunction with a PaCO₂ of 5.9kPa

Brainstem death is defined by the Department of Health as 'irreversible loss of capacity for consciousness, combined with irreversible loss of the capacity to breathe'. It is established as follows:

Preconditions

There must be an identifiable pathology causing brain damage in a deeply unconscious patient. Hypothermia, depressant drugs (narcotics, neuromuscular blockade, tranquilizers, and recreational variants thereof), and reversible circulatory, metabolic, and endocrine disturbances must have been excluded. The patient should be apnoeic and require mechanical ventilation under the following conditions.

The test conditions

The test should be carried out by two doctors with a minimum of five-years General Medical Council registration, one of whom is a consultant. Both should be experienced in the testing protocol and not part of the transplant team. Two sets of tests should be performed. There is no defined time interval between these tests, but it should be sufficient to inform the next of kin.

Testing protocol

- Pupils must be fixed in diameter and not responsive to light (CN II, III)
- There must be no corneal reflex (CN V, VII)
- Vestibulo-cochlear reflexes are absent—the caloric reflex is used, elicited by injecting 50ml of ice-cold water into each ear over a minute. Access to the tympanic membrane is confirmed by otoscopy (CN VIII, III)
- No motor response in the cranial distribution should occur as a result of stimulation of a somatic area. No limb movement to supraorbital stimulation (CN V, VII).
- No gag reflex in response to posterior pharyngeal wall stimulation (CN IX)
- No cough or other reflex in response to bronchial stimulation passing a catheter down the endotracheal tube (CN X)
- No respiratory movement should occur in response to disconnection of the ventilator. Hypoxia should be prevented by pre-oxygenation of the patient. This tests the response to hypercarbia, thus it is critical to confirm, using arterial blood gases, that the $PaCO_2$ is greater than 6.65kPa.

Academy of Medical Royal Colleges (2008). 'A Code of Practice for the Diagnosis and Confirmation of Death'. <http://www.aomrc.org.uk>.

4. d) The completion of the first set of brainstem death tests

A full discourse on the diagnosis and confirmation of death including brainstem death testing can be found on the British Transplant Society's website.

British Transplantation Society. <https://bts.org.uk/information-resources/publications/>.

5. c) Reversal of peripheral neuropathy

Successful SPK transplantation provides insulin independence and freedom from hypoglycemia. 5-year insulin independence is 75% for SPK. Adjusted 10-year survival for SPK is 67%, with a relative risk of death at 5 years of 0.4, compared to patients who remain on dialysis. Hypoglycemic unawareness is an indication for transplantation in itself and improves through successful transplantation. With successful transplantation the patient should be free of dietary restrictions.

Although reversal of diabetic neuropathy can occur through transplantation, this is not guaranteed. Nerve conduction studies often demonstrate early improvement, although clinically relevant recovery can take many months. Obesity, continued smoking, and advanced neuropathy are predictive of poor recovery.

Forsythe JLR (ed.). *Transplantation: A Companion to Specialist Surgical Practice*, 5th edn. Philadelphia, PA: Saunders Ltd, 2013.

Smets TYC et al. Effect of simultaneous pancreas–kidney transplantation on mortality of patients with Type 1 diabetes and end stage renal failure. *Lancet* 1999; 353:1915–20.

6. e) Seroma

Sirolimus is an mTOR (mammalian target of rapamycin) inhibitor. It prevents activation of T- and B-cells by inhibiting the production of interleukin-2. Like all immunosuppressive drugs, sirolimus increases the risk of infection (though deep-seated wound infections remain uncommon) and certain malignancies. Sirolimus is also diabetogenic, nephrotoxic, and promotes fluid retention and hypertension. However, the major complications associated with sirolimus are poor wound healing and seroma formation. Significant wound complications occur in 25–50% of patients on sirolimus undergoing surgery. For this reason, many advocate that sirolimus should not be used as initial maintenance immunosuppression following transplantation (instead switching to sirolimus after wound healing has occurred).

For elective surgery, it is advised that surgery is delayed and consideration given to switching to an alternative immunosuppressant agent for three months prior to and following surgery.

Other factors to consider when performing elective surgery in renal transplant recipients include ensuring adequate hydration (either via intravenous fluids or minimizing the fasting period), an increased cardiovascular risk in patients with end-stage renal disease (even post-transplantation), and the risk of adrenal insufficiency and need for additional steroid cover in patients on long-term steroid treatment.

Morath C et al. Sirolimus in renal transplantation. *Nephrology Dialysis Transplantation* 2007; 22 (Suppl. 8):viii61–5.

7. a) Banff 1A

Renal transplant biopsy is the gold standard in diagnosis of allograft rejection in renal transplant dysfunction. The Banff working classification of renal allograft pathology has standardized the interpretation and reporting of transplant biopsies internationally. Acute allograft rejection is divided into two categories: T-cell-mediated rejection (TCMR) and antibody-mediated rejection (ABMR), although the two can coexist. The classification of T-cell-mediated rejection is shown.

- Banff 1A Significant interstitial inflammation and moderate tubulitis
- Banff 1B Significant interstitial inflammation and severe tubulitis
- Banff 2A Mild or moderate intimal arteritis, with or without interstitial inflammation or tubulitis
- Banff 2B Severe intimal arteritis, with or without interstitial inflammation or tubulitis
- Banff 3 Transmural arteritis +/− fibrinoid necrosis[2]

In the case described there is no evidence of any vascular involvement, therefore categories 2 and 3 are incorrect. The tubulitis is moderate only and so the biopsy would be described as Banff classification 1A.

Solez K et al. Banff 07 classification of renal allograft pathology: updates and future directions. *American Journal of Translational Research* 2008; 8(4):753.

[2] Adapted from American Journal of Transplantation, 8, Solez K, Colvin RB, Racusen C, Haas B et al. *Banff 07 Classification of Renal Allograft Pathology: Updates and Future Directions*, pp. 753–60. Copyright (2008) The Authors Journal compilation © 2008 The American Society of Transplantation and the American Society of Transplant Surgeons.

8. d) Tacrolimus toxicity

The patient in this scenario is displaying signs and symptoms of tacrolimus toxicity (tremor and nephrotoxicity). Tacrolimus is a drug that requires regular drug monitoring to maintain levels within a tight therapeutic range. It is metabolized via the cytochrome P450 pathway.

The bioavailability of tacrolimus is underlined: increased by concomitant administration of drugs that inhibit the cytochrome P450 CYP3A pathway (e.g. clarithromycin, erythromycin, anti-fungals, calcium-channel blockers, anticonvulsants, and grapefruit juice). In this case clarithromycin has been given to treat a chest infection. A working knowledge of these drug interactions is necessary as they may lead to clinically important side effects or acute rejection.

Acute rejection and urinary tract infection must be considered in the differential diagnosis for this patient. However, the presence of tremor is suggestive for tacrolimus toxicity. Measurement of a serum tacrolimus trough level will assist in making the diagnosis.

van Gelder T. Drug interactions with tacrolimus. *Drug Safety* 2002; 25(10):707–12.

9. b) Mycophenolate mofetil

Mycophenolic acid (the active metabolite in mycophenolate mofetil (MMF)) is an anti-proliferative agent with action against both T- and B-cells. Gastrointestinal side effects of mycophenolate (particularly diarrhoea) are common and typically respond to dose reduction. Other side effects of MMF include arthralgia and bone marrow suppression (anaemia and leukopenia).

Gastrointestinal side effects may also occur with calcineurin inhibitors (e.g. tacrolimus), however tremor and nephrotoxicity are more common. The side effects of steroid treatment include weight gain, fluid retention, hypertension, and weight gain. Both steroids and tacrolimus are diabetogenic. Valganciclovir and co-trimoxazole are commonly given as prophylaxis against cytomegalovirus (CMV) and pneumocystis carinii pneumonia (PCP) respectively. Both may cause a leukopenia.

Transplant patients are also vulnerable to opportunistic infections causing diarrhoea. Persisting gastrointestinal symptoms should not simply be ascribed to the side effects of medication. Further investigation for potential infectious causes of diarrhoea should be carried out.

10. d) Cytomegalovirus

Cytomegalovirus (CMV) is a herpes virus that is highly prevalent within the general population with approximately two-thirds of adults in the United Kingdom exhibiting CMV IgG seropositivity. In most immunocompetent hosts, the initial viral infection is either asymptomatic or presents as a mild flu-like illness. With immunosuppression following solid organ transplantation, the virus can reactivate in a previous CMV IgG-positive host. It can also be acquired from a CMV IgG-positive donor or, rarely, be acquired as a *de novo* infection. CMV infection post-transplant confers a threefold increased risk of death by four years post-transplant in affected individuals.

Risk factors for CMV infection following transplantation include the use of lymphocyte-depleting drugs, older recipient age, and poor graft function. CMV IgG-negative recipients of organs from CMV IgG-positive donors are also at increased risk of a donor-derived infection.

High-risk recipients commonly receive valganciclovir prophylaxis for six months. The Improved Protection Against CMV in Transplant (IMPACT) trial demonstrated that a 200-day course of prophylactic valganciclovir reduced the incidence of CMV disease in high-risk (CMV D+/R−) recipients to 16.1% at 12 months post-transplant.

Sagedal S et al. Impact of early cytomegalovirus infection and disease in long-term recipient and kidney graft survival. *Kidney International* 2004; 66(1):329–37.

Humar A et al. Extended valganciclovir prophylaxis in D+/R− kidney transplant recipients is associated with long-term reduction in cytomegalovirus disease: two-year results of the IMPACT study. *Transplantation* 2010; 90(12):427–31.

11. e) Reduction in immunosuppression

Merkel cell cancer?)

The case describes BK nephropathy. The BK virus is a polyomavirus with a seroprevalence of 60–80% in the general population. BK reactivation following transplantation is common but it rarely causes clinically significant disease. Presentation tends to occur within the first year of transplantation (though may occur at any time) with deterioration in renal function secondary to BK nephropathy or with ureteric strictures.

The diagnosis is made with positive PCR (polymerase chain reaction) for BKV DNA and a transplant biopsy showing viral cytopathic changes and non-specific inflammation. Immunohistochemistry is positive for SV40. BK viraemia occurs as a result of over-immunosuppression. Therefore, the mainstay of treatment is minimization of immunosuppression. If this fails, treatment with leflunomide may be considered.

The differential diagnosis in this case is acute rejection or urinary tract infection. Urinary tract infection is the commonest cause for deterioration in graft function in the early months following transplantation. It can normally be treated simply with oral antibiotics. A diagnosis of acute rejection (either antibody or cell-mediated) is made on transplant biopsy. The diagnostic features of acute rejection on biopsy are inflammation (tubulitis and arteritis) and C4d positive staining suggests the possibility of antibody-mediated rejection. *Banff category*

Memon IA and Brennan DC. Cytomegalovirus, Epstein–Barr virus and BK virus infection following solid organ transplantation. In: Forsythe JLR (ed.). *Transplantation: A Companion to Specialist Surgical Practice*, 4th edn. Philadelphia, PA: Elsevier, 2009, pp. 235–67.

12. d) Urinary tract infection

Urinary tract infection is the most common infection following renal transplantation, occurring in >75% of transplant recipients. It commonly presents with mild transplant dysfunction in the absence of other symptoms. Frank haematuria is not uncommon, particularly in patients who still have a stent in their transplant ureter.

Acute rejection presents with deterioration in transplant function. However, aside from hyperacute rejection, which is rare and presents in the early post-operative period, haematuria is uncommon.

Arterial thrombosis normally presents in the early post-operative period (<24–48hrs post-transplantation) with a sudden decline in urine output +/− pain over the transplant kidney. Urgent transplant ultrasound will make the diagnosis with absent arterial flow in the transplant kidney. Immediate exploration is required to prevent graft loss.

Venous thrombosis typically presents three to seven days post-transplantation with a decline in urine output, pain over the transplant kidney, or occasionally frank haematuria. Again, transplant ultrasound makes the diagnosis (with high-resistance arterial waveforms within the renal parenchyma due to occlusion of the outflow from the kidney) and urgent re-exploration is required.

13. d) Reinsert urinary catheter

Perinephric collections and wound complications are not uncommon following renal transplantation. Normally such collections reflect perinephric haematoma or seromas. In this case, however, the high level of creatinine within the fluid compared to the patient's serum, is consistent with urine leak. This is an uncommon complication following renal transplantation, affecting 2–3% of patients.

The most common cause for ureteric complications is technical error, followed by ischaemia of the distal ureter.

First-line management of urine leak is to decompress the bladder with a urinary catheter. If this fails to control the problem, re-exploration and re-implantation of the transplant ureter may be required. If the urine leak is delayed, percutaneous nephrostomy followed by antegrade ureteric stenting may be possible and allow control prior to considering delayed re-implantation.

14. b) HIV infection with CD4 count <200/μL

Renal transplantation is indicated for all patients with stage 5 CKD (eGFR <15ml/min/1.73m^2) or who are anticipated to require renal replacement therapy within 6 months for whom transplantation is anticipated will confer a survival benefit.

There are few absolute contraindications to renal transplantation. These include:

- Uncontrolled cancer
- Active systemic infection
- Any condition with a life expectancy less than two years

Relative contraindications include:

- Predicted survival less than five years:
  - ◆ Malignant disease not amenable to curative treatment
  - ◆ HIV infection not treated with highly active antiretroviral therapy (HAART) or already progressed to AIDS
  - ◆ Cardiovascular disease—ischaemic heart disease, the prognosis of which cannot be improved with revascularization and/or cardiac failure with predicted risk of death >50% at 5 years
- Predicted graft loss >50% at 1 year
- Patients unable or unlikely to adhere to immunosuppressive requirements
- Immunosuppression likely to cause life-threatening complication

In the case of HIV, uncontrolled infection with T-cell levels <200cells/μL or detectable HIV RNA, multi-drug resistance, and non-concordance with treatment are absolute contraindications.

BMI is not an absolute contraindication to transplantation, although some guidelines advocate avoiding transplantation in patients with a BMI >35kg/m^2. A past history of any malignancy is not a contraindication to transplantation, though patients must be appropriately counselled. Certain underlying renal diseases (including IgA nephropathy) are at risk of recurrence within the transplanted kidney. However, so long as this risk does not exceed 50%, it should not be considered a contraindication to transplantation.

UK Renal Association Clinical Practice Guidelines. Assessment for Transplantation, 5th edn. 2010.

NHS Blood and Transplant (Kidney Advisory Group) Patient Selection for Deceased Donor Kidney Only Transplantation. February 2016. <http://www.odt.nhs.uk/pdf/kidney_selection_policy.pdf>.

British Transplantation Society. UK Guidelines for Kidney and Pancreas Transplantation in Patients with HIV. March 2015. <http://www.bts.org.uk/Documents/Guidelines/Active/Kidney%20Txp%20in%20HIV%20Guidelines%20-%20Mar%202015%20FINAL.pdf>.

15. a) Heterotopic allograft

Orthotopic refers to transplantation of an organ into its normal anatomical position (e.g. liver or heart) whilst heterotopic refers to an organ transplanted into an abnormal anatomical position (e.g. kidney or pancreas).

An autograft is a tissue or organ taken from one part of a person's body and transplanted into another part (e.g. skin graft). An allograft (or homograft) is tissue or an organ taken from one person and transplanted into another whilst a xenograft comes from another species. An isograft is a transplant from a genetically identical donor (i.e. identical twin). Theoretically, such a transplant would not require immunosuppression.

16. c) A virtual crossmatch after discussion with a consultant clinical scientist

The three commonly used methods for assessing HLA-specific antibody levels are the complement dependent cytotoxic crossmatch (CDC), the flow cytometry crossmatch (FC), and HLA antibody microbead analysis. For a conventional antibody-compatible transplant, donor/recipient compatibility is characterized by negative CDC and FC and low or undetectable donor-specific antibodies (DSA) by microbead analysis.

A virtual crossmatch is an assessment undertaken by a Histocompatibility and Immunology professional that allows determination of the presence of donor HLA specific antibodies in a patient. This is done by comparing the potential recipient's HLA antibody profile to the HLA profile of the proposed donor without carrying out a CDC or flow crossmatch prior to the transplant procedure.

A virtual crossmatch is appropriate in this example as this patient has up-to-date HLA antibody monitoring and no recent sensitizing events such as a blood transfusion. In females it is important to exclude recent pregnancies or miscarriages as potential sensitizing events. Other sensitizing events include previous transplantation.

An individual with blood group AB has no anti-A or anti-B antibodies and this is a blood group-compatible transplant. There is no necessity for any blood group antibody titres.

Taylor CJ et al. Ten-year experience of selective omission of the pretransplant crossmatch test in deceased donor kidney transplantation. *Transplantation* 2010; 89:185–93.

17. b) Male friend 45 years, blood group A (subtype A2), negative HLA crossmatch

Due to this patient's pregnancies, she has become sensitized as demonstrated by her calculated reaction frequency of 77%. This is calculated by NHS Blood and Transplant as the percentage incidence, among a pool of 10,000 ABO compatible organ donors, of HLA antigen-incompatible donors with patient defined HLA-specific antibody(s). In this instance this potential recipient would be incompatible due to HLA antibody to 77% of donors in the United Kingdom. This is reflected in that there is a positive CDC crossmatch with three potential live donors. The remaining two donors are HLA compatible but are ABO-incompatible. The relevance of the A1/2 subtype relates to risk level in any subsequent ABOi incompatible transplant. Grafts from blood group A2 donors appear to be at lower risk than those from A1 donors, as the antigen is expressed at lower levels on tissue. Nevertheless, rejection and graft loss can still occur. The maximum period of risk is during the initial two-week post-operative period and those transplants that last greater than two weeks without ABMR have a similar survival to standard transplants.

The outcomes of ABO-incompatible transplantation from large European, Japanese, and American studies demonstrate a slightly higher risk of early graft loss due to acute antibody-mediated rejection.

None of these potential recipients are a straightforward HLA- or ABO-compatible transplant and in this instance one or all could complete their live donor assessment and be entered into the national Living Kidney Donor Sharing scheme. If this is not feasible, donor B is the most appropriate to take forward. It is generally recommended that incompatible pairs go through two matching runs of the sharing scheme prior to proceeding with an incompatible transplant due to the additional risks of augmented immunosuppression/antibody depletion.

Antibody-incompatible transplantation guidelines of the British Transplant Society. <http://www.bts.org.uk/BTS/Guidelines_Standards/Current/BTS/Guidelines_Standards/Current_Guidelines.aspx?hkey=e285ca32-5920-4613-ac08-fa9fd90915b5>.

18. e) Age over 65 years

Potential live kidney donors undergo an initial medical screening questionnaire followed by initial blood group and renal function assessment. Thereafter they undergo full medical history and clinical examination, combined with formal assessment of the GFR (glomerular filtration rate), cardiovascular system, and relevant anatomy.

Well-controlled hypertension is not a contraindication to donation (even if taking one or two medications). That said, hypertension is the commonest finding in assessment that requires further investigation. There are two concerns. First, that hypertension presents a risk for perioperative morbidity and mortality. Second, that pre-existing hypertension in the donor will deteriorate post-nephrectomy.

All donors have a fasting blood glucose checked and proceed to oral glucose tolerance test (OGTT) if indicated. Traditional guidance has suggested that individuals with diabetes should not donate. Those with impaired glucose tolerance need careful lifetime risk assessment.

Donor coercion is an absolute contraindication to donation.

Older age is not an absolute contraindication to donation but the medical work-up of older donors must be particularly rigorous to ensure suitability.

19. b) Extrahepatic malignancy

Liver transplant is a lifesaving procedure in a variety of acute and chronic indications. These include patients with hepatitis B and C, either as a single cause or co-factor. The presence of portal vein thrombosis is a relative rather than an absolute contraindication. The presence of a single hepatocellular carcinoma of <5cm, or <3 lesions of 3cm, is not a contraindication. However, potential recipients are listed in conjunction with other adjuvant treatments such as TACE/ablation. They also undergo an assessment of extrahepatic disease radiologically and/or laparoscopically. Evidence of extrahepatic malignancy is an absolute contraindication to transplantation.

Forsythe JLR (ed.). *Transplantation: A Companion to Specialist Surgical Practice*, 5th edn. Philadelphia, PA: Elsevier, 2013.

20. e) Check the wound fluid for urea and electrolytes

In this scenario, the patient's serum creatinine remains elevated post-transplant. Potential diagnoses include delayed graft function, urine leak, or early rejection. This was an immunologically low-risk transplant and primary function is likely with a young donor and short cold ischaemic time.

Renal transplant biopsy may be required but is generally not performed before day 5 post-operatively. Whilst a renal transplant ultrasound is indicated, the most important diagnosis to make is that of a urine leak. The most appropriate investigation is to check the urea and electrolytes in the wound fluid. CT with IV contrast and MRI are inappropriate investigations at this stage.

Extended Matching Items

Simultaneous pancreas/kidney transplant

1. H. Acute haemorrhage

Bleeding is the commonest reason for re-exploration in SPK transplantation. Leakage of pancreatic exocrine secretions over the body of the pancreas that come into contact with thrombus-sealed small vessels or anastomoses and can cause breakdown and haemorrhage. Despite frequent re-operation for this complication (25%), only 1% of pancreas transplants are lost to bleeding.

2. B. Renal vein thrombosis

Renal vein thrombosis is uncommon (approximately 1–3% of transplants). In contrast to renal artery thrombosis, obstruction of the venous outflow causes significant swelling of the kidney. If left untreated catastrophic haemorrhage can occur. Transplant nephrectomy is almost inevitable. The diagnosis can be confirmed by ultrasound. Reversed diastolic arterial flow and an absence of flow in the renal vein can be seen. It is unlikely to be rejection in this case as the amylase is normal. Discordant rejection can occur but only accounts for 5–10% of rejection episodes.

3. G. Graft pancreatitis

Pancreas thrombosis is the commonest cause of early graft loss, usually secondary to venous thrombosis. Predisposing factors include donor age and BMI as well as prolonged cold ischaemic time. Once diagnosed it requires prompt laparotomy and removal of the pancreas.

In this question, with a normal PI in a well-functioning renal transplant, graft pancreatitis is more likely than rejection. Monitoring of the pancreas for rejection is difficult but amylase is routinely used as a non-specific marker. Long-term surveillance relies almost completely on following the course of the renal transplant through serial creatinine measurements and/or biopsy. The exocrine pancreas is normally first affected by rejection; thus amylase elevation can occur before deterioration of glucose control in rejection.

Forsythe JLR (ed.). *Transplantation: A Companion to Specialist Surgical Practice*, 5th edn. Philadelphia, PA: Elsevier, 2013.

Complications of renal transplantation

4. J. BK nephropathy

Renal transplantation is now established as the optimum treatment for patients with end-stage renal failure. The benefits of renal transplantation are of improved survival, correction of the metabolic consequences of chronic kidney disease and their associated dietary restrictions, freedom from uraemic symptoms, correction of anaemia, and vitamin D and calcium metabolism. Furthermore, there is a significant improvement in patient's quality of life, exercise capacity, ability to work, and be fertile. Transplantation is also substantially cheaper than maintenance haemodialysis. Studies both in Europe and the United States have demonstrated a significant reduction in mortality with transplantation versus wait-listed dialysis patients. Renal transplantation can be complicated by universal risks of surgery such as bleeding (life-threatening haemorrhage is rare) or wound complications (7%). Specific vascular complications such as graft thrombosis can be secondary to either renal vein thrombosis or renal artery thrombosis. Renal vein thrombosis (3%) is slightly more common than arterial thrombosis (1%) but together they are the commonest cause of early graft loss. Rarely can a graft be salvaged and usually by the time the diagnosis is made the graft has sustained irreversible damage leading to graft nephrectomy.

Ureteric complications include urine leak or ureteric obstruction. Most obstructions (80%) are due to the presence of distal ureteric ischaemia with subsequent stricturing.

Other complications include delayed graft function (30–40% of deceased donor transplants, 50–70% if DCD), post-operative lymphocele (1–20%), acute rejection (10–25%), and urinary tract infections.

BK nephropathy is caused by a polyomavirus which is endemic in the human population. BK virus nephropathy occurs in 2.1% of UK patients. The greatest risk factor for BK nephropathy is the intensity of immunosuppression. It is not attributable to any particular drug or drug level; rather, the overall burden of immunosuppression (i.e. T-cell-depleting induction with full-dose tacrolimus, MMF, and steroids)

Wolfe RA et al. Comparison of mortality in all patients on dialysis, patients on dialysis awaiting transplantation and recipients of a first cadaveric transplant. *New England Journal of Medicine* 1999; 341:1725–30.

Torpey N et al. (eds). *Renal Transplantation*. Oxford: Oxford University Press, 2010.

5. E. Post-transplant diabetes mellitus

Post-transplant diabetes mellitus (PTDM) is a common and serious complication after kidney transplantation. It has a multifactorial aetiology. Risk factors include the specific immunosuppressive regimen, ethnicity, elderly patients, and a high body mass index. Among these, calcineurin inhibitors (ciclosporin, pimecrolimus, and tacrolimus) and steroid use seems to be particularly relevant. Both patient and graft survival is significantly reduced in recipients affected by PTDM.

Salvadori M et al. Post-transplant diabetes mellitus. *Journal of Nephrology* 2003; 16(5):626–34.

6. F. Transplant renal artery stenosis

Transplant renal arterial stenosis (TRAS) is a well-recognized vascular complication after kidney transplant. It occurs most frequently in the first six months after kidney transplant and is one of the major causes of graft loss and premature death in transplant recipients. There is a wide range in the reported incidence (1–25%), perhaps in part due to differences in diagnostic modalities. However, it appears to occur more frequently than renal artery thrombosis (6%). It can occur at the anastomotic site but more commonly in the donor artery. The clinical features are of unexplained renal dysfunction, severe hypertension, and, rarely, flash pulmonary oedema. The latter condition can develop in patients with critical bilateral renal artery stenosis or renal artery stenosis in a solitary or transplant kidney (Pickering syndrome). Most can be managed with an interventional radiology approach with angioplasty +/– stent.

Chen W et al. Transplant renal artery stenosis: clinical manifestations, diagnosis and therapy. *Clinical Kidney Journal* 2015; 8(1):71–8.

7. C. Acute antibody-mediated rejection

Antibody-mediated rejection (AMR) is an important cause of acute and chronic allograft dysfunction and graft loss. AMR can occur as three separate entities:

- Hyperacute AMR is mediated by preformed donor-specific antibodies (DSA) and presents as very early graft failure (can occur within minutes of transplant but sometimes may be delayed for a few days). This type of rejection is extremely rare because of the universal adoption of pre-transplantation crossmatching.

- Acute AMR presents with graft dysfunction over a few days following transplantation. It is mediated by DSAs that may either be preformed or develop *de novo* after transplantation. It occurs in about 5–7% of all kidney transplants and is responsible for 20–48% of acute rejection episodes among pre-sensitized positive crossmatch patients. The cardinal histopathologic features are of an antibody-mediated endothelial injury. There may be evidence of endothelial cell swelling, neutrophilic infiltration of glomeruli and peritubular capillaries, interstitial oedema, and haemorrhage. Routine C4d-staining in biopsies has led to better and more accurate diagnosis of AMR.
- Chronic AMR is an important cause of chronic allograft injury which typically manifests as transplant glomerulopathy. Patients may be asymptomatic in the early stages although the condition may progress to nephrotic range proteinuria, hypertension, and allograft dysfunction. Rapid progression can sometimes occur, especially against a background of ongoing acute AMR, resulting in graft failure within months. Transplant glomerulopathy is seen in protocol biopsies with an incidence of 5% at 1 year and 20% at 5 years.

Puttarajappa C et al. Antibody-mediated rejection in kidney transplantation: a review. *Journal of Transplantation* 2012: 193724.

8. B. Primary non-function

The causes of liver transplant dysfunction can be broadly classified into the following categories:

- Preservation/ischaemic reperfusion injury manifesting as primary non-function (PNF)
- Rejection
- Technical: hepatic artery thrombosis/portal vein thrombosis/venous outflow obstruction/bile leak or stricture
- Infection: bacterial/viral/fungal
- Disease recurrence: viral hepatitis/alcohol recidivism/autoimmune disease/PSC/PBC

The timing and severity of graft dysfunction influences investigations and diagnosis. In this scenario the transplant liver is not working but is being perfused, which describes the situation of primary non-function. This is an indication for urgent re-transplantation.

Callaghan CJ et al. Outcomes of transplantation of livers from donation after circulatory death donors in the UK: a cohort study. *British Medical Journal* Open 2013; 3:e003287.

9. D. Ischaemic cholangiopathy

There has been a significant expansion in donor-after-circulatory-death (DCD) liver transplantation as a consequence of increased demand. DCD transplants now account for 17% of all UK adult liver transplants. However, both graft and patient survival are poorer with DCD transplantation. The incidence of biliary complications after DCD transplantation ranges between 25–60% compared to 10–30% observed in donor-after-brain-death (DBD) orthotopic liver transplants. The most common biliary complication requiring re-transplantation is ischaemic cholangiopathy. It is diagnosed when there is evidence of intrahepatic or extrahepatic biliary strictures (not related to the anastomosis) in the presence of a patent hepatic artery. It frequently results in significant morbidity including biliary sepsis and/or multiple endoscopic or percutaneous biliary procedures.

10. F. Bile duct anastomotic stricture

Bile leaks occur in 5–10% of cases and, if anastomotic, are technical or ischaemic in nature. Non-anastomotic bile leaks are usually due to aberrant ducts or from the cut surface of split or reduced grafts. Biliary strictures occur in 5–15% of liver transplants and are more likely in the context of a previous bile leak. Management consists of drainage of the biliary tree, management of sepsis, and imaging. If not associated with hepatic artery thrombosis and extrahepatic in nature, reconstructive surgery with a Roux-en-Y hepaticojejunostomy can be considered.

Callaghan CJ et al. Outcomes of transplantation of livers from donation after circulatory death donors in the UK: a cohort study. *British Medical Journal* Open 2013; 3:e003287.

Organic donation

11. C. Donor after circulatory death

Deceased donors are categorized as either donors after brainstem death (DBD) or after circulatory death (DCD). In the context of donor after brainstem death (DBD), the donor is transferred to theatre whist still ventilated and on any additional support to maintain stability. The retrieval of organs occurs whilst the donor still has circulating blood and hence there is no additional warm ischaemia prior to organ perfusion as observed in DCD donation.

The current scenario describes the process whereby life-sustaining treatment is withdrawn in the context of donation after circulatory death (usually withdrawal of ventilatory and/or inotropic support) and the patient dies. After a period of five minutes after asystole the patient is rapidly transferred to theatre for laparotomy and organ retrieval.

12. E. Directed altruistic donor

Directed altruistic donation is where an organ is donated by a healthy person and contact between the donor and recipient has been made because the recipient requires a transplant. The HTA classifies them within two categories discussed as follows:

1. Genetic relationship but no emotional relationship
2. No pre-existing relationship prior to identification of the recipient's need for transplant (i.e. via social media)

13. F. Non-directed altruistic donor

Living donation of kidneys has changed dramatically in the last 10–15 years. The Human Tissue Authority (HTA) was established as the regulatory body under the 2004 Act. The HTA regulates the removal, storage, use, and disposal of human bodies, organs, and tissue from the deceased and the storage of human organs and tissue from the living. The HTA is responsible for assessing all applications for organ donation from living people. This involves an independent assessment process. All donors and recipients see an independent assessor (IA) who is trained and accredited by the HTA and acts on their behalf to ensure that the donor has given valid consent and that reward is not a motivating factor in the donation.

In September 2012 the HTA published a revised legal framework which specifies the types of relationships that are permitted between the living donor and recipient under the Human Tissue Acts.

Directed donation:

i) Genetically related donation: where the donor is a blood relative of the recipient
ii) Emotionally related donation: where the potential donor has a relationship with the potential recipient (e.g. spouse, partner, or friend)

iii) Paired donation: where a relative, friend, or partner is fit and able to donate but is incompatible with the potential recipient and they are matched with another donor and recipient in a similar situation

iv) Pooled donation: a form of paired donation where more than two donor/recipient pairs are involved (e.g. a three-way swap or a long chain donation)[3]

Non-directed altruistic donation is where an organ or part of an organ is donated by a healthy person who does not have a relationship with the recipient and who is not informed who the recipient will be.

Living Donor Kidney Transplantation British Transplant Society Guidelines. <http://www.bts. org.uk/BTS/Guidelines_Standards/Current/BTS/Guidelines_Standards/Current_Guidelines. aspx?hkey=e285ca32-5920-4613-ac08-fa9fd90915b5>.

Organ preservation

14. A. University of Wisconsin solution

At organ retrieval, potential organs for transplantation are perfused with cold, acellular, balanced electrolyte solutions to prevent intravascular thrombosis and to rapidly cool the organ and slow metabolism. University of Wisconsin solution (UW) is a more effective preservation solution for kidneys stored >24hrs compared to HTK. HTK is not used for perfusion of the pancreas.

Finger EB. Organ preservation. Medscape online article. <http://emedicine.medscape.com/article/ 431140-overview>.

15. C. Hypothermic pulsatile perfusion

Most kidneys retrieved are stored in preservation fluid and on ice (static cold storage). A proportion of kidneys (more frequently DCD or extended criteria kidneys) are stored in hypothermic pulsatile perfusion using several commercially available perfusion systems. A large randomized controlled trial suggested a reduction in delayed graft function with their use. This was not observed in a UK trial, although methodological differences may account for this.

Moers C et al. Machine perfusion or cold storage in deceased donor kidney transplantation. *New England Journal of Medicine* 2009; 360(1):7–16.

Watson CJ et al. Cold machine perfusion versus static cold storage of kidneys donated after cardiac death: a UK multicentre randomized controlled trial. *American Journal of Translational Research* 2010; 10(9):1191–9.

16. D. Normothermic regional perfusion

Normothermic regional perfusion (NRP) is performed *in situ* at the retrieval procedure for donors after circulatory death for a two-hour period. The regional perfusion is performed upon cannulation of the aorta and IVC, which allows perfusion of abdominal organs using an extracorporeal membrane oxygenator circuit at 37°C. The aim is to restore ATP levels and facilitate *in situ* recovery after the period of warm ischaemia in the agonal phase and after death.

Oniscu GC et al. *In situ* normothermic regional perfusion for controlled donation after circulatory death: the UK experience. *American Journal of Translational Research* 2014; 14(12):2846–54.

---

[3] Source data from Guidance to Transplant Teams and Independent Assessors, March 2015.

Immunosuppressive drug therapy

17. D. Interleukin-2 (IL-2) receptor blocker

Basiliximab is a chimeric monoclonal antibody to the interleukin-2 (IL-2) receptor on T-lymphocytes. It inhibits T-cell activation and prevents the body from mounting an immune response against the transplanted organ. It is used as an induction agent, given prior to the transplant, to reduce the risk of early acute rejection, whereas calcineurin inhibitors such as tacrolimus form the mainstay of most maintenance immunosuppressive regimens. See Figure 9.2.

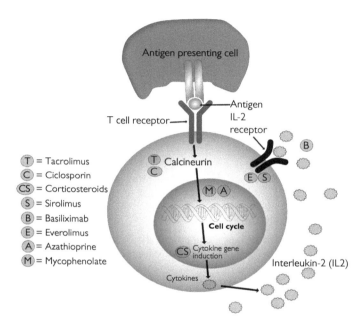

Fig. 9.2 Mode of action of immunosuppressive drugs used in renal transplantation

Halloran PF. Immunosuppressive drugs from kidney transplantation. *New England Journal of Medicine* 2004; 351:2715–29.

18. B. Monoclonal antibody to CD-52

Alemtuzumab is a monoclonal antibody to CD52, an antigen present on the surface of both B and T cells as well as monocytes, macrophages, and natural killer (NK) cells. It is used as an induction agent, given prior to the transplant to reduce the risk of early acute rejection.

19. C. Anti-CD20 antibody

Rituximab is a monoclonal antibody to CD20 on the surface of B-cells. Along with asiliximab, alemtuxumab, and ATG, rituximab is used as an induction agent, given prior to the transplant to reduce the risk of early acute rejection.

20. E. Inhibitor of inosine monophosphate dehydrogenase (IMPDH)

Mycophenolate mofetil (MMF) is a prodrug of mycophenolic acid (MPA), an inhibitor of inosine monophosphate dehydrogenase (IMPDH). This is the rate-limiting enzyme in *de novo* synthesis of guanosine nucleotides. T- and B-lymphocytes are more dependent on this pathway than other cell types. MMF suppresses T-lymphocytic responses to allogeneic cells and other antigens. The drug also suppresses primary, but not secondary, antibody responses.

VASCULAR SURGERY

QUESTIONS

Single Best Answers

1. **Concerning dialysis-associated steal syndrome, which of the following statements is correct:**
    a) The majority of cases are related to a high-flow situation alone in the fistula
    b) Symptoms commonly occur in the immediate post-operative period with pain and paraesthesia being foremost
    c) Ligation of the radial artery distal to the anastomosis in a radio-cephalic fistula may resolve steal symptoms in a high-flow situation with patent ipsilateral ulnar artery and palmar arch
    d) The presence of retrograde flow in the artery distal to the anastomosis is a good predictor of steal syndrome
    e) The presence of steal requires intervention

2. **A 74 year old male smoker with diabetes presents with a sudden deterioration in his calf claudication distance to 50m. His claudication distance over the last 18 months had been 400m. He has only a femoral pulse palpable. The most likely diagnosis is:**
    a) Atherosclerotic arterial disease with thrombosis *in situ*
    b) Popliteal artery entrapment
    c) Cystic adventitial disease
    d) Persistent sciatic artery
    e) Acute arterial embolism

3. **A 69 year old female patient with diabetes presents with a 10-month history of pain in her left calf which stops her walking at 100m. The pain is quickly relieved at rest. Her ankle-brachial pressure index (ABPI) at rest is 0.88 on the left and 0.96 on the right, with monophasic pedal signals bilaterally. The most likely diagnosis is:**
    a) Cystic adventitial disease
    b) Atherosclerotic arterial disease
    c) Deep venous thrombosis
    d) Musculoskeletal back pain
    e) Peripheral neuropathy

4. **A 28 year old male who injects heroin presents with a 4-day history of increasing pain in the left groin and pyrexia. On examination he has a swollen, tender left thigh with raised inflammatory markers (CRP 240 and WCC 18). The most appropriate initial management is:**
    a) Admit for limb elevation and intravenous antibiotics
    b) Admit for exclusion of a deep venous thrombosis
    c) Admit for limb elevation and low molecular weight heparin
    d) Admit for intravenous antibiotics and a contrast-enhanced CT scan
    e) Admit for thigh compartment pressures

5. **A 65 year old male patient presents to the clinic with a screen-detected abdominal aortic aneurysm (AAA) measuring 6.4cm in AP (anteroposterior) diameter. He has a fullness in his right popliteal fossa with a strong, bounding popliteal pulse. Which statement concerning popliteal artery aneurysms is correct?**
    a) Popliteal artery aneurysms are treated to prevent rupture in the majority of patients
    b) 40% of patients with a popliteal artery aneurysm will have an AAA
    c) 15% of patients with a popliteal artery aneurysm will have an AAA
    d) 70% of patients with popliteal artery aneurysm will have bilateral aneurysms
    e) Popliteal artery aneurysms should be preferentially treated by an endovascular approach

6. **A 70 year old male with a known abdominal aortic aneurysm attends the outpatient clinic. The patient has been referred from the surveillance programme with an increase in the AP diameter of his aneurysm from 4.5cm to 5.4cm (9mm) over 6 months. He remains asymptomatic. The most appropriate management plan is:**
    a) Repeat aortic duplex in six months
    b) CT angiogram to re-assess AP diameter
    c) CT angiogram + physiological testing with a view to urgent intervention
    d) Repeat duplex in three months
    e) MR angiogram to assess aortic characteristics

7. **While inserting a peritoneal dialysis catheter using a laparoscopic technique, you notice a small enterotomy in the distal ileum with spillage of enteric contents. What is the appropriate management?**
    a) Laparotomy, repair of the enterotomy, lavage, and insertion of the PD (peritoneal dialysis) catheter
    b) Laparoscopic repair of the enterotomy, lavage, and insertion of the PD catheter
    c) Abandon PD catheter insertion, repair the enterotomy, and lavage the abdomen
    d) Exteriorize the ileum, lavage, and insertion of the PD catheter
    e) Laparoscopic repair of the enterotomy, insertion of the PD catheter, and drain

8. **A patient with a brachio-basilic transposition fistula is admitted from the dialysis unit with no thrill noted in the fistula. Clinical and duplex examination confirms an occluded fistula 3cm distal to the anastomosis. The central basilic vein is patent. No prior problems with the fistula were reported. What would be the most appropriate course of management?**
   a) Open thrombectomy with fistulogram performed at a later date
   b) Formation of new fistula
   c) Percutaneous thrombectomy + fistulogram +/− fistuloplasty at same sitting
   d) Open thrombectomy alone
   e) No intervention

9. **A 33 year old female patient who injects drugs presents with a painful swelling in the left groin. Imaging demonstrates a pseudoaneurysm of the distal left common femoral artery. There is a surrounding soft tissue collection containing gas. The most appropriate management of this pseudoaneurysm is:**
   a) Placement of a covered stent
   b) Primary suture repair with prolene
   c) Arterial reconstruction with an ileo-femoral vein graft
   d) Observation
   e) Ligation of the femoral artery and debridement

10. **Regarding peritoneal dialysis catheters, what is the incidence of exit site infection/peritonitis within the first two weeks post-insertion?**
    a) 0%
    b) <5%
    c) 20%
    d) 40%
    e) 60%

11. **A 56 year old male smoker presents to the vascular clinic with a history of right calf claudication at 50 yards. The history suggests which pattern of arterial disease?**
    a) A 4cm occlusion of the right common iliac artery
    b) A full-length occlusion of the right posterior tibial artery
    c) A 10cm occlusion of the right superficial femoral artery
    d) A full-length occlusion of the right anterior and posterior tibial artery
    e) A full-length iliac system occlusion

12. A 48 year old male presents with persistent hypertension despite treatment with three antihypertensives. His resistant hypertension is suspected to be due to renovascular disease. Imaging demonstrates an 80% stenosis in the right renal artery and other secondary causes have been excluded. The most appropriate treatment for this patient is:

a) Angioplasty of the right renal artery

b) Best medical therapy

c) Denervation of the right renal artery

d) Right nephrectomy

e) Stenting of the right renal artery

13. A 62 year old female presents as an emergency with a 24-hour history of central abdominal pain, increasing in severity, and on a background of post-prandial pain and weight loss. The pain is out of proportion to the physical signs. Haematological investigations demonstrate a WCC of 14 and CRP of 50 with normal blood gases. CT imaging demonstrates thickening of the small bowel, a heavily calcified aorta, an occluded left common iliac artery, an occluded superior mesenteric artery, and coeliac axis. Please select the most appropriate management plan from the following list:

a) Active observation and repeat imaging in 48hrs

b) Anticoagulation

c) Endovascular stenting of her visceral vessels

d) Endovascular stenting of the visceral vessels followed by laparotomy

e) Laparotomy, left ilio to superior mesenteric bypass

14. Which of the following is not a recognized complication of warfarin therapy?

a) Euphoria

b) Haemorrhage

c) Purple toe syndrome

d) Purpura

e) Skin necrosis

15. Concerning lower limb trauma, which statement is correct?

a) The presence of a pedal pulse excludes proximal arterial trauma

b) Manipulation of a fracture with return of a distal pulse excludes arterial trauma

c) A pedal pulse may be palpable in the presence of arterial intimal damage

d) A non-pulsatile haematoma excludes arterial trauma

e) The presence of audible pedal Doppler signals excludes arterial trauma

16. **A patient presents with a penetrating neck injury. There is a suspicion of carotid trauma. Which of the following is correct?**
    a) Zone I is classed as an injury above the mandible
    b) Zone III injuries can be simply observed with no imaging required
    c) Zone II is classed as an injury between the cricoid cartilage and the mandible
    d) Zone III injuries will require thoracotomy for active haemorrhage proven on CT angiogram
    e) Zone II injuries with occlusion of the carotid artery and dense neurological deficit require immediate exploration

17. **Concerning acute mesenteric ischaemia, select the correct statement from the following:**
    a) Arterial embolism accounts for 50% of cases
    b) Laparotomy is not indicated following successful endovascular revascularization
    c) Mesenteric venous thrombus accounts for 50% of cases
    d) Non-occlusive mesenteric ischaemia has a mortality of less than 20%
    e) The Arc of Riolan is synonymous with the marginal artery of Drummond

18. **Concerning visceral aneurysms, aneurysms of the splenic artery**
    a) Are the most common visceral artery aneurysms
    b) Should always be treated due to their risk of thrombosis
    c) Require no further follow-up if found incidentally on imaging
    d) Are mycotic in nature in more than 60% of cases
    e) Have a risk of death from rupture of less than 5% due to endovascular treatments

19. **A 78 year old male presents with a 12-hour history of a sudden onset, painful, cold leg. The patient has known atrial fibrillation and is taking aspirin. On examination there is loss of sensation from the mid-calf to the foot. There is loss of motor function in the foot with absent capillary return and fixed mottling. Which of the following are correct?**
    a) The leg is threatened but still viable if treated within four hours
    b) The leg is threatened but still viable if treated within 12 hours
    c) The leg is threatened but still viable, although the patient may have residual neurological deficit if treated
    d) The leg is irreversibly damaged and amputation/palliation should be considered
    e) If amputation is required, this would take the form of a hip disarticulation

20. **An 81 year old female patient presents with an acutely ischaemic left leg and undergoes successful left femoral embolectomy. Her risk of peri-operative mortality is**
    a) Less than 1%
    b) Less than 5%
    c) 20–30%
    d) 50%
    e) 90%

21. **A 56 year old male patient with diabetes has an eGFR of 29ml/ min/1.73m². The patient is taking aspirin, ramipril, and amlodipine. He is scheduled to have a CT angiogram to investigate symptoms and signs suggestive of lower limb ischaemia. What complication are you most worried about in this patient?**
    a) Contrast-induced nephropathy
    b) Contrast allergy
    c) Contrast extravasation into surrounding tissue
    d) Fluid overload
    e) Nephrogenic systemic fibrosis

22. **A 65 year old male patient is now 5 years following an abdominal aortic aneurysm repair with a bifurcated graft. He presents to the Emergency department with a small episode of melaena followed six hours later by a large haematemesis. The most likely diagnosis is:**
    a) Aorto-enteric fistula
    b) Ischaemic colitis
    c) Pancreatic malignancy
    d) Peptic ulceration
    e) Rupture of cystic artery aneurysm

23. **The most likely site of an aorto-enteric fistula secondary to aortic surgery with an aorto-bifemoral graft is**
    a) Duodenum
    b) Jejunum
    c) Pancreatic duct
    d) Sigmoid colon
    e) Stomach

24. **A 10 year old boy falls from the roof of a garden shed and sustains a displaced supracondylar fracture. His arm is cold, white, and painful with paraesthesia to his fingertips. The arm does not improve following manipulation of the fracture. What is the most appropriate management plan?**
    a) Catheter (digital subtraction) angiogram
    b) CT angiogram under anaesthesia
    c) Intravenous heparin and observe
    d) MR to image the brachial plexus
    e) MR angiogram

25. **Dysphagia lusoria is defined as compression of the oesophagus by**
    a) The aortic arch
    b) The left subclavian artery
    c) The right subclavian artery
    d) The left axillary artery
    e) The right axillary artery

26. **The dialysis nurse calls you with regard to a 58 year old female patient who has been dialysing with no issues for the last 2 years through a superficial femoral artery-to-superficial femoral vein PTFE (polytetrafluoroethylene) graft. The patient returned to the dialysis unit one day post-dialysis with pyrexia and a painful diffuse swelling of the mid thigh (not localized to the last needle site). The skin overlying the graft is erythematous and hot to the touch. What complication are you most concerned about?**
    a) Deep venous thrombosis
    b) Graft infection
    c) Graft occlusion
    d) Ischaemic monomelic neuropathy
    e) Steal

27. **The vascular access nurse calls you regarding which needling technique you wish for a patient with a standard brachio-axillary PTFE graft fashioned six weeks ago. Which of the following is the most appropriate technique?**
    a) Buttonhole technique
    b) Single needle dialysis
    c) Rope ladder technique
    d) Area puncture technique
    e) Not to use the arteriovenous graft yet

Extended Matching Items

Vascular access

A. Brachio-cephalic fistula
B. Radio-basilic fistula
C. Brachio-axillary PTFE arteriovenous graft
D. Axillary–axillary necklace graft
E. Peritoneal dialysis catheter
F. Brachio-basilic transposition fistula
G. Thigh loop PTFE arteriovenous graft
H. Tunnelled central venous catheter
I. Ulnar-cephalic fistula

For each of the following scenarios, select the single most likely vascular access from the list. Each option may be used once, more than once, or not at all.

1. A 33 year old male patient with diabetes has been referred for access planning pre-dialysis. He has had multiple laparotomies for Crohn's disease. Duplex scanning demonstrates good quality brachial arteries in the upper limbs, with small diameter (1.5mm) calcified radial and ulnar arteries. The cephalic and basilic veins are excellent with no obvious central vein stenosis.

2. A 69 year old male patient with known bilateral iliac artery occlusive disease resulting in a 300-yard claudication distance. The patient required emergency dialysis and is currently dialysing through a femoral line. The renal team is keen for urgent vascular access creation. Both brachial systolic pressures are approximately 80mmHg and duplex suggests bilateral subclavian vein stenoses.

Extra-cranial carotid disease

A. Best medical therapy
B. Bilateral carotid endarterectomy within two weeks
C. Bilateral carotid endarterectomy within six weeks
D. Carotid to carotid bypass
E. Left carotid endarterectomy within two weeks
F. Left carotid endarterectomy within six weeks
G. Left carotid subclavian bypass
H. Right carotid endarterectomy within two weeks
I. Right carotid endarterectomy within six weeks
J. Right carotid subclavian bypass

For the following scenarios, select the most appropriate management strategy from the list.

3. A 60 year old, right-handed, female smoker presents to the stroke physicians with a history of right-sided arm weakness of 1 hour duration. She experienced left amaurosis fugax two days before her presentation. A carotid duplex ultrasound scan demonstrates bilateral internal carotid artery stenosis of >80%, with normal vertebral arteries.

4. A 72 year old diabetic female presents to the stroke physicians with a history of left arm and leg weakness (of 3hr duration), two weeks prior. A carotid duplex ultrasound shows

a 50% right internal carotid artery stenosis and an 80% left internal carotid artery stenosis, with antegrade flow in both vertebral arteries.

5. A 53 year old male smoker presents to the stroke clinic with a history of right arm and leg weakness which occurred 10 days prior and is gradually resolving. A carotid duplex ultrasound demonstrates an occluded left internal carotid artery and a 40% stenosis in the right internal carotid artery, with normal vertebral arteries bilaterally.

Aortic pathology

A. Type A aortic dissection (Stanford classification)
B. Type B aortic dissection (Stanford classification)
C. Type A (Stanford) dissecting aortic aneurysm
D. Type B (Stanford) dissecting aortic aneurysm
E. DeBakey Type II aortic dissection
F. DeBakey Type III aortic dissection
G. Infra-renal abdominal aortic aneurysm
H. Juxta-renal abdominal aortic aneurysm
I. Modified Crawford type IV
J. Modified Crawford type V

For the following scenarios, select the most appropriate diagnosis from the list of options

6. A 69 year old male presents with a sudden onset of inter-scapular pain and marked hypertension (systolic >200mmHg). CT imaging with contrast shows a thoracic aortic dissection with an entry point distal to the left subclavian artery. The dissection extends proximally to the brachiocephalic artery and distally to the level of the coeliac axis. The maximum aortic diameter is 2.5cm. What is the diagnosis?

7. A 58 year old female has an incidental finding on contrast CT of an aortic aneurysm extending from the diaphragm, involving the visceral aortic segment down to the aortic bifurcation. What is the correct diagnosis?

General vascular

A. Acute aortic occlusion
B. Acute arterial embolism
C. Chronic arterial occlusion
D. Compartment syndrome
E. Distal embolization (trashing)
F. Persistent sciatic artery
G. Phlegmasia alba dolens
H. Phlegmasia cerulea dolens
I. Popliteal entrapment syndrome
J. Klippel–Trenaunay syndrome

For the following scenarios, select the most appropriate diagnosis from the list.

8. A 60 year old female patient is 10 days after an open left hemicolectomy for malignancy and develops a swollen, tender left thigh and calf, with patchy mottling throughout and a cool foot.

9. A 23 year old female presents with long-standing marked varicose veins on the lateral aspect of her left leg with a capillary malformation on the same leg.

10. A 70 year old female, with a known 4cm infra-renal aortic aneurysm, presents with painful toes on the left with patches of dusky skin on the tips of the toes and strong pedal pulses.

11. A 30 year old male with alcohol dependence is found to have collapsed at home. They present with an acute kidney injury and a swollen, tender right thigh and calf with a cool and dusky foot. A venous duplex scan demonstrated no DVT.

12. A 23 year old female with active ulcerative colitis undergoing medical treatment, presents with a sudden onset painful, cold left leg and a dusky left foot.

Venous pathology

A. Anticoagulation alone
B. Anticoagulation, thrombolysis, and first rib resection
C. Anticoagulation, thrombolysis, and balloon venoplasty
D. Elevation, compression therapy, and mobilization
E. Foam sclerotherapy to the long saphenous vein
F. Antibiotics, compression, and elevation
G. High saphenous tie, stripping of the long saphenous vein, and stab avulsions
H. Non-steroidal anti-inflammatories, compression, and elevation
I. Radiofrequency ablation of the long saphenous vein
J. Three-layer elasticated compression bandaging

For the following scenarios, select the most appropriate initial management from the list.

13. A 50 year old female patient with marked ulceration around her medial malleolus. Her ABPI is 0.85 bilaterally with biphasic waveforms and there is duplex evidence of deep venous reflux.

14. A 30 year old male, with known varicose veins, presents with tender, erythematous skin overlying the long saphenous vein. Duplex confirms superficial thrombophlebitis.

15. A 44 year old female patient has a past history of a left-sided DVT following gynaecological surgery. She now has left varicose veins with associated skin changes. A venous duplex demonstrates a patent but significantly refluxing deep venous system with reflux into the long saphenous system.

16. A 28 year old male Commonwealth weightlifter presents with a 3-day history of a swollen tender and dusky right arm. Imaging confirms a subclavian vein DVT and no cervical rib.

Anticoagulant mode of action

A. Enhance action of antithrombin III
B. Factor Xa inhibitor
C. Direct thrombin inhibitor
D. Cox-2 inhibitor
E. Direct factor Xa inhibitor
F. Inhibits vitamin K-dependent synthesis of clotting factors II, VII, IX, and X
G. Inhibits vitamin K-dependent synthesis of clotting factors II, VII, VIII, and X
H. Calcium channel blocker
I. Antifibrinolytic

Concerning the following pharmaceutical agents, select the method of action on the clotting cascade:

17. Rivaroxaban
18. Dabigatran
19. Warfarin

Vascular syndromes

A. May–Thurner syndrome
B. Klippel–Trenaunay syndrome
C. Paget–Schroetter syndrome
D. Ehlers–Danlos syndrome
E. Postphlebitic syndrome
F. Antiphospholipid syndrome
G. Marfan syndrome
H. Neurological thoracic outlet syndrome
I. Subclavian steal syndrome
J. Gardner syndrome

For the following scenarios, select the most appropriate diagnosis from the list.

20. A 38 year old obese female typist presents with a few months' history of paraesthesia to her left hand on exertion. She develops weakness in the arm especially when her arm is being used in the overhead position.
21. A 63 year old male smoker presents with a few months' history of pain in his left forearm and hand on exertion, associated syncopal episodes, and weakness in the affected limb.
22. A 43 year old female who presents with an unprovoked right ileo-femoral DVT, her third DVT in 10 years.

Vasculitides

A. Kawasaki disease
B. Giant cell arteritis
C. Thromboangiitis obliterans
D. Polyarteritis nodosa
E. Wegener's granulomatosis
F. Behçet's disease
G. Fibromuscular dysplasia
H. Cogan syndrome
I. Churg–Strauss syndrome
J. Takayasu's arteritis

For the following scenarios, select the most appropriate diagnosis from the list.

23. A 38 year old female, non smoker, presents with weight loss and claudication of her left arm. CT angiography demonstrates a non-atherosclerotic stenosis in the left subclavian artery, aneurysmal dilation of her brachio-cephalic artery, and stenosis of her distal descending aorta.

24. A 33 year old female patient has hypertension which is refractory to three anti-hypertensive medications. A CT scan carried out for an unrelated reason has demonstrated multi-segment areas of focal dilation/stenosis of the left renal artery.

25. A 78 year old male presents with a 2-week history of jaw claudication and transient visual disturbance.

Single Best Answers

1. c) Ligation of the radial artery distal to the anastomosis in a radio-cephalic fistula may resolve steal symptoms in a high-flow situation with patent ipsilateral ulnar artery and palmar arch

Distal radial artery ligation requires a patent ulnar artery and intact palmar arch. The majority of steal cases are related to poor distal run off, significant arterial inflow stenosis, or a combination of both. Steal symptoms develop over time as the arterial inflow and venous outflow dilate (resulting in increased flows). The immediate occurrence of such symptoms should alert the physician to other diagnoses such as nerve compression secondary to haematoma formation, iatrogenic damage to the nerves, and ischaemic monomelic neuropathy. The majority of patients with an arteriovenous fistula (AVF) have some degree of symptoms or signs of steal. Not all of these patients require intervention.

2. a) Atherosclerotic arterial disease with thrombosis *in situ*

Given the patient's demographics (age, diabetes) and past history of claudication, it is most likely that the deterioration in his claudication distance is related to progression of his atherosclerotic disease (thrombosis *in situ* within native arterial disease).

Popliteal artery entrapment is a rare cause of claudication and chronic lower leg ischaemia. It often affects a younger age group without risk factors associated with atherosclerosis. It is caused by compression of the popliteal artery by muscular or tendinous insertions in the popliteal fossa and can lead to stenosis, occlusion, or aneurysmal dilation. It is seen particularly in athletic individuals with well-developed muscles such as professional sportspeople and military personnel.

Cystic adventitial disease is another more rare cause of claudication (approx. 1 in 1200 cases). It commonly presents in male patients in middle-age, with cysts developing in the adventitial layer causing luminal compression and progressive claudication. The popliteal artery is the most frequently affected but it can involve the iliac, femoral, radial, and ulnar arteries.

A persistent sciatic artery (PSA) is a rare anomaly caused by failure of embryological involution. There is a variety of different anatomical variants. The sciatic artery may be the dominant supply to the leg and the femoral artery may be absent, or the femoral artery may still be the dominant artery with an incomplete PSA. Complications such as ischaemia or aneurysm formation occur in the majority of patients.

Flanigan DP et al. Summary of cases of adventitial cystic disease of the popliteal artery. *Annals of Surgery* 1979; 189:165–75.

Van Hooft IM et al. The persistent sciatic artery. *European Journal of Vascular and Endovascular Surgery* 2009; 37(5):585–91.

3. b) Atheroslcerotic arterial disease

The history is consistent with atherosclerotic arterial disease resulting in intermittent claudication. Although the ABPIs appear normal, the pedal flow signals are monophasic, implying the ABPI may be falsely elevated due to calcified vessels. ABPIs must be interpreted in conjunction with the waveforms of the distal vessels. Normal waveforms are triphasic or biphasic. Monophasic signals imply dampening of the flow upstream secondary to occlusive disease. Post-exercise ABPIs are essential and would demonstrate a drop in pressure ratio if significant stenotic/occlusive arterial disease were present (resting ABPIs can on occasion be relatively normal despite peripheral vascular disease).

4. d) Admit for intravenous antibiotics and a contrast-enhanced CT scan

The patient has clear evidence of sepsis with pain, swelling, tenderness, and raised inflammatory markers. For this reason, initial management should include blood cultures followed by early administration of antibiotic treatment. A high index of suspicion for a necrotizing soft tissue infection and vessel involvement (arterial pseudoaneurysm) or an infected deep venous thrombosis has to be considered. The patient should be admitted to hospital for treatment of sepsis and rapid imaging (preferentially CT with arterial/venous phase contrast). This will allow delineation of any collections and determine the presence and extent of muscle necrosis and any vessel involvement. In patients such as this, imaging is recommended prior to surgical intervention to allow specialist vascular involvement if required.

5. b) 40% of patients with a popliteal artery aneurysm will have an AAA

Popliteal artery aneurysms are the most common peripheral aneurysm. Unlike abdominal aortic aneurysms rupture is rare. The rationale for treating popliteal artery aneurysms in the elective setting is primarily to prevent thrombosis and distal trashing/embolization. 10–15% of patients with a known AAA will have a popliteal artery aneurysm or, put another way, 40% of patients with a popliteal artery aneurysm will have an abdominal aortic aneurysm. Approximately half of all those with a popliteal artery aneurysm will have bilateral aneurysms. Treatment is dependent on numerous factors: age, symptoms, size, site of aneurysm in relation to vessel bifurcation, physiological fitness for surgery, diameter and length of normal vessel proximal and distal to the aneurysm. Open surgical intervention includes bypass of the affected segment with ligation of the aneurysmal segment or endovascular stenting.

Dawson J et al. Update on aneurysm disease: current insights and controversies: peripheral aneurysms: when to intervene—is rupture really a danger? *Progress in Cardiovascular Diseases* 2013; 56(1):26–35.

6. c) CT angiogram + physiological testing with a view to urgent intervention

The UK prevalence of AAA is approximately 5% in men aged 65–74. Mortality for patients suffering a ruptured AAA remains very high at between 70–80%. There is a 53% reduction in risk of aneurysm-related death for patients who attend the screening programme. The UK AAA screening programme is offered to men at the age of 65 involving an initial ultrasound assessment. The aorta is defined as being aneurysmal once the AP diameter is ≥3cm.

The indications for intervention include size (≥5.5cm AP diameter in an asymptomatic patient), rapid growth (>5mm in 6 months, or 1cm/year), symptomatic patients, and rupture. This patient has not reached the threshold of 5.5cm AP diameter but has had a rapid expansion in size over 6 months, a concerning feature. Studies assessing timing of surgery in asymptomatic aneurysms have based their AP sizing on duplex ultrasound and not CT. CT itself may overestimate the AP diameter in comparison to ultrasound measurements.

Ashton HA et al. The Multicentre Aneurysm Screening Study (MASS) into the effect of abdominal aortic aneurysm screening on mortality in men: a randomized controlled trial. *Lancet* 2002; 360(9345):1531–9.

The UK Small Aneurysm Trial Participants. Mortality results for randomized controlled trial of early elective surgery or ultrasound surveillance for small abdominal aortic aneurysms. *Lancet* 1998; 352(9141):1649–55.

Filardo G et al. Surgery for small asymptomatic abdominal aortic aneurysms. *Cochrane Database of Systematic Reviews* 2015; 8(2):CD001835.

7. c) Abandon PD catheter insertion, repair the enterotomy, and lavage the abdomen

Approximately one-third of patients with end-stage renal disease (ESRD) are managed by peritoneal dialysis. The benefits compared to haemodialysis are particularly related to patient mobility and independence. Several techniques have been described for placement of the peritoneal dialysis catheter including open, laparoscopic, and percutaneous approaches. The laparoscopic approach is popular as it allows precise catheter placement and can be combined with adhesiolysis if required. While percutaneous placement may be less invasive and provides logistical benefits, there is a risk of iatrogenic injury and poor catheter placement.

Spillage of enteric contents during insertion of a peritoneal dialysis catheter necessitates repair of the enterotomy and lavage of the peritoneal cavity. The catheter should not be left in due to the high risk of infection (enteric contents in the presence of a prosthesis). Risk of bowel perforation during PD catheter insertion is low with the audit standard being <1%. Perforation should be suspected in patients with significant post-operative abdominal pain or hypotension. Urgent re-exploration of the abdomen should be carried out with removal of the catheter and antibiotic therapy instituted.

8. c) Percutaneous thrombectomy +fistulogram +/– fistuloplasty at same sitting

A fistula occludes for a reason, namely a significant stenosis. The ideal management is a combined thrombectomy (either open or percutaneous) and fistulogram so that any underlying occlusive issue can be identified and treated at the same sitting. As this is a brachio-basilic fistula (more complex access than a brachio-cephalic), this implies the patient is running out of autologous options in the upper limbs. For this reason, salvage of the fistula should be paramount.

9. e) Ligation of the femoral artery and debridement

In this instance the history and imaging are suggestive of an infected pseudoaneurysm of the femoral artery. This is the most common arterial complication in IV drug users. Placement of a covered stent (prosthetic material) into infected tissue is not advised, nor is primary repair (high risk of repair breakdown and re-bleed). An ileo-femoral vein graft can be considered at a later date once the sepsis is controlled and depending on the patient's symptoms. An infected pseudoaneurysm, unlike an iatrogenic, non-infected pseudoaneurysm, does not tend to spontaneously thrombose and the patient can deteriorate rapidly from sepsis/rupture.

Mittapalli D et al. Necrotizing soft tissue infections in intravenous drug users: a vascular surgical emergency. *European Journal of Vascular and Endovascular Surgery* 2015; 49(5):593–9.

10. b) <5%

Placement of peritoneal dialysis catheters should be carried out with the involvement of a multi-disciplinary team experienced in the different aspects of access placement. Clear perioperative catheter care protocols should be in place to minimize the risk of complications. Prophylactic antibiotics should be used to reduce the incidence of catheter-related infections and wound sepsis. The incidence of exit site infection/peritonitis within the first 2 weeks post-insertion should be less than 5%. Regular audit is required to monitor outcomes and performance. Long-term catheter patency of 80% at 1 year is also suggested as a marker of successful outcome.

Figueiredo A et al. Clinical practice guidelines for peritoneal access. *Peritoneal Dialysis International* 2010; 30(4):424–9.

11. c) A 10cm occlusion of the right superficial femoral artery

Claudication, pain, or cramping in the leg due to inadequate blood flow, is one of the most common manifestations of peripheral arterial occlusive disease. The prevalence of intermittent claudication in men aged 55–74 years is 4.5%. The prognosis for claudicants is generally benign.

Superficial femoral artery (SFA) occlusions are a common cause of claudication and typically lead to claudication in the calf region (no involvement of the thigh or buttock). Proximal iliac artery occlusions tend to result in buttock, thigh, and possibly calf claudication. Crural vessel disease usually results in distal calf/foot problems.

12. b) Best medical treatment

Atherosclerosis is the most common cause of renovascular disease and is associated with chronic kidney disease (CKD), hypertension, and end-stage renal failure. It is usually a reflection of diffuse atherosclerosis rather than being an isolated finding. There have been numerous studies looking at intervention for renovascular disease in order to improve renal function and cardiovascular outcomes. The two landmark studies (ASTRAL and CORAL) have demonstrated that elective intervention on renal artery stenosis does not confer benefit in treating hypertension, renal function, or on clinical events. Of note, intervention for renal artery stenoses does not come without risk, with up to 10% of patients suffering a significant complication. Indications for intervention include flash pulmonary oedema in the setting of significant renal artery stenosis, fibromuscular dysplasia, as part of an open aortic procedure and renal artery stenosis in a transplanted kidney.

ASTRAL Investigators. Revascularization versus medical therapy for renal-artery stenosis. *New England Journal of Medicine* 2009; 361(20):1953–62.

CORAL Investigators. Stenting and medical therapy for atherosclerotic renal-artery stenosis. *New England Journal of Medicine* 2014; 370:13–22.

Davies MG et al. The long-term outcomes of percutaneous therapy for renal artery fibromuscular dysplasia. *Journal of Vascular Surgery* 2008; 48:865–71.

13. d) Endovascular stenting of the visceral vessels followed by laparotomy

Alternative options for this patient include aorto-mesenteric bypass (probably not in this case due to aortic calcification) and right ilio-mesenteric bypass (left side occluded). These procedures require open surgery in the form of a laparotomy, thereby allowing inspection of the GI tract. CT findings demonstrating an abnormal GI tract in the presence of acute on chronic mesenteric ischaemia usually occur late in the process of mesenteric ischaemia (i.e. the GI tract may already be irreversibly damaged) so the clinician needs a high index of suspicion. There should be a very low threshold for inspecting the GI tract after arterial intervention in such patients.

Zhao Y et al. Management of acute mesenteric ischemia: a critical review and treatment algorithm. *Vascular and Endovascular Surgery* 2016; 50(3):183–92.

Douard R et al. Clinical interest of digestive arterial trunk anastomoses. *Surgical and Radiologic Anatomy* 2006; 28(3):219–27.

14. a) Euphoria

Haemorrhage is the most common complication of warfarin therapy (annual rate approximately 1–3%) with haemorrhagic stroke being perhaps the most significant. The risk of bleeding increases dramatically with rising INR (international normalized ratio). Bleeding risk is also increased with age, drug interactions, hypertension, history of stroke, history of previous bleeds, and alcohol misuse.

Warfarin can induce skin necrosis related to acquired protein C deficiency. The protein C deficiency leads to a temporary hyper-coagulable state, particularly during initiation of warfarin therapy, leading to skin necrosis in certain individuals.

Purple toe syndrome is a rare but recognized complication and is thought to be related to cholesterol micro emboli, the mechanism for which is still to be elucidated (either via an insult directly from the anticoagulation or via haemorrhage into areas of atherosclerotic plaques).

Stewart A et al. Warfarin induced skin necrosis. *Postgraduate Medical Journal* 1999; 75:233–5.

Cakebread H et al. Warfarin induced purple toe syndrome successfully treated with apixaban. *British Medical Journal Case Reports* 12 June 2014.

15. c) A pedal pulse may be palpable in the presence of arterial intimal damage

Intimal damage may result in a localized stenosis/dissection with impedance to flow but still detectable pulses distally. Doppler examination must be undertaken with caution and appropriate interpretation because as in chronic arterial occlusions, signals can still be heard distal to long arterial occlusions. In this situation analysis of the waveform is paramount (or perform ABPI).

16. c) Zone II is classed as an injury between the cricoid cartilage and the mandible

Zone I extends from the clavicle to the cricoid cartilage. Zone II is between the cricoid cartilage and the mandible. Zone III encompasses injuries above the mandible. Imaging should be performed for all suspected carotid artery injuries. Either CT or MRI with contrast should be considered for Zone I and III injuries. Duplex ultrasound by an experienced ultrasonographer can be helpful in Zone II injuries. The disadvantage of Duplex is that it will not identify other non-arterial injuries as accurately as contrast imaging. Any injury of the carotid with complete occlusion of the carotid and dense neurological deficit, especially in the presence of proven infarct, have a grave prognosis regardless of treatment. See Figure 10.1.

17. a) Arterial embolism accounts for 50% of cases

Causes of acute mesenteric ischaemia include arterial embolism (50%), non-occlusive mesenteric ischaemia (20%), venous thrombosis (5–10%), and arterial thrombosis *in situ* on the background of atherosclerotic plaque (25%). Arterial embolism is often related to arrhythmia (e.g. atrial fibrillation) and is more common in females. Sources include atrial thrombi, mural thrombi following myocardial infarction, vegetations on the heart valves, or atherosclerotic plaques affecting the aorta. There is often a history of previous embolic episodes. The superior mesenteric artery (SMA) is the most common of the visceral arteries to be affected. The inferior mesenteric artery territory may be protected by better collateral circulation.

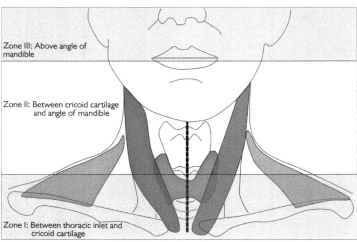

Fig. 10.1 Zones of neck trauma

Non-occlusive mesenteric ischaemia is caused by reduced mesenteric perfusion related to shock states such as cardiac, septic, or hypovolaemic shock. It can also be caused by vasopressors used in the setting of the critically ill patient. The mortality from non-occlusive mesenteric ischaemia is higher than other causes of mesenteric ischaemia at between 70–90%. This is most likely due to the severity of the precipitating conditions.

Numerous collaterals exist between the three major visceral vessels: the marginal artery of Drummond between the SMA and IMA (inferior mesenteric artery) running peripherally along the inner border of the left colon; the Arc of Riolan (mesenteric meandering artery), if present, classically runs from the middle colic to the left colic branch of the IMA, running close along the root of the mesentery; and the Arc of Bruhler, if present (1–4%), connects the coeliac axis and the superior mesenteric artery. The Arc of Barkow is another arterial-to-arterial communication between the right gastro-epiploic and the left gastro-epiploic arteries, supplying the transverse colon with multiple ascending branches.

18. a) Are the most common visceral artery aneurysms

The splenic artery is the most common site for visceral artery aneurysm (60%), followed by the hepatic artery (20%), the superior mesenteric artery (5%), and the coeliac artery (4%). Splenic artery aneurysms can be multiple, arise more commonly in the distal one-third of the artery and are usually saccular in nature. They occur more commonly in females. Rapidly enlarging, symptomatic, or ruptured aneurysms require intervention as do false aneurysms. The mortality from a rupture is in the region of 50%. They require follow-up with serial imaging due to their propensity to enlarge (especially in younger patients). Of particular concern are splenic artery aneurysms in young pregnant females as there is a high rate of rupture, especially during the third trimester (70% maternal death, 95% foetal death).

The vast majority of visceral artery aneurysms are true aneurysms, but they can arise secondary to trauma, iatrogenic injury, infection, (pancreatitis, post-surgery) fibromuscular dysplasia, and connective tissue disorders (e.g. Ehlers–Danlos syndrome).

Lakin RO et al. The contemporary management of splenic artery aneurysms. *Journal of Vascular Surgery* 2011; 53(4):958–65.

19. d) The leg is irreversibly damaged and amputation/palliation should be considered

The duration and onset of symptoms, in conjunction with the history, are consistent with acute lower limb ischaemia. The presence of complete paralysis and loss of sensation implies severe muscle and nerve ischaemia. In combination with fixed mottling, this implies a non-salvageable limb and revascularization is likely to result in massive reperfusion injury and death. Amputation or palliation should be considered. Hip disarticulation would be unnecessary as the thigh muscles are not involved.   *Acute limb Rutherford 3 classification.*
NO) viable.

20. c) 20–30%

Patients with acute limb ischaemia secondary to embolism have a high mortality as a result of their underlying cardiac disease. Up to 90% of embolisms will have a cardiac source with most related to atrial fibrillation. Embolism from more distal sources such as aortic atherosclerotic plaques carry a worse prognosis as embolectomy is less effective. Following embolectomy most surgeons perform an on-table arteriogram to confirm that the distal blood flow is adequate. In the post-operative period consideration should be given to anticoagulation. Limb loss rates range from 5–7% during the initial admission to 15% overall. Up to 20% of patients die within a year of presentation, commonly as a result of the medical comorbidities which put them at risk of acute limb ischaemia.

21. a) Contrast-induced nephropathy

This patient has significant risk factors, including diabetes and potentially nephrotoxic medication, as well as evidence of renal dysfunction, with a reduced EGFR. In this setting the risk of contrast-induced nephropathy should be of major concern. Iodinated contrast media used for radiological investigation have a good safety record and the risk of adverse events is low. The risk of severe contrast reaction is approximately 0.2%. The risk of adverse reaction is increased in patients who have had a previous reaction, patients with allergies, and patients with asthma.

The risk of contrast-induced nephropathy specifically is increased five to ten times in patients with pre-existing renal dysfunction, such as in this case. Patients with diabetic nephropathy carry the greatest risk. Other risk factors include nephrotoxic drugs (e.g. NSAIDs, aminoglycosides), heart failure, dehydration, and large doses of contrast or repeated doses over a short space of time.

Contrast extravasation is a recognized complication which occurs in approximately 0.5% of examinations. Symptoms include pain, swelling, and erythema which are usually self-limiting. Management involves rapid recognition, discontinuing the infusion, and elevation of the limb with a cold compress. More serious sequelae such as skin ulceration or compartment syndrome may require specialist surgical input.

In the setting of either acute or chronic renal failure the volume of contrast media can exacerbate fluid overload. The volume of both oral and IV contrast should be included in any overall fluid intake. Just because a patient is on dialysis does not mean that IV contrast does not carry additional risks.

Nephrogenic systemic fibrosis is a complication of the MRI contrast agent Gadolinium in patients with renal dysfunction.

22. d) Peptic ulceration

The clinician must be concerned regarding an aorta-enteric fistula in any patient who has undergone prior aortic surgery. Although the incidence of secondary aorto-enteric fistula is more common after open repair it should also be considered in relation to endovascular surgery. The most common cause of secondary aorto-enteric fistulae is infection around the graft leading to erosion into the duodenum. Patients can present from a few months to many years after the initial aortic surgery. However, the incidence of such fistulae following aortic procedures is low (0.3–2%), meaning peptic ulceration is still the top of the diagnostic list. Pancreatic malignancy and cystic artery aneurysms are much rarer causes of upper GI bleeding and ischaemic colitis typically presents with rectal bleeding associated with abdominal pain.

23. a) Duodenum

The most common site for an aorta-enteric fistula secondary to aortic surgery is the duodenum. The fistula is often located at the third part of the duodenum as it crosses the aorta at the level of the aortic anastomosis in most aortic repairs. Failure to separate the duodenum from the graft by closing the aortic wall/retroperitoneum/aneurysm sac over the graft means the anastomosis apposes the intestinal tract. This can lead to erosion of the GI tract, with spillage of enteric contents around the graft, which may result in breakdown of the anastomosis, graft infection, and massive haemorrhage. There is usually a small 'herald' bleed prior to massive exsanguinating haemorrhage.

24. b) CT angiogram under anaesthesia

Supracondylar fracture of the humerus is the most common paediatric fracture at the elbow and is a usually the consequence of a fall onto an outstretched hand. The fracture has a high complication rate with around 4–14% of children suffering a vascular injury. The brachial artery is the most commonly affected vessel, and injury ranges from contusion and intimal damage to complete transection. The sequelae to vascular injury include compartment syndrome, limb threat, contracture, or late claudication.

CT with contrast allows rapid, non-invasive imaging allowing delineation of the arterial trauma and planning of reconstruction. Imaging will require the support of the anaesthetic team due to the risk of restlessness secondary to pain and the requirement for high-quality imaging. MR angiogram takes considerably longer than CT (an important factor in trauma), although it does not involve a radiation dose.

Campbell CC et al. Neurovascular injury and displacement in type III supracondylar humerus fractures. *Journal of Pediatric Orthopedics* 1995; 15(1):47–52.

25. c) The right subclavian artery

Compression of the oesophagus by an aberrant right subclavian artery may result in dysphagia (dysphagia lusoria). An aberrant right subclavian artery occurs in 0.5% of the population. The right subclavian artery arises as the fourth branch of the aortic arch and then passes either behind or in front of the oesophagus to supply the right arm. This anomaly is probably asymptomatic in the majority of cases. It can be associated with congenital cardiac disease. Diagnosis is usually made by a combination of barium swallow and CT. Endoscopic diagnosis is rare. Treatment depends on the degree of symptoms and ranges from dietary modification to surgical intervention.

26. b) Graft infection

The commonest cause of hospital admissions and mortality amongst dialysis patients is infection, especially with prosthetic graft in situ. Venous access for haemodialysis is achieved either by central venous access, autologous arteriovenous fistula (AVF) or an arteriovenous fistula using prosthetic graft. An autologous fistula has clear benefits in terms of durability and reduced infective complications. However, arteriovenous grafts (AVG) may be required for patients where the venous anatomy is insufficient to support an AVF or who have had previous failed AVFs.

Infection affects up to 20% of AVGs and is 10 times more likely than with an AVF. The risk is further increased in thigh grafts, such as in this patient, compared to upper limb grafts. For this reason, upper limb graft is preferred and suggests this patient may have limited alternative options for access. The risk factors for infection are numerous including: previous history of infections; repeated cannulations; poor aseptic technique; venipuncture technique; diabetes; hypoalbuminaemia; obesity; previous failed/thrombosed grafts.

The potential consequences of graft infection are significant and include central line use with associated complications, graft loss, prolonged hospital stay, septicaemia, and mortality. Prevention of infection with proper technique should be the focus. Infections are most commonly caused by Staphylococcus aureus. Treatment, after blood cultures, consists of initially empirical broad-spectrum antibiotics with Gram-positive and Gram-negative cover. The spectrum can be narrowed once culture results are available with treatment likely to be prolonged. Infection is often difficult to clear in the setting of prosthetic material. Intervention is frequently required and may ultimately involve partial or complete graft excision.

Buttonhole AVF.

27. c) Rope ladder technique

The buttonhole technique involves needling the fistula in exactly the same spot and at the same angle every time. This creates a track which can eventually be accessed using a blunt needle. This may be less painful for the patient and reduce haematomas. There is a risk of septic complications and this technique is used for AVFs and not for an AVG such as in this patient.

Single needle dialysis is required when concerns arise regarding the length of usable access and recent traumatic cannulations.

The rope ladder technique is the most frequently used cannulation technique. It describes rotating the needle site each time the fistula is cannulated to give the previous sites time to heal. Alternative puncture techniques result in repetitive trauma to a localized segment of the graft leading to graft disruption/infection. Standard PTFE arteriovenous grafts can be needled four to six weeks after insertion—there are concerns with regards to haematoma or infection along the graft until it is incorporated into the soft tissues. Rapid cannulation PTFE grafts are available allowing cannulation immediately upon creation.

Rope ladder most common

Extended Matching Items

Vascular access

1. A. Brachio-cephalic fistula

The patient is not a candidate for peritoneal dialysis due to intra-abdominal pathology and prior laparotomies. Access should be created as distal as possible in the non-dominant hand, preferably with autologous material (as there is no requirement for immediate dialysis).

2. E. Peritoneal dialysis catheter

The patient requires urgent removal of the femoral line to reduce the risk of septic complications. His iliac disease precludes lower limb fistulae and his upper limb arteries would not sustain a fistula or PTFE graft. The best option for this patient would be for peritoneal dialysis.

Extra-cranial carotid disease

3. E. Left carotid endarterectomy within two weeks

The factors involved in decision-making for carotid surgery include symptoms, the age and gender of the patient, timing of the event, recovery from the event, and the degree of stenosis. The side of surgery is based on the site of the cerebral event. The patient in this scenario has suffered a transient ischaemic attack (TIA) affecting the right arm (indicating a left-sided cerebral event). Amaurosis fugax on the left is consistent with a left-sided athero-embolic event. The maximum benefit to be gained from carotid endarterectomy is within the first two weeks after the event.

4. A. Best medical therapy

Left-sided symptoms indicate a right-sided cerebral event, implicating the right carotid territory. With symptoms for more than 2 weeks prior to the presentation in a carotid with 50% stenosis in a female, the evidence suggests this patient is best treated with medical therapy.

5. A. Best medical therapy

Right-sided symptoms indicate a left-sided cerebral event, implicating the left carotid artery. There is no evidence to suggest that performing an endarterectomy on an occluded ICA (intracranial carotid artery) in this circumstance would confer any benefit in stroke prevention.

Benefit for carotid endarterectomy in symptomatic patients can be split into:

Males

- 50–70% stenosis of the ICA—surgery as soon as possible, ideally within 2 weeks of the event (no benefit thereafter)
- 70–99% stenosis of the ICA—surgery as soon as possible, ideally within 2 weeks of the event, but benefit from carotid surgery present up to 12 weeks after the event

Females

- 50–70% stenosis of the ICA—no benefit from carotid surgery
- 70–99% stenosis of the ICA—surgery as soon as possible, ideally within 2 weeks of the event (no benefit after 4 weeks)

Males/Females

- occluded ICA or trickle flow (near occlusion)—no benefit from carotid surgery

Rothwell P et al. Endarterectomy for symptomatic carotid stenosis in relation to clinical subgroups and timing of surgery. *Lancet* 2004; 363(9413):915–24.

Rothwell P et al. Analysis of pooled data from the randomised controlled trials of endarterectomy for symptomatic carotid stenosis. *Lancet* 2003; 363:107–16.

Naylor R. Time is brain—an update. *Expert Reviews in Cardiovascular Therapy* 2015; 13(10):1111–26.

Aortic pathology

6. A. Type A Aortic Dissection (Stanford Classification)

The majority of the vascular community use the Stanford classification of thoracic aortic dissection—Type A and B. Type A dissection always involves the aorta proximal to the left subclavian, irrespective of where the entry tear or the distal endpoint of the dissection is. Type B dissection involves the descending thoracic aorta, from the left subclavian distally. See Figure 10.2.

2010 ACCF/AHA/AATS/ACR/ASA/SCA/SCAI/SIR/STS/SVM Guidelines for the Diagnosis and Management of Patients with Thoracic Aortic Disease: Executive Summary Circulation. 2010; 121:1544–79. <http://circ.ahajournals.org/content/circulationaha/121/13/1544.full.pdf>.

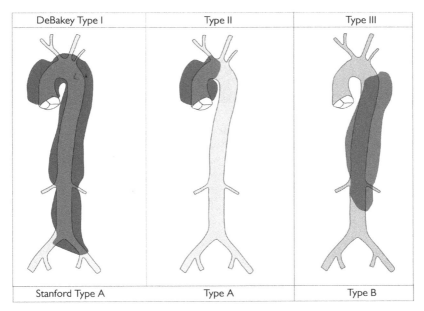

Fig. 10.2 Classification of dissection thoracic aneurysms

7. 1. Modified Crawford type IV

An Extent IV aneurysm extends from the diaphragm down to the aortic bifurcation, involving the visceral vessels. Extent I, II, III, and IV thoraco-abdominal aneurysms are pictorially represented in Figure 10.3.

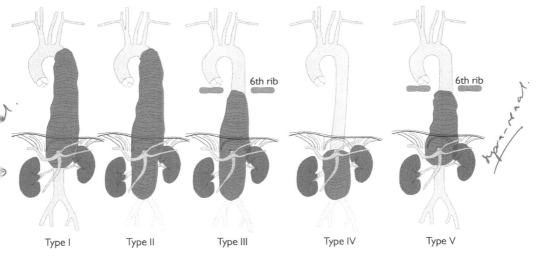

Fig. 10.3 Classification of Thoraco-abdominal aortic aneurysms

Muss F et al. Acute aortic dissection and intramural hematoma—a systematic review. *Journal of the American Medical Association* 2016; 316(7):754–63.

General vascular

8. H. Phlegmasia cerulea dolens

The history is consistent with an extensive ilio-femoral deep vein thrombosis. The findings correlate with Phlegmasia cerulea dolens.

Phlegmasia cerulea dolens is a rare but severe form of deep venous thrombosis caused by extensive thrombosis of the venous system. It is often associated with malignancy such as in the patient described. The risk of pulmonary embolism is high, even with systemic anticoagulation. The extent of thrombosis can lead to ischaemia and venous gangrene.

Phlegmasia alba dolens is an earlier presentation of deep venous thrombosis caused by occlusion of the deep venous system. Because the superficial system is still patent and allows some outflow, oedema predominates leading to a white, painful, swollen leg. If left untreated this can progress to ischaemia.

An ischaemic leg secondary to arterial occlusion is not swollen in the immediate presentation.

9. J. Klippel–Trenaunay syndrome

Klippel–Trenaunay syndrome is a rare condition consisting of capillary malformations/port-wine stains (>90% of patients), severe varicose veins (70% of patients), and limb hypertrophy (60% of patients). The genetic basis for the condition is currently unclear (PIK3CA gene mutations in some patients) but it does not follow a direct inheritance pattern (usually sporadic). Although the port-wine stain may be identified at birth, the condition is often not diagnosed until later in childhood as the varicose veins or limb hypertrophy develop. The leg is much more commonly involved and the capillary malformation is usually on the same side as the affected limb. Venous malformations include hypoplasia/aplasia of the deep system and valve absence or incompetence. There is an increased risk of venous thromboembolism due to the venous changes. Varicose veins and limb hypertrophy can cause pain and are managed initially with compression therapy to alleviate symptoms. Bony and soft tissue hypertrophy can be managed using orthotics while orthopaedic surgical interventions are reserved for more severe cases.

10. E. Distal embolization (trashing)

The picture in the foot is classic of distal embolization. The emboli may arise from the thrombus load within the aortic aneurysm or may be from another source entirely (i.e. cardiac). Distal embolization is also seen related to both open and endovascular interventions with an incidence of approximately 1–2%. Treatment is supportive with analgesia and antibiotics for signs of infection. Debridement or amputation may be required for necrosis.

11. D. Compartment syndrome

Compartment syndrome results when pressure rises within a confined space in the body, commonly the fascial compartment of a limb, resulting in tissue ischaemia. This may be as a consequence of muscle swelling or bleeding into the compartment. Causes include fractures, burns, haemorrhage (trauma/iatrogenic), re-perfusion injury, crush/prolonged compression (such as in the patient described), deep venous thrombosis, plaster casts, and vigorous exercise. Initial signs include swelling and paraesthesia, while motor loss and reduced/absent pulses are a later development. Release of compartment pressure by opening the skin and fascial compartment should be carried out expeditiously to avoid irreversible damage to muscles and nerves resulting in Volkmann's ischaemic contracture

The patient's history in the described scenario (collapse, lying on floor for unknown duration) and the concomitant acute kidney injury points to compartment syndrome complicated by rhabdomyolosis. The muscle injury leads to myoglobin being present in the urine giving it a dark red or brown colour. Excess levels of myoglobin cause acute kidney injury, electrolyte disturbance, and renal failure.

12. B. Acute arterial embolism

The history and findings are consistent with arterial occlusion (acute). Arterial embolisms have been associated with active inflammatory bowel disease. Meta-analysis suggests a modest increased risk in arterial embolism compared with the greater risk of VTE in IBD. The risk particularly applies to female patients and those under the age of 40 years. There is no difference in risk between patients with Crohn's disease and ulcerative colitis. Embolism may occur spontaneously or in the perioperative period in patients undergoing surgery for active disease.

Kuy S et al. The increasing incidence of thromboembolic events among hospitalized patients with inflammatory bowel disease. *Vascular* 2015;23(3):260–4.

Venous pathology

13. J. Three-layer elasticated compression bandaging

The history and duplex findings are consistent with venous ulceration. With ABPI >0.8 and biphasic waveforms, compression should form the mainstay of the initial treatment. 70–90% of venous ulcers will heal with graduated compression dressings alone. Compression can be by either bandaging or stockings with the pressure highest at the ankle reducing venous pooling and improving outflow. Compression stocking are contraindicated in patients with peripheral vascular disease. Superficial venous surgery does not significantly improve the healing rate of venous ulcers but may reduce recurrence.

14. H. Non-steroidal anti-inflammatories, compression, and elevation

Superficial thrombophlebitis most commonly affects varicose veins (90% of cases). Other causes include pregnancy, venous surgery/ablation, hypercoagulable states, malignancy, and Buerger's disease. It is usually a self-limiting, inflammatory condition and as such, anti-inflammatories, elevation, and compression are the mainstays of initial management. Duplex ultrasound should be considered in thrombophlebitis of the larger, axial superficial veins to exclude deep venous thrombosis. It should also be considered in patients with progressive symptoms or signs. There is a well-established increase in the risk of VTE in patients with superficial thrombophlebitis which is greatest in the first three months. Anticoagulation is reserved for patients with proven DVT or where superficial thrombus propagates close to the deep system.

15. D. Elevation, compression therapy, and mobilization

Post-phlebitic syndrome can occur in up to 50% of patients following deep venous thrombosis, with 10% being severely affected. It can lead to deep venous insufficiency (with associated symptoms and skin changes) and venous ulceration. Severe post-thrombotic syndrome significantly impacts quality of life. Treating varicose veins in the presence of deep venous reflux can lead to worsening of symptoms/skin changes, with a high incidence of recurrence.

16. B. Anticoagulation, thrombolysis, and first rib resection

The patient in this scenario has symptoms and signs consistent with Paget–Schroetter disease or venous thoracic outlet syndrome. The classic presentation is of sudden severe upper limb pain and swelling after exercise in a young healthy patient. Primary DVT of the upper limb is rare and is usually due to damage to the axillo-subclavian vein by bony compression (e.g. cervical rib, callus formation) or musculo-tendinous impingement (e.g. congenital anomalies, muscular hypertrophy from repetitive lifting). The majority of upper limb DVTs are secondary to other causes (i.e. central venous catheters, trauma, malignancy).

While anticoagulation with compression and elevation is potential option, especially in the immediate management, given the short duration of symptoms, aggressive management with thrombolysis and first rib resection should be considered. Active management is suggested to improve long-term outcomes and in particular post-phlebitic symptoms. This is an important consideration given the career of the patient in the scenario. Conservative management with anticoagulation and elevation may be more appropriate in mild cases or where presentation is delayed.

Anticoagulant mode of action

17. E. Direct factor Xa inhibitor

Rivaroxaban's mode of action is by direct inhibition of both free and bound factor Xa. It is rapidly absorbed via the oral route with high bioavailability (maximal plasma concentrations in two to four hours) The maximal anticoagulant effect is seen at one to four hours and it is reported to be predictable from a pharmacokinetic perspective. It does not accumulate and has a half-life of 7–11 hours. The half-life is particularly important, as no reversal agent exists. In life-threatening haemorrhage, prothrombin complex concentrate (e.g. octaplex/beriplex and/or tranexamic acid) may help although there is no clear evidence of efficacy.

18. C. Direct thrombin inhibitor

Dabigatran works by binding and directly inhibiting thrombin. This prevents thrombin from converting fibrinogen to fibrin. It has a predictable dose-related response with peak plasma concentrations achieved two hours after oral administration. The half-life is 14–17 hours. The pharmacokinetics of these new agents also mean that attention should be paid to the fact that the timing of cessation is usually only 48 hours before surgery, and conversely the reintroduction when compared to warfarin should be lengthened.

There is a direct antidote—Praxbind® (idarucizumab). It is reported to result in 100% reversal of the drug effect as it is a direct antibody to the drug.

It is used in the prevention of strokes in patients with non-valvular atrial fibrillation. It appears to be as effective as warfarin in preventing non-haemorrhagic strokes and embolic events in such patients.

It is also used to treat DVTs and pulmonary emboli if patients have undergone an initial five to ten-day treatment with low molecular weight heparin. When compared to patients who are anticoagulated with warfarin, dabigatran causes fewer life-threatening gastrointestinal bleeds and intracranial bleeds but there does appear to be a higher overall risk of gastrointestinal bleeding. It can be associated with dyspepsia as the oral preparation contains an acid to facilitate absorption. It has been hypothesized that this may play a role in the increased risk of gastrointestinal bleeding.

Lip GH and Douketis JD. Perioperative management of patients receiving anticoagulants. *UpToDate* article, September 2016. <https://www.uptodate.com/contents/perioperative-management-of-patients-receiving-anticoagulants>.

19. F. Inhibits vitamin K-dependent synthesis of clotting factors II, VII, IX, and X

Warfarin inhibits the vitamin K-dependent clotting factors. It also has an inhibitory effect on protein C and S. The anticoagulant effect is unpredictable varying from 24–96 hours. Monitoring of PT/APTTr (or INR) is required. The usual half-life for a single dose of warfarin is two to five days and will increase as doses overlap.

If reversal is not urgent then allowing the INR to slowly normalize is acceptable (stop five days prior to surgical procedures, check INR one to two days prior to the procedure). Vitamin K is the main route for active reversal of warfarin. If the procedure can wait up to 24 hours, then reversal with 5–10mg vitamin K is appropriate. If it is necessary to reverse the drug immediately, then FFP (fresh frozen plasma) or prothrombin complex concentrates (e.g. octaplex/beriplex) can be administered. Warfarin resistance can occur with high doses of vitamin K administration making it difficult to re-establish treatment.

Vascular syndromes

20. H. Neurological thoracic outlet syndrome

In the majority of thoracic outlet syndromes, the symptoms are neurological (90%), with pain and weakness in the upper limb. Compression of the nerves may occur between the first rib and the clavicle or may be compressed by anatomical variants such as a fibromuscular band, cervical rib, and abnormalities of the scalene muscles. Traction can also cause damage to the brachial plexus. Management is more commonly conservative with analgesia and gentle physiotherapy.

21. I. Subclavian steal syndrome

This syndrome occurs when there is significant subclavian/brachiocephalic artery stenosis/ occlusions proximal to the origin of the vertebral artery. This results in reversed flow in the vertebral artery, depriving the posterior intracranial circulation in order to preserve flow down the affected limb. Neurological symptoms are vertebra-basilar in origin. Classically, the syndrome is characterized by neurological symptoms when the upper limb is exercised, but this only exists in a small number of patients.

22. F. Antiphospholipid syndrome

Investigation into the underlying cause of an unprovoked DVT is paramount, especially in the setting of a third DVT. A full thrombophilia screen should be performed along with a full history and examination (malignancy, pelvic compression of veins, venous lines as a neonate).

Antiphospholipid syndrome (previously known as Lupus anticoagulant) is an autoimmune condition which leads to an increased risk of thrombosis and fetal loss. The exact mechanism of thrombosis is unclear but it may account for 10–15% of all DVTs. It is much more common in women than men and up to 50% of patients have another autoimmune condition. Treatment includes risk factor modification, anticoagulation, and/or antiplatelet agents.

Illig K et al. A comprehensive review of Paget Schroetter Syndrome. *Journal of Vascular Surgery* 2010; 51(6):1538–47.

Negrini S et al. The antiphospholipid syndrome: from pathophysiology to treatment. *Clinical and Experimental Medicine* 20176; 17(3):257–67.

National Institute of Health and Care Excellence. Venous thromboembolic diseases: diagnosis, management and thrombophilia testing. NICE Clinical Guidelines [CG144] November 2015. <https://www.nice.org.uk/guidance/cg144>.

Vasculitides

23. J. Takayasu's arteritis

Takayasu's arteritis (TA), fibromuscular dysplasia (FMD), and giant cell arteritis (GCA) are considered large vessel vasculitides (inflammatory conditions of the vessel wall). Vasculitides can be classified by either primary or secondary causes and further subdivided by the size of the vessels involved (large, medium, and small vessel vasculitides). Many patients with vasculitides initially present with non-specific constitutional symptoms. More specific/distinctive symptoms develop at a later date. Takayasu's arteritis classically affects the aorta and its major branches, has a predilection for women (F:M 8:1) and is mainly a disease of younger people (<40yrs). It can lead to non-atherosclerotic arterial stenosis/occlusion and aneurysm formation.

24. G. Fibromuscular dysplasia

Fibromuscular dysplasia is a large vessel vasculitis, classically affecting younger patients (women of child-bearing age). It is the most common cause for secondary hypertension in this age group. It has a predilection for certain arterial segments, namely renal involvement (60–75%), cerebrovascular involvement (25–30%, predominantly the internal carotid artery), visceral involvement (9%), and limb vasculature involvement (5%). The common renal variant classically demonstrates multiple areas of focal dilation within the renal arteries ('string of beads' sign) on angiography. Treatment of renal FMD may be indicated for refractory hypertension or worsening renal function and usually involves balloon angioplasty in the first instance combined with antiplatelet therapy.

25. B. Giant cell arteritis (GCA)

GCA, is the most common of the large vessel vasculitides, mainly affecting those >50yrs, with a slight female preponderance. The inflammation commonly affects the superficial temporal, ophthalmic, and vertebral arteries, with the most frequent symptoms being headaches and jaw claudication. More severe complications include anterior ischaemic optic neuropathy (visual disturbance, can be permanent in up to 20%), and ischaemic stroke. Diagnosis is based on the American College of Rheumatologists' Scoring system (age >50yrs, new onset headache, increased ESR, abnormal artery biopsy), with the presence of three or more of these yielding >90% sensitivity and specificity for GCA.

Polyarteritis nodosa (medium vessel vasculitis) may be associated with hepatitis B infection and characterized by systemic symptoms (weight loss, fever), myalgia, mono/polyneuropathy, arterial stenosis/occlusion, or aneurysm formation unrelated to atherosclerosis or FMD.

Wegener's granulomatosis (polyangiitis) and Churg–Strauss Syndrome (small vessel vasculitis) are known as anti-neutrophil cytoplasmic autoantibody-associated vasculitides. Wegener's granulomatosis is defined (Chapel Hill Consensus Conference) as granulomatous inflammation involving the respiratory tract and necrotizing vasculitis affecting small vessels with renal involvement (necrotizing glomerulonephritis is common). Churg–Strauss syndrome is defined as an eosinophil-rich and granulomatous inflammation involving the respiratory tract and necrotizing vasculitis affecting small vessels. It may be associated with asthma and blood eosinophilia.

Behçet's disease is a small vessel systemic vasculitis of younger persons (age 20–40yrs) and affecting multiple systems—the oral/genital mucous membranes (ulcers/scarring), eyes (optic neuropathy/uveitis), skin (erythema nodosum), arthropathy, cardiovascular system (pulmonary artery aneurysms, superficial thrombophlebitis, coronary vasculitis, endo/myo/pericarditis), gastrointestinal tract (bleeding, ulceration), and the central nervous system.

Kawasaki disease (medium vessel vasculitis) is a rare vasculitis affecting children, commonly affecting the coronary arteries which may lead to aneurysm formation. It presents with fever, rash, 'strawberry' tongue, cracked lips, lymphadenopathy, and oedema of the hands and feet.

Cogan syndrome is a rare vasculitis affecting the younger age group (20–30yrs) with no predilection for either sex. It is characterized by hearing loss, vertigo, and inflammation of the eyes and medium-sized vessels.

Thromboangiitis obliterans, also known as Buerger's disease, is a segmental occlusive inflammatory condition affecting the small and medium sized arteries, more common in males. Onset usually occurs before 45yrs of age and is strongly associated with smoking. Classical angiographic appearances are those of 'corkscrewing' arterial collaterals. Smoking cessation is paramount. It may lead to distal ischaemia and limb loss.

Gallagher KA et al. Vascular arteritides in women. *Journal of Vascular Surgery* 2013; 57 (4 suppl):27S–36S.

Scovell SD. Giant cell and Takayasu arteritis. *Scientific American Vascular and Endovascular Surgery* 2015;1–15. doi 10.2310/7800.3031.

Vasculitides

MR scan way = Key mode of diagnosis imaging helps.

Large vessel
- Takayasu = <40; F
  Upper limb / aorta.
- focal fibromuscular dysplasia = most common in <40; F
  = stroke; renal, 'string beads'
- Giant cell arteritis

medium = PAN - hep B.

Small - Wegener's. = kidney + small vessel PANCA

- Churg-Strauss = lungs PANCA. Similar to UC/PSC.

- Burgers = thromboangitis obliterans <40 : Male : smoker.

- Kawasaki = children.

INDEX

Notes:
Abbreviations used are as in xi-xx
Tables and figures are indicated by an italic *t* or *f* following the page number.